Clinical Obesity Genetics

Mieke van Haelst • Erica van den Akker
Editors

Clinical Obesity Genetics

Springer

Editors
Mieke van Haelst
Department of Human Genetics, Section Clinical Genetics
Amsterdam University Medical Center
Amsterdam, The Netherlands

Erica van den Akker
Department of Pediatric Endocrinology
Erasmus University Medical Center
Rotterdam, The Netherlands

ISBN 978-3-032-04094-7 ISBN 978-3-032-04095-4 (eBook)
https://doi.org/10.1007/978-3-032-04095-4

This Springer imprint is published by the registered company Springer Nature Switzerland AG
The registered company address is: Gewerbestrasse 11, 6330 Cham, Switzerland

Preface

Dear colleagues,

With great pleasure, we introduce the first edition of the Clinical Obesity Genetics textbook. Obesity is one of the most pressing public health challenges of the twenty-first century. While environmental factors such as sedentary behavior and high-calorie diets play undeniable roles, it has become increasingly clear that genetic predisposition exerts a profound influence on individual susceptibility to obesity.

The study of obesity genetics has evolved from early family-based studies and twin cohorts to modern genome-wide association studies (GWAS), rare variant discovery, and epi- and polygenetic contribution. These advances have moved our understanding from descriptive epidemiology to biologically grounded mechanisms. Although the heritability of body mass index (BMI) is estimated to be as high as 40–70%, we still cannot explain the majority of cases with suspected genetic obesity.

In this textbook, we provide a comprehensive overview of the rapidly expanding genetic technologies and their practical implications in clinical medicine. This first edition explores how genetic insights can guide risk prediction, prevention strategies, therapeutic decisions, and personalized care. The chapters are organized around key genetic pathways, syndromic and non-syndromic obesity, methodologies in genetic discovery, and future applications such as genetic therapies and pharmacogenomics also visualized in Figure 1.

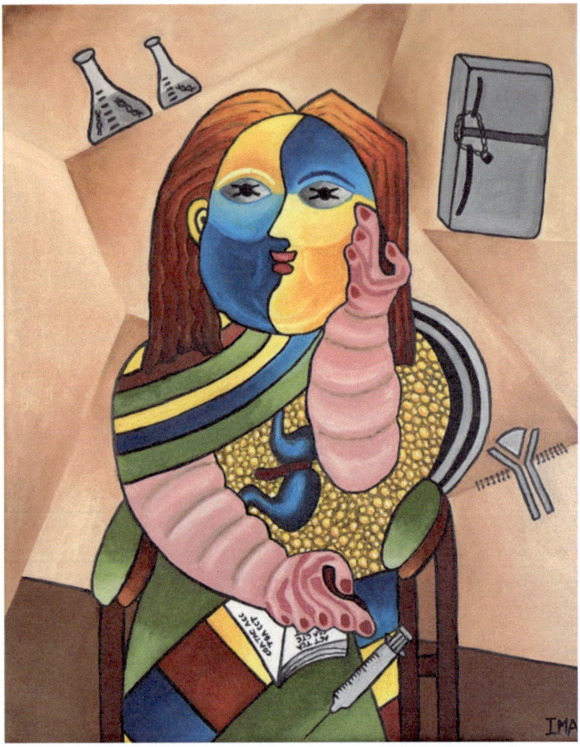

Fig. 1 Painting by Inge Mathijssen illustrating Genetic obesity characteristics. Patients have an *increased number of fat cells. Red hair* and *extra fingers* (polydactyly) can be indicative of syndromic obesity. The *DNA code* in the book on the patient's lap and the Erlenmeyer flask containing DNA strands at the top-left corner symbolize the search for genetic causes. The 'locked refrigerator' symbolizes the *extreme insatiability* (hyperphagia) caused by gene defects affecting the *leptin receptor*. While gastric bands have long been a known *metabolic surgery treatment*, an increasing number of *medications* is becoming available. The syringe refers to *MC4R-agonist*, *medication* that normalizes disturbance of the leptin melanocortin pathway

As we have entered a new era of precision healthcare, understanding the genetic contribution to obesity disorders is no longer an academic task; it is a clinical skill! This book provides clinicians, researchers, and students a comprehensive guide to the past, present, and future of the clinical implications of obesity genetics (Fig. 1).

Amsterdam, The Netherlands — Mieke van Haelst
Rotterdam, The Netherlands — Erica van den Akker

Contents

About This Book

This book provides a concise and practical overview of clinical obesity genetics for both clinicians and scientists in need of a single resource on the topic. Clinical genetic obesity disorders, genetic analysis, clinical treatment, and future directions are discussed in detail, with new insights and approaches to personalized medicine highlighted throughout the book.

About the Editors

Mieke van Haelst is Head of Clinical Genetics at the Department of Human Genetics, Amsterdam University Medical Centers. After her specialist training at Erasmus MC, Rotterdam, and Great Ormond Street Hospital, London, she worked as a clinical geneticist in London and Utrecht. Her translational research focusses on the identification of (novel) gene defects and unravelling the pathogenicity of obesity-related disorders. As co-director of Emma Center for Personalized Medicine at Amsterdam UMC, she works on the identification and understanding of causal (epi) genetic factors that result in rare diseases. She integrates knowledge and methods of diverse disciplines to accelerate the development of personalized treatment for rare genetic disorders. She has established genetic clinics, research, and education programs at the departments of paediatrics in the Dutch Caribbean and aims to provide equal genetic care for diverse populations. Together with co-editor Erica van den Akker, she established the Dutch national center of expertise for genetic obesity disorders.

Erica van den Akker is Head of Pediatric Endocrinology at the Department of Pediatrics, Erasmus MC-Sophia Children's Hospital, Rotterdam, the Netherlands. She is Lecturer at the Faculty of Medicine, Erasmus University, and Cofounder of the Obesity Clinic CGG, which is a European Association Studies of Obesity Center of Management (EASO-COM) and a Dutch national center of expertise in diagnosis and treatment of children and adolescents with genetic obesity. Dr. van den Akker's research focuses on clinical and translational projects in the diagnostics and treatment of (genetic) obesity. She is member of the European Society of Pediatric Endocrinology Clinical Practice Committee, the RareEndo European Reference Network main thematic group on growth and obesity.

Introduction

General Introduction to Obesity Genetics and Genomics

Philip Jansen, Jorrit van Uhm, and Mieke van Haelst

1 Introduction

Genetic studies of obesity have a long history that range from early twin studies to recent gene identification studies that successfully found genetic variants influencing body weight [1] (Fig. 1). Predisposition to develop obesity is often a combination of environmental, behavioural and heritable factors. Twin studies have shown heritability estimates (i.e. variation explained by genetic differences) of 47–90% for BMI [1, 2], suggesting that genetic variation is a major contributor to its aetiology. Advances in DNA technologies, such as genotyping arrays and next-generation sequencing (NGS), have allowed researchers to identify genetic variants that predispose to obesity and molecular mechanisms through which these variants affect body weight regulation. It is now known that genetic predisposition for obesity covers a spectrum that can be subdivided in common genetic variation (e.g. genetic variants with a frequency of >1% in the population) with typical small individual effects on obesity, and rare variants with strong effects on obesity that follow a Mendelian inheritance pattern. These rare monogenic variants play an important role in current genetic diagnostics in the clinic, which can help in individual risk assessment, counselling of family members, improve acceptance by the patient and his or her environment and facilitate personalized treatment options. Research on both ends on this variant frequency spectrum hold promises to better understand the biological factors underlying obesity pathophysiology. With the development of larger genetic

P. Jansen (✉) · M. van Haelst
Department of Human Genetics, Section Clinical Genetics, Amsterdam University Medical Center, Amsterdam, the Netherlands
e-mail: p.jansen3@amsterdamumc.nl; m.vanhaelst@amsterdamumc.nl

J. van Uhm
Department of Pediatrics, Erasmus University Medical Center, Rotterdam, the Netherlands
e-mail: j.vanuhm@erasmusmc.nl

M. van Haelst, E. van den Akker (eds.), *Clinical Obesity Genetics*,
https://doi.org/10.1007/978-3-032-04095-4_1

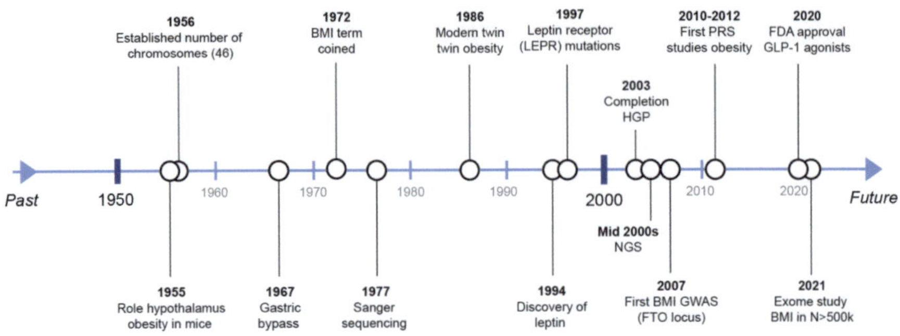

Fig. 1 Timeline of major milestones in obesity genetics research. BMI body-mass index, HGP Human Genome Project, NGS next-generation sequencing, PRS polygenic risk scores

datasets and more accurate genetic technologies, it is expected that we will identify even more variants that contribute to obesity, elucidate how genetics and the environment shape obesity, and develop more effective interventions tailored to an individual's genetic profile.

2 Structure of the Genome

The discovery of the double helix structure of the genome in 1953 by Watson and Crick [3] marks an important milestone in genetics. Not only does this iconic structure account for a mechanism for both storing and replicating genetic information, it also finally gave geneticist an 'organ' to study and explain the long-known heredity of disease. Understanding the structure of the genome from largest to smallest scale is vital in understanding how genetic variation relates to obesity through different dimensions of system biology.

2.1 Chromosomes

A term first coined by German scientist Wilhelm Waldeyer in 1888 [4], *chromosomes* are structures found in the nucleus of each cell that contain the genetic material of an organism. Chromosomes are made up of long strands of DNA that are tightly coiled and packaged into a compact structure (*chromatin*). Each chromosome contains hundreds or thousands of genes, which are the instructions for producing proteins that serve several functions in the human body. Chromosomes can be subdivided into autosomes 1 to 22 (same for both sexes), largely ordered by chromosome length, and sex chromosomes (X and Y).

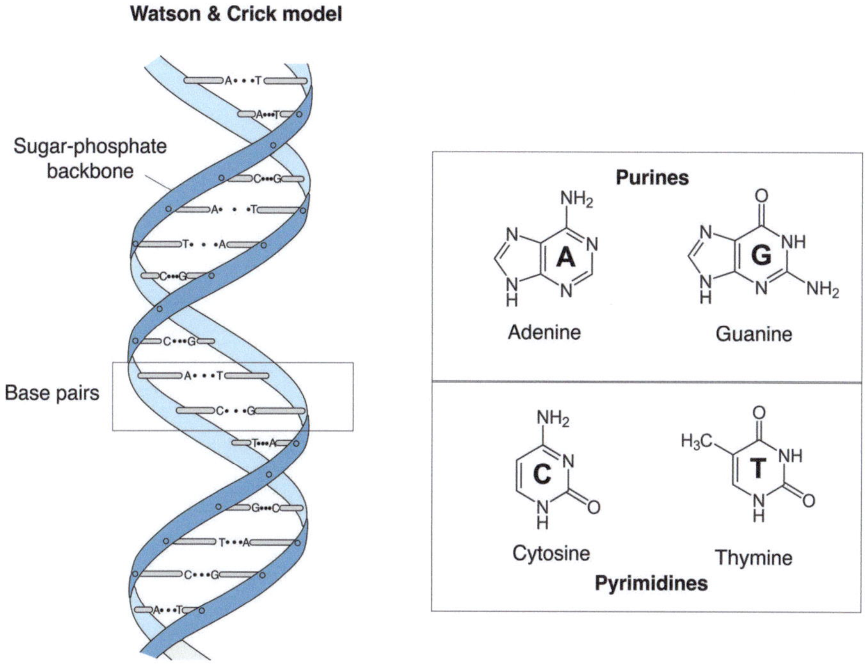

Fig. 2 Structure of the DNA molecule

2.2 *DNA*

Deoxyribonucleic acid, or *DNA*, is the genetic material that carries the instructions for the development and function of all living organisms. DNA is a long, linear molecule made up of *nucleotides* (Fig. 2), which are themselves composed of a sugar (*deoxyribose*), a *phosphate* group, and a nitrogenous base (adenine (A), cytosine (C), guanine (G), or thymine (T)). The DNA backbone is composed of alternating sugar and phosphate groups. The arrangement of the sugar-phosphate backbone and the nitrogenous bases gives DNA its characteristic double helix structure [3].

2.3 *Epigenetic Regulation*

Epigenetics concerns the regulation of gene expression without changing the underlying DNA sequence. Together with genetic variation, epigenetic differences have shown to be an important mechanism that contributes to obesity susceptibility [1]. Epigenetic regulation has effects on gene-expression through *histone modifcations and DNA modification.* Histones are the proteins that package DNA into open or dense structures. Through addition or removal of chemical groups, such as acetyl,

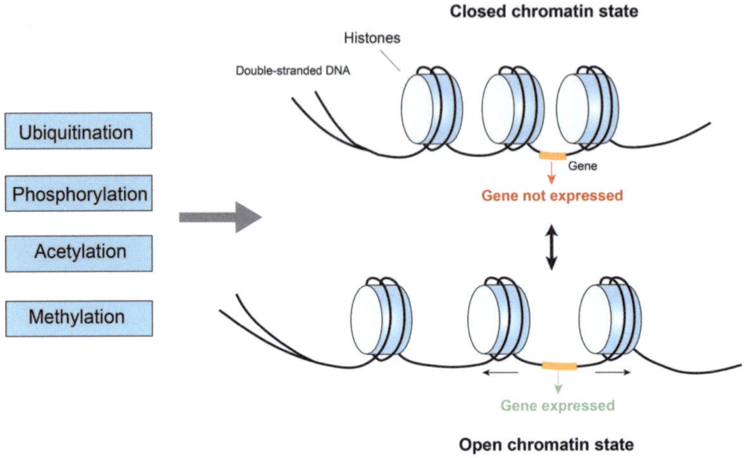

Fig. 3 Epigenetic regulation of gene-expression by histone modification through methylation, acetylation, ubiquitination and phosphorylation

ubiquitin, methyl, or phosphate groups, the accessibility of the DNA for transcription is altered by opening and closing of the chromatin. There are several mechanisms that are responsible for epigenetic regulation (Fig. 3), including:

- *Methylation:* The most common epigenetic modifications include DNA methylation and histone methylation. DNA methylation adds a methyl group (CH3) to cytosine (C) bases of the DNA, typically at cytosine bases that are followed by a guanine base (G), known as *CpG dinucleotides.* Methylation of the promoter region of a gene usually leads to a lower expression of the gene. Alternatively, gene expression can be influenced by methylation of specific histones (histone methylation). Methylation also plays an important role in imprinting, a physiological process that causes genes to be silenced depending on the parent of origin. Environmental exposures such as smoking [5], stress [6]) have also been associated with characteristic changes in DNA-methylation patterns, for example at specific CpG sites [7].
- *Acetylation:* adds an acetyl group (C2H3O) to the histone, which activates gene expression by making chromatin more accessible for transcription factors.
- *Phosphorylation:* adds a phosphor group (PO4) to the histone which makes chromatin more- or less accessible for gene-expression.
- *Ubiquitination:* involves attaching ubiquitin to other proteins. Ubiquitination regulates gene expression by modifying proteins involved in the transcription of genes or signalling them to be degraded. It can also modify histones to change to a more open and transcription-accessible chromatin formation.

3 From DNA to Protein

3.1 Transcription

The sequence of DNA stores information about the structure of well over 20,000 proteins. *Transcription* is the first step to convert this information into synthesis of proteins, through the intermediate step of producing messenger RNA (mRNA) from DNA. In contrast to DNA, RNA molecules are single-stranded instead of double-stranded, have a different sugar (ribose) in their nucleotide units and contains uracil (U) instead of thymine (T).

Transcription starts at a specific site on the DNA molecule, known as the *transcription start site* (TSS). *Promoters* are specific sequences of DNA that are recognized by transcription factors, which bind to DNA and form a complex to initiate transcription. The RNA polymerase enzyme subsequently moves along the DNA template, synthesizing RNA that complements the DNA template, until termination is reached at the transcription stop site. Before mRNA is used for *translation* into proteins, the pre-mRNA needs to undergo RNA modifications to become mature mRNA (Fig. 4): *splicing* removes intronic RNA, *capping* adds a cap to the mRNA 5′ ends, and *polyadenylation* adds a large string of adenine (poly-AAA tail) to the 3′ end for stability. Mature RNA can now be transported to the ribosomes to start the translation process into proteins.

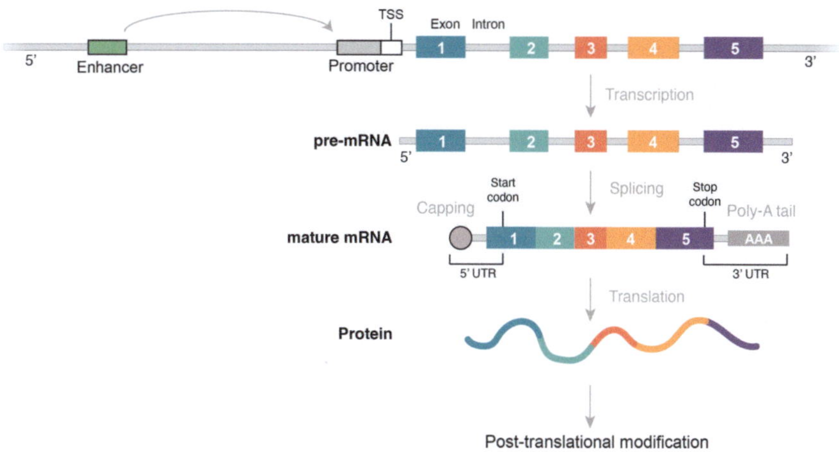

Fig. 4 From DNA to protein: transcription and translation

3.2 Translation

Translation is the next step to produce protein from the intermediate mRNA at the *ribosomes*, small organelles composed of ribosomal RNA (rRNA). Translation starts at a specific site on the mature mRNA, known as the *start codon* (bases AUG) which codes the amino acid *methionine*. The sequence of nucleotide bases in the mRNA molecule specifies the sequence of amino acids in the protein. A ribosome moves along the mRNA and adds a new amino acid to the chain that makes up the protein, using transfer RNA (tRNA) molecules that carry the amino acids to be incorporated. Every three bases of the mRNA form a *codon* which codes for one of many amino acids, and is complementary to a codon on the tRNA. Translation is terminated at a *stop codon* (coded by either UAA, UAG or UGA). The ribosome releases the newly synthesized protein, which is now ready to perform its various functions in the cell.

3.3 DNA Replication

In addition to protein synthesis, *DNA replication* is the process that leads to an accurate duplication of DNA information from one cell to the other. Replication at specific locations called origins of replication, where the double helix is unwound by helicase enzymes, creating a replication fork (Fig. 5). The *leading strand* is synthesized continuously in the 5′ to 3′ direction *by DNA polymerase*. In contrast, the lagging strand is synthesized discontinuously in short segments called Okazaki fragments, also in the 5′ to 3′ direction, but moving away from the replication fork. These fragments are later joined together by the enzyme DNA ligase, creating a continuous strand. After successful replication, the complete set of genetic information can be transferred to the new cell, containing a nearly identical copy of the set of genes.

4 From Gene to Disease

4.1 Inheritance

The inheritance of disease (e.g. the transmission of risk alleles across generations) has traditionally been divided into *monogenic* and *polygenic* inheritance, based on the number, frequency and effect of risk genes involved. On one end of the spectrum, monogenic disorders have a straightforward *Mendelian* pattern of inheritance, and the risk of inheriting the disorder can often be accurately predicted based on a single gene mutation. The search for monogenic disease genes has been highly successful [8], with over 3000 monogenic disorders genes that have been identified for

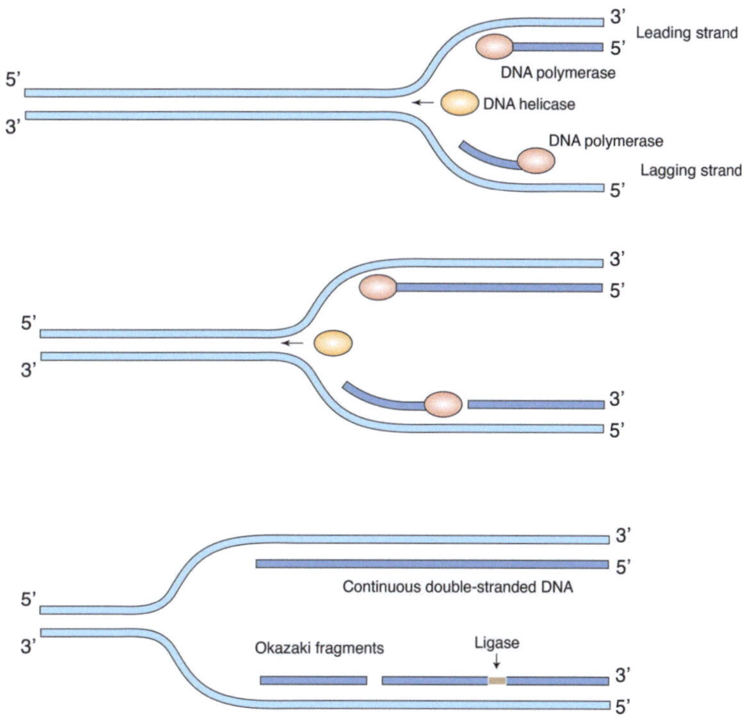

Fig. 5 The process of DNA replication

diseases such as cystic fibrosis, sickle cell anaemia, and Huntington's disease. On the other end, *complex* or *polygenic disorders* refers to a group of traits or disorders in which multiple genes are involved. These genes interact with each other and with environmental factors, and collectively determine disease risk. According to the *common disease-common trait hypothesis*, any common disorder has, at least partially, such a *polygenic* component. These common genetic variants (most often single-nucleotide polymorphisms, or SNPs) involved in complex traits such as BMI almost always have a low relative risk per individual SNP. This correlation of lower effect-sizes for more frequent variants results in part from negative selection pressures on deleterious alleles that affect fitness and transmission in the population, pushing them to the rarer end of the frequency spectrum. In practise, the monogenic-polygenic distinction is in fact much less clear, since disease risk of monogenic disease (i.e. *penetrance*) can be modified by common variants [9]. For obesity, this picture is shown to be equally complex, with both rare single coding variants and multiple common variants having been identified. Common genetic variants for obesity have shown to influence risk from monogenic causes of obesity [10] (such as *MC4R*), or interact with relevant environmental factors [11]. In this chapter, we further focus on (the diagnosis of) monogenic genetics of obesity, whereas in Chapter 23 we further discuss the role of common variation in obesity.

4.2 Mendelian Inheritance

Based on an individual's family history and family tree, a clinician can recognize a certain *inheritance pattern* for certain traits or disorders in the family. Some of these patterns were first described by Mendel based on pea plant experiments, where he observed that certain traits reappeared in future generations after crossing for certain phenotypes (e.g. recessive pattern), far before genes and mutations were known. Several *Mendelian inheritance patterns* can now be distinguished (Fig. 6):

- *Autosomal dominant:* having a disease predisposing (e.g. pathogenic) DNA variant on one of the two alleles is sufficient to develop the disorder. The particular genetic disorder appears in subsequent generations.
- *Autosomal recessive:* the disease only occurs when a pathogenic variant is present in both alleles of the gene. Healthy parents of the index are often carriers. The

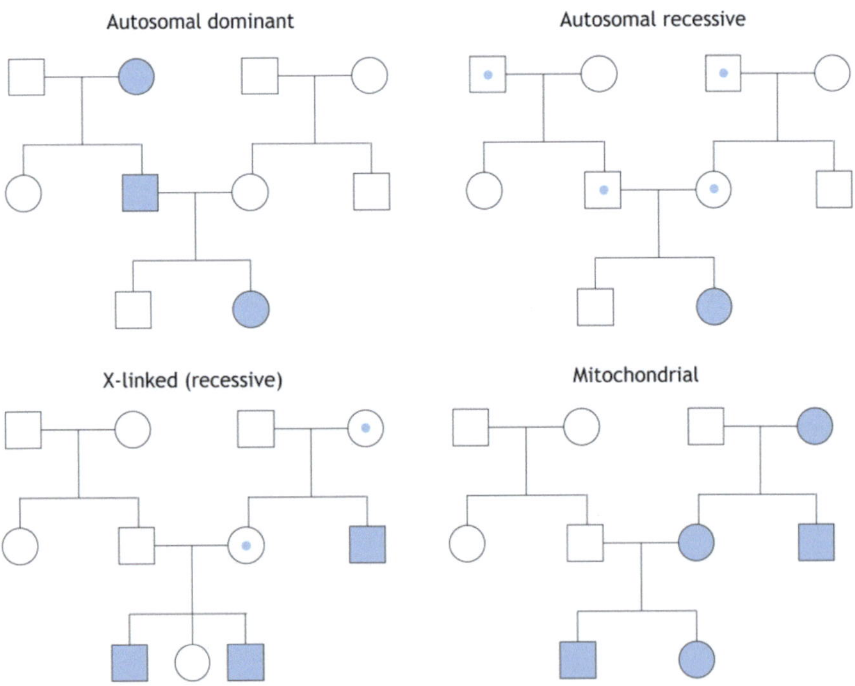

Fig. 6 Different types of inheritance patterns based on an individual's family history. Filled circles and squares represent affected individuals, whereas dots represent (asymptomatic) carriers of a pathogenic variant

risk for offspring of a carrier couple is 25%. The probability that two individuals are both a carrier of the same disease is elevated when they are related (consanguineous). Family history in previous generations is often negative for the disorder.

- *X-linked:* the pathogenic variant is located on the X-chromosome. Females are often asymptomatic, but can transmit the gene variant to males who are then affected. Due to scewed inactivation of the X-chromosome in females, they may have (mild) symptoms themselves. A typical X-linked family tree however, shows only affected males and no affected females.
- *Mitochondrial:* In mitochondrial disorders, the pathogenic variant is present in the mitochondrial DNA (mtDNA) located in the mitochondrium. This mtDNA is transmitted through the oocyte of the female. Thus females will transmit the genetic predisposition to all of their children, and males will not transmit the disease.

4.3 Monogenic Variants

Gene variants can change the DNA sequence of a gene that can result in changes to the protein that is produced. There are several types of monogenic gene variants depending on how they change the DNA sequence, including:

- *Single nucleotide variants (SNVs)*: are single base pair changes in the DNA sequence. Point mutations can be *missense*, *nonsense* or *synonymous*, depending on whether they change the amino acid sequence of the protein (Fig. 7). In *missense* variants, the point mutation causes one amino acid to be replaced by another amino acid. In *nonsense* mutations, the amino acid is replaced by a stop codon, causing translation of the protein to terminate, possibly resulting in a truncated protein. The abnormal mRNA containing a premature stop codon is often degraded through *nonsense-mediated decay*, leading to no protein at all from that specific allele. *Synonymous* mutations cause the amino acid to be replaced by the exact same amino acid. Although synonymous mutations thus do not alter the amino acid sequence of the codon, they may still lead to abnormal *splicing* of the mRNA and thus still affect the final protein product.
- *Insertions/deletions* of one or more base pairs of the DNA sequence. This can cause an incorrect or shortened protein, or no protein at all. If the number of inserted or deleted base pairs cannot be divided by three, the mutation results in a *frame-shift*. The reading frame in the translation process is shifted, and often a new stop codon is created, causing both an abnormal and shortened composition of the protein. When the reading frame is not affected, this results in a *inframe deletion* or *insertion.*
- *Copy number variants:* are large-scale deletions or duplications within chromosomes approximately larger than 50 basepairs, often spanning multiple or large sets of genes.

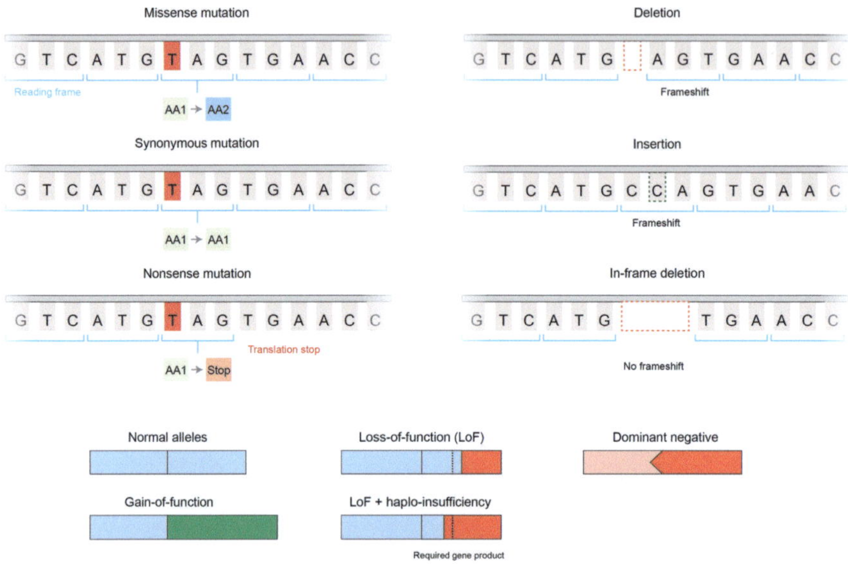

Fig. 7 Types of DNA mutations and mutation mechanisms that are observed in human disease. AA amino acid

Loss-of-function mutations are mutations that result in the complete or partial loss of function of a gene. Loss-of-function mutations are often truncating mutations (such as deletions or nonsense mutations) that can result in the complete absence of a protein or a reduction in its function (Fig. 7). If the loss-of-function leads to insufficient normal functioning protein, there is *haploinsufficiency* of that gene. *Gain-of-function* mutations are mutations that result in the acquisition of a new function or an increase in the function of a gene. These types of mutations can occur in any part of the gene, including the promoter, coding region, or regulatory elements. In *dominant-negative* mutations, the mutated allele interferes with the functioning of the other (normal) allele, causing proteins from both alleles to be affected.

4.4 Epigenetic Mutations

Beyond alterations in the sequence of the genome, changes in epigenome are responsible for *epigenetic disorders*. These epigenetic mutations, which include both *hyper-* and *hypomethylation*, are typically not inherited from one of the parents (unless caused by a DNA mutation), as the methylation parental gametes transmitted via the sperm- or egg cell undergo a reset of the epigenetic profile during gametogenesis. Disruptions in epigenetic processes are linked to a wide variety of diseases and syndromes, ranging from developmental disorders [12] to complex diseases such as cancer [13]. There are specific obesity disorders that are resulting from imprinting disturbances. One example is Temple syndrome, characterized by intra-uterine growth restriction, early puberty and childhood obesity. Temple syndrome mostly originates from two copies of a chromosome from one parent in the child (uniparental disomy, UPD), in this case of chromosome 14 (UPD14), causing loss of expression of genes on the paternal allele and overexpression of genes on the maternal allele [14]. Alternatively, methylation disorders can be caused by DNA variants in genes involved in epigenetic processes such as methylation and histone modification. This can disrupt the enzymes or regulatory factors responsible for these processes and the normal pattern of gene expression, leading to developmental abnormalities. Examples include mutations in *DNMT3A* which codes for a DNA methyl transferase protein, causing Tatton-Brown-Rahman syndrome, of which obesity is a feature. Epigenetic alterations caused by genetic variants involved in epigenetic regulation can be identified by methylation profiling (see Sect. 5.3).

4.5 Variant Interpretation

Every person carries on average five million genetic variants [15] (i.e. variants that differ from a reference genome), of which up to a 100 are not inherited from one of both parents (i.e. *de novo*) [16]. The vast majority of genetic variants have no known impact on health, however a small proportion of variants can have significant consequences. It can be challenging to determine which genetic variants are likely to be *pathogenic* (disease-causing) and which are *benign* (harmless). Variant interpretation is a complex process that requires a good understanding of the human genome and the potential impacts of genetic variations on an individual's health. The *American College for Medical Genetics (ACMG)* have provided criteria that aid in classifying genetic variants in genetic diagnostics [17], classifying variants in five scales along an increasing likelihood of pathogenicity: class 1 ('benign'), class 2 ('likely benign'), class 3 ('uncertain significance'), class 4 ('likely pathogenic'), and class 5 ('pathogenic').

Several variant characteristics are in use in clinical practise that support the categorisation of variants:

- *Domain:* certain gene domains are more sensitive to genetic variants or have a domain-specific effect (e.g. certain gain-of-function mutations) which can make pathogenicity more likely.
- *Conservation*: variants located in conserved sequences of DNA that are relatively unchanged through evolution history are more likely to be pathogenic.
- *Biochemical change*: missense variants that lead to amino acid changes with large differences in biochemical properties are more likely to be pathogenic. These changes are expressed in Grantham score [18] (range: 5-215).
- *Prediction algorithms:* several prediction algorithms have been developed that can suggest pathogenicity based on variant characteristics, such as SIFT [19] and PolyPhen [20].

- *Population frequencies*: genetic variants that appear in higher frequencies in population databases such as gnomAD [21] are less likely to be pathogenic.

The classification of these variants is a dynamic process during which certain variants can switch between categories (e.g. a class 3 variant can be upgraded to class 4 or vice versa), as is the case for *MC4R* variants, an important monogenic obesity gene. For this gene (and other genes), online databases register whether known variants can be classified as pathogenic or benign (or even protective), such as the MCR4 website https://www.mc4r.org.uk/. Other regularly used databases that register pathogenicity of gene variants are GnomAD [21] and ClinVar [22]. More recently, artificial intelligence (AI) tools are being developed that can possibly aid in the interpretation of variants and automating this process [23].

5 Genetic Diagnostics

5.1 Chromosomal Diagnostics

Chromosomal abnormalities are changes in the number or structure of chromosomes that can have serious consequences for an individual's health. Chromosomal abnormalities can be associated with a range of health problems, including birth defects, developmental delay and intellectual disability. For obesity, deletions such as 16p11.2 are known syndromes associated overweight and obesity [24]. There are several diagnostic techniques that are used to detect chromosomal abnormalities, including:

- *Karyotyping*: A karyogram is a visual representation of all 46 chromosomes arranged in order according to size, shape, and band patterns. A karyotype can be used to identify abnormalities in the number or structure of chromosomes, such as missing or extra chromosomes (monosomy/trisomy). Also, in contrast to most other techniques, karyotyping can detect chromosomal translocations (exchange of chromosome segments) that remain undetected by chromosome analyses using e.g. SNP array. Klinefelter syndrome (46, XXY karyotype) is among the disorders that can be detected by karyotyping.
- *Fluorescent in situ hybridization (FISH)*: uses fluorescent probes to detect specific chromosomal regions or genes. FISH can be used to identify chromosomal abnormalities, such as missing or extra copies of specific genes, and can be performed on cells from a variety of tissues, including blood, bone marrow, and amniotic fluid. The 16p11.2 deletions are among the abnormalities that can be detected by FISH probes for this region, which are often too small to be detected by regular karyotyping.
- *SNP array/array CGH*: Single-nucleotide polymorphism (SNP) array technique and comparative genomic hybridization (CGH) arrays are techniques designed to detect small chromosomal abnormalities, including deletions and duplications.

These array techniques were developed and implemented in the early to mid 2000s and provided a much higher resolution than karyotyping chromosomal abnormalities. The size of CNVs that array technologies can detect, are from the 5-50 kb range up to whole-chromosome level abnormalities. This means that we can now identify abnormalities (microdeletions or duplications) that were missed by regular karyotyping. For detection of deletions related to obesity (16p11.2 deletions, Prader-Willi syndrome) these are often first detected using SNP array testing.

- *NIPT/NIPD*: Chromosomal analysis can be done in the prenatal setting as well. Non-invasive techniques such as NIPT (*non-invasive prenatal test*) are specifically developed to test the unborn foetus for chromosomal abnormalities, detected from cell-free DNA in the blood circulation of the pregnant mother. NIPD (*non-invasive prenatal diagnostics)* is an extension of NIPT, where the circulating foetal DNA is tested for specific mutations. NIPT and NIPD provide non-invasive alternatives to more invasive procedures chorion biopsy or amniocentesis, and it is expected that more information can be derived from cell-free DNA when these techniques develop further. This more recent prenatal test sometimes leads to the potential detection of CNVs related to obesity already in the prenatal phase (e.g. 2q37 deletions) as a secondary finding.

5.2 Sequencing Technologies

Sequencing technologies are used to determine the order of nucleotide bases A,C,T and G of DNA. These technologies have greatly advanced the field of genomics by allowing researchers and clinicians to quickly and accurately determine the sequence of DNA, which has important contributions to gene discovery and more rapid genetic diagnosis. Several different types of sequencing technologies that are used in daily clinical practise, including:

- *Sanger sequencing*: the traditional method of DNA sequencing, developed in 1977, initially used to sequence single genes. Sanger sequencing is still being used to sequence shorter fragments and is considered a gold standard for mutation detection. In obesity diagnostics, Sanger sequencing may be used to confirm genetic variants found by more rapid sequencing techniques.
- *Next-generation sequencing (NGS):* NGS technologies (also called second generation sequencing) can sequence multiple DNA fragments simultaneously, which allows for rapid and cost-effective sequencing of large amounts of DNA. NGS has revolutionized the identification of disease genes by enabling the rapid analysis of entire genomes and discover *novel* mutations and variants associated with genetic disorders. NGS has become available in the mid 2000s, and can be used to sequence the full coding region of the genome (whole-exome sequencing (WES)) or the entire genome (whole-genome sequencing, WGS). Often, NGS is used to sequence specific *gene-panels*, which contain sets of genes

related to a specific symptom or disorder. NGS with an obesity gene-panel in patients with suspected monogenic obesity (caused by a single pathogenic variant in an obesity gene) characterized by early onset obesity, currently leads to a diagnosis in 5–15% of the patients with the clinical phenotype [25, 26]. NGS is mostly based on short reading sequencing technologies, which refers to the length in DNA fragments that are sequenced. Short-read sequencing technologies produce reads of typically up to 300 base pairs (bp) in length). These technologies are highly accurate and can quickly and at a low cost produce large mounts of sequence data.
- *Third generation sequencing*: Whereas second generation sequencing is based on short read sequencing, *long-read sequencing technologies* (sequenced fragments up to one million bp reads) have the advantage of producing long uninterrupted reads, which can be useful for certain applications. Examples include difficult to sequence regions of the DNA, improving identification of certain variations, such as large insertions/deletions, inversions and DNA repeats. Although short-read sequencing is established in genetic diagnostics, the benefit of long read sequencing in obesity over short read has yet to be fully established.

5.3 Epigenetic Tests

Epigenetic abnormalities, such as abnormal DNA methylation patterns can be detected by epigenetic tests, including:

- *Epigenetic signature testing:* Several disease genes are known to influence the methylation and expression pattern of other genes (see Sect. 4.4). Variants in these genes lead to certain 'epigenetic signatures': characteristic patterns of methylated genes. These methylation patterns can be detected using an epigenetic signature test ('episignature', Fig. 8, see also Chapter "Anti-obesity Pharmacotherapy for Patients with Genetic Obesity Disorders"), which detects DNA methylation at multiple sites in the genome [27]. An observed methylation pattern can then be compared to methylation signatures of patients with confirmed genetic syndromes. An episignature test can aid in solving a case when no DNA variant is found or help interpret variants of unknown significance (VUS). In obesity diagnostics, mutations in the *GNAS* gene associated pseudohypoparathyroidism type IA/B (obesity, endocrine abnormalities) can lead to methylation patterns of other genes, which are detectable by episignature testing or detected using GNAS gene sequencing.
- *Methylation-Specific Multiplex Ligation-dependent Probe Amplification (MS-MLPA):* This technique combines the principles of MLPA (detection of variants by using oligonucleotide probes) and methylation-specific analysis to detect and quantify methylation of specific gene regions, often used for diagnosis disorders like Prader-Willi and Angelman syndromes (both in the 15p region).

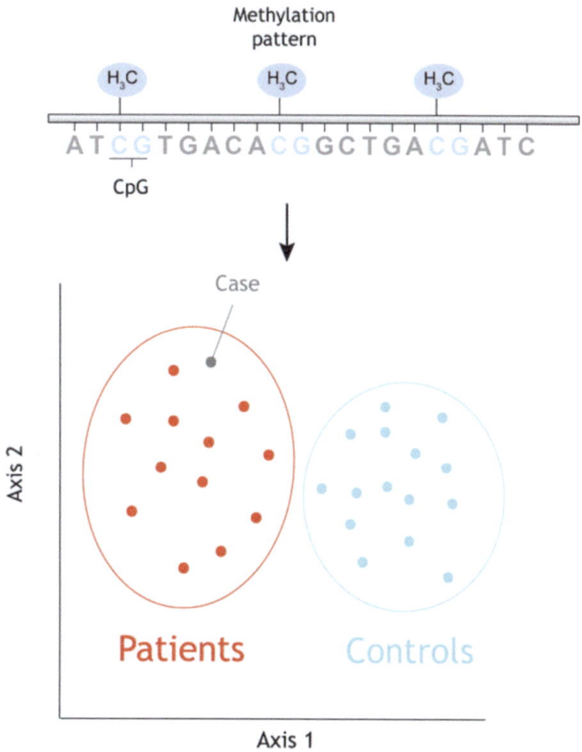

Fig. 8 Epigenetic signature test to detect patterns of methylation anomalies. Methylation patterns of the index case are compared with patient cases and controls. The methylation of the index case can then be detected by clusters of patients and controls on the main axes of variation in methylation. If a pattern is observed that resembles cases, a suspicion of this particular syndrome in the index cases is raised (for more in depth discussion see also Chapter "Anti-obesity Pharmacotherapy for Patients with Genetic Obesity Disorders")

6 Conclusions

In conclusion, advancements in genetic technologies have tremendously expanded our ability to study the genome at the smallest scale. These innovations have facilitated a deeper understanding of the genetic underpinnings of obesity, allowing for more precise identification of genetic variants associated with this complex condition. Understanding these genetic factors requires a foundational knowledge of genetics and genomics, highlighting the importance of integrating these disciplines into obesity research. Ultimately, an improved knowledge of these genetic factors will contribute to an improved risk prediction and treatment of obesity, and eventually improved patient outcomes.

References

1. Loos RJF, Yeo GSH. The genetics of obesity: from discovery to biology. Nat Rev Genet. 2022;23:120–33.
2. Elks CE, et al. Variability in the heritability of body mass index: a systematic review and meta-regression. Front Endocrinol (Lausanne). 2012;3:29.

3. Watson JD, Crick FHC. Molecular structure of nucleic acids: a structure for deoxyribose nucleic acid. Nature. 1953;171:737–8.
4. Waldeyer W. Über Karyokinese und ihre Beziehungen zu den Befruchtungsvorgängen. Arch für mikroskopische Anat. 1888;32:1–122.
5. Gao X, Jia M, Zhang Y, Breitling LP, Brenner H. DNA methylation changes of whole blood cells in response to active smoking exposure in adults: a systematic review of DNA methylation studies. Clin Epigenetics. 2015;7:1–10.
6. Vinkers CH, et al. Traumatic stress and human DNA methylation: a critical review. Epigenomics. 2015;7:593–608.
7. Robertson KD. DNA methylation and human disease. Nat Rev Genet. 2005;6:597–610.
8. Claussnitzer M, et al. A brief history of human disease genetics. Nature. 2020;577:179–89.
9. Moss DJH, et al. Identification of genetic variants associated with Huntington's disease progression: a genome-wide association study. Lancet Neurol. 2017;16:701–11.
10. Akbari P, et al. Sequencing of 640,000 exomes identifies GPR75 variants associated with protection from obesity. Science (80-.). 2021;373:eabf8683.
11. Dashti HS, et al. Interaction of obesity polygenic score with lifestyle risk factors in an electronic health record biobank. BMC Med. 2022;20:1–12.
12. Berdasco M, Esteller M. Genetic syndromes caused by mutations in epigenetic genes. Hum Genet. 2013;132:359–83.
13. Esteller M. Epigenetics in cancer. N Engl J Med. 2008;358:1148–59.
14. Juriaans AF, et al. Temple syndrome: clinical findings, body composition and cognition in 15 patients. J Clin Med. 2022;11:6289.
15. Consortium, 1000 Genomes Project. An integrated map of genetic variation from 1,092 human genomes. Nature. 2012;491:56.
16. Jónsson H, et al. Parental influence on human germline de novo mutations in 1,548 trios from Iceland. Nature. 2017;549:519–22.
17. Richards S, et al. Standards and guidelines for the interpretation of sequence variants: a joint consensus recommendation of the American College of Medical Genetics and Genomics and the Association for Molecular Pathology. Genet Med. 2015;17:405–23.
18. Grantham R. Amino acid difference formula to help explain protein evolution. Science (80-). 1974;185:862–4.
19. Sim N-L, et al. SIFT web server: predicting effects of amino acid substitutions on proteins. Nucleic Acids Res. 2012;40:W452–7.
20. Adzhubei I, Jordan DM, Sunyaev SR. Predicting functional effect of human missense mutations using PolyPhen-2. Curr Protoc Hum Genet. 2013;76:7–20.
21. Koch L. Exploring human genomic diversity with gnomAD. Nat Rev Genet. 2020;21:448.
22. Landrum MJ, et al. ClinVar: public archive of interpretations of clinically relevant variants. Nucleic Acids Res. 2016;44:D862–8.
23. Dias R, Torkamani A. Artificial intelligence in clinical and genomic diagnostics. Genome Med. 2019;11:70.
24. Chung WK, Roberts TPL, Sherr EH, Snyder LG, Spiro JE. 16p11. 2 deletion syndrome. Curr Opin Genet Dev. 2021;68:49–56.
25. Kleinendorst L, et al. Identifying underlying medical causes of pediatric obesity: results of a systematic diagnostic approach in a pediatric obesity center. PLoS One. 2020;15:e0232990.
26. Kleinendorst L, et al. Genetic obesity: next-generation sequencing results of 1230 patients with obesity. J Med Genet. 2018;55:578–86.
27. Sadikovic B, et al. Clinical epigenomics: genome-wide DNA methylation analysis for the diagnosis of Mendelian disorders. Genet Med. 2021;23:1065–74.

General Introduction Obesity in Children and Adults

Erica van den Akker

1 Obesity as a Global Health Challenge

Obesity is a chronic, relapsing disease characterized by excessive adiposity that impairs health. It has emerged as a global health challenge, with its prevalence escalating significantly over the past decades. The global obesity rate increased from 4.7% (~1 in 20 people) in 1975, to 1 in 8 people in the world in 2022 were living with obesity [1]. Projections of the World Obesity Atlas 2025 suggest that by 2035, the prevalence of overweight or obesity will rise to 54% (~1 in 2 people) among adults and 37% (~1 in 3) among children with around half of them being obese [2]. Especially in adolescents, the increase is notable in high income, as well as in low income countries (Fig. 1) [3]. As the rate of spontaneous remission of obesity to a healthy weight is low; at least 90% of the adolescents with obesity will have overweight or obesity in young adulthood [4]. In the Netherlands, the prevalence of obesity among Dutch adults, doubled from 6.1% in 1990 to 16.0% in 2024 and in children (<18 years) rose from 2.5% in 2009 to 3,7% in 2024, with a notable increase among adolescents aged 12–17 years [5]. Despite its widespread impact, many countries remain inadequately prepared to address the rising health burden of obesity.

E. van den Akker (✉)
Department of Pediatrics, Division Pediatric Endocrinology, Obesity Center CGG, Center of expertise genetic obesity, Erasmus University Medical Center – Sophia Children's Hospital, Rotterdam, The Netherlands
e-mail: e.l.t.vandenakker@erasmusmc.nl

M. van Haelst, E. van den Akker (eds.), *Clinical Obesity Genetics*,
https://doi.org/10.1007/978-3-032-04095-4_2

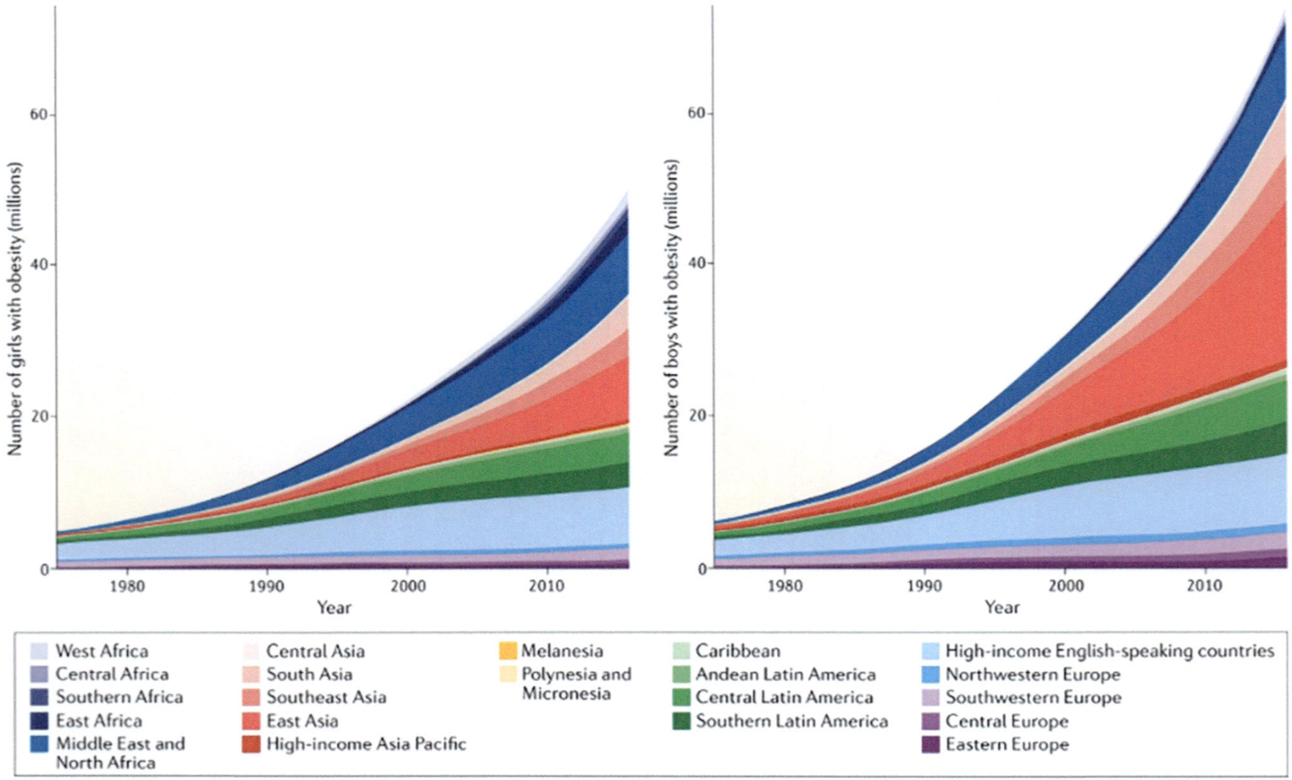

Fig. 1 Increase in the number of children and adolescents affected by obesity over more than four decades. (Adapted from NCD Risk Factor Collaboration (NCD-RisC). Worldwide trends in body-mass index, underweight, overweight, and obesity from 1975 to 2016: a pooled analysis of 2416 population-based measurement studies in 128.9 million children, adolescents, and adults. Lancet 390, 2627–2642 (2017) reprinted under a CC-BY-4.0 licence. Steinbeck et al. [3])

2 Definition and Diagnosis of Obesity

The diagnosis of obesity is traditionally established by using body mass index (BMI). BMI is calculated by weight in kilograms divided by height in meters squared (kg/m^2). For adults, a healthy BMI ranges from 18.5 to 24.99 kg/m^2. Higher BMI values are categorized as overweight (BMI of 25.0 to <30.0 kg/m^2), obesity grade 1 (BMI of 30.0 to <35.0 kg/m^2), obesity grade 2 (BMI of 35.0 to <40.0 kg/m^2), and obesity grade 3 (BMI of ≥40 kg/m^2). In children 2–18 years of age, BMI is adjusted for age and sex, resulting in BMI standard deviation scores (BMI-SDS) that align with adult obesity categories. For children <2 years of age, World Health Organization definition of obesity is defined by a weight-for-height SDS of 3.0 or above [6].

While BMI provides an easy screening method with a high correlation to fat mass, it should be noted that it does not account for variations fat distribution, muscle mass, and metabolic health. Recently, the Lancet Diabetes & Endocrinology Commission proposed a new diagnostic framework [7]. To increase diagnostic accuracy, this commission advised to incorporate additional measures of body fat (distribution) to BMI, such as waist circumference or a direct assessment for example by using a DEXA scan. For individuals with a BMI grade 3 (i.e., >40 kg/m^2), excess adiposity can pragmatically be assumed without further confirmation.

Further, this report proposed to make a distinction between “preclinical” and “clinical” obesity. Clinical obesity is characterized by ongoing organ dysfunction due to excess adiposity, and “preclinical obesity,” is associated with elevated health risks. The commission suggests that the diagnosis of ‘clinical obesity’ requires evidence of reduced organ or tissue function due to obesity (i.e., signs, symptoms, or diagnostic tests showing abnormalities in the function of one or more tissue or organ systems) or substantial, age-adjusted limitations of daily activities reflecting the specific effect of obesity on mobility and other basic activities of daily living (e.g., bathing, dressing, toileting, continence, and eating). The recommendations in this report are a start of an important conversation on how these will be conferred to clinical practice.

3 Etiology of Obesity and Its Health Burden

Obesity arises from a complex interplay of environmental, genetic, behavioral, and biological factors (Fig. 2). Environmental factors such as high-calorie diets, rich in processed foods and sedentary lifestyles are primary drivers of obesity by dysregulating energy homeostasis. Genetic predisposition can influence appetite regulation, energy expenditure, and fat storage. Excess caloric intake leads to adipocyte hypertrophy and hyperplasia. Adipose tissue dysfunction triggers chronic low-grade inflammation and hormonal imbalances that contribute to insulin resistance, dyslipidemia, and systemic complications such as cardiovascular disease. Thus, the

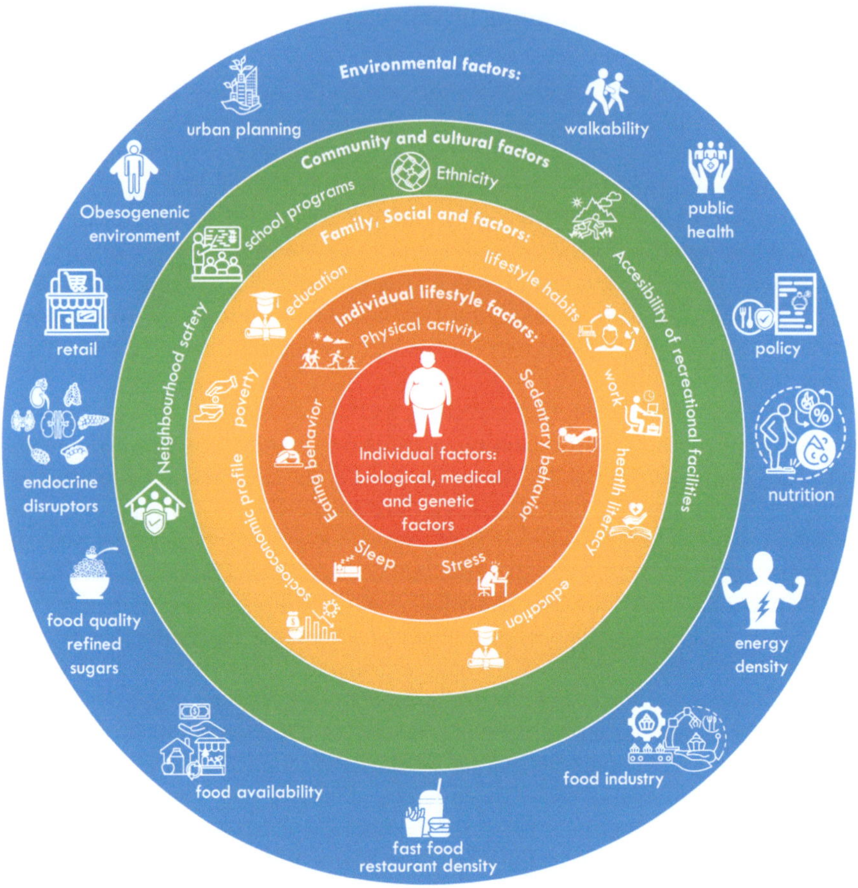

Fig. 2 Obesity is a wicked problem resulting from a complex interplay of environmental, genetic, behavioral, and biological factors

accumulation of excess fat in obesity is associated with numerous health risks (Fig. 3). First, obesity is a disease in itself, leading to complaints of shortness of breath, tiredness, joint pain, reduced quality of life by impairing physical activity, sleep, and mental health. Additionally, obesity significantly increases the risk of non-communicable diseases (NCDs) such as type 2 diabetes, cardiovascular disease, certain cancers, and musculoskeletal disorders. These risks are exacerbated in higher body mass index (BMI) categories, leading to a reduction in life expectancy. For instance, life expectancy is predicted to decrease by 8.1–10.3 years for women and 5.6–7.6 years for men with obesity aged 20–29 years. Consequently, there is an urgent need for effective prevention and treatment strategies to mitigate these health risks.

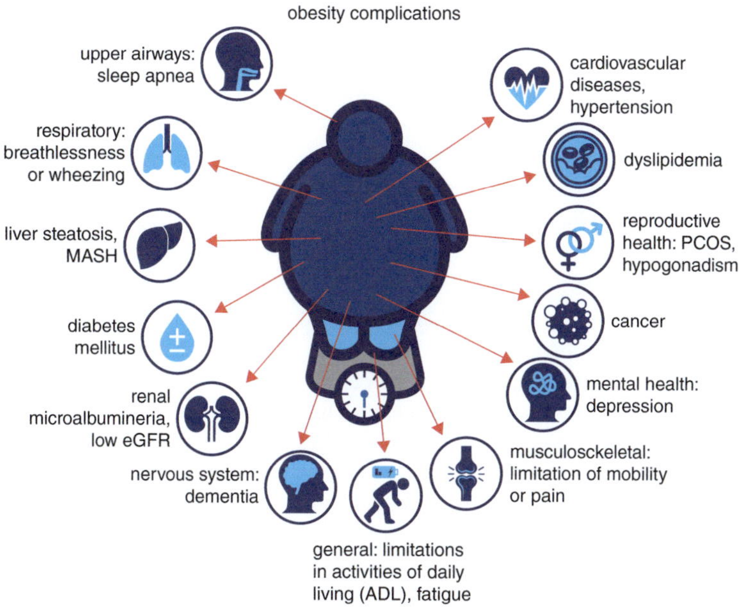

Fig. 3 Obesity complications. *MASH* metabolic dysfunction associated steato-hepatitis (formerly NASH), *eGFR* glomerular filtration rate, *ADL* activities of daily life, *PCOS* polycystic ovary syndrome

4 Individual Underlying Causes and Contributing Factors

Obesity typically has a multifactorial etiology, resulting from the combined effects of environmental factors (the obesogenic environment), genetic predisposition, and lifestyle behaviors. Unhealthy lifestyle factors such as poor dietary habits, reduced physical activity, inadequate sleep, stress, and socioeconomic and cultural factors, act together with genetic predisposition and environmental factors. Less common causes include weight-inducing medication, endocrine disorders, hypothalamic dysfunction and rare genetic obesity disorders. Identifying potential underlying medical causes is crucial for understanding obesity, reducing stigmatization, and providing personalized treatment advice. Recently the open access tool www.checkcausesobesity.com was launched, a digital open access tool, supporting health care professionals to identify potential underlying causes of obesity. This webtool contains a questionnaire that can be filled in by a person with obesity. The results can be downloaded or printed to be taken to their doctor or nurse specialist, providing an overview of possible underlying causes and contributing factors to the obesity of this individual.

5 Obesity Treatment

Individuals with obesity should receive timely, evidence-based treatment aimed at improving clinical manifestations of obesity and preventing progression to end-organ damage. The treatment of obesity has evolved significantly over the past few decades, from incorporating a combination of lifestyle intervention, to pharmacotherapy and surgical interventions [8].

The cornerstone of obesity treatment is, and remains lifestyle interventions, which consists of a multidisciplinary integrative approach aimed towards healthier lifestyle behaviors. These include dietary adjustments, increased physical activity, and behavioral counseling to address psychological barriers to weight loss. Effective dietary strategies often focus on reducing caloric intake, improving nutritional quality, and promoting sustainable healthy eating habits. Physical activity recommendations typically include both aerobic and resistance exercises to enhance weight loss and improve metabolic health. The impact of these lifestyle modifications extends beyond weight loss, promoting long-term health benefits both physical and mental wellbeing. The efficacy of these interventions differs per individual, acknowledging the unique needs and challenges faced by each individual. Therefore, a personalized strategy has the best chance to achieve sustainable lifestyle changes on long term. A weight loss of ≥5% is associated with significant improvements in cardiometabolic risk factors. Weight loss targets should be defined individually based on clinical profiles, with progress measured in the context of health outcomes rather than weight loss alone.

Pharmacotherapy has become an increasingly important component of obesity management, particularly for individuals who do not achieve sufficient weight loss through lifestyle modifications alone. Several medications have been approved for long-term use in obesity treatment (Fig. 4).

Pharmacological interventions targeting that have proved to be effective are GLP-1 Receptor agonists,: liratglutide, semaglutide, tirzepatide, show significant reduction of body weight (~5%, 10%, 20%) by mimicking the gut hormone GLP-1, which regulates appetite and food intake. Dual agonists, which are medications combining different mechanisms of action, such as phentermine-topiramate and naltrexone-bupropion, or GLP-1ra and GIP offer additional options for patients. Semaglutide and tirzepatide do not only promote weight loss but also reduce cardiovascular risks (See Chapter 15 Anti-obesity Pharmacotherapy for patients with genetic obesity).

Surgical interventions. For patients with severe obesity or those who have not responded to other treatments, metabolic (bariatric) surgery can be highly effective (~ 35% weight loss). Although little is know about the effect in patients with genetic obesity, procedures such as gastric bypass or sleeve gastrectomy, have demonstrated substantial and sustained weight loss, along with improvements in obesity-related comorbidities (See Chapter 16 Metabolic Bariatric Surgery).

The landscape of obesity treatment continues to evolve with ongoing research and development. Emerging therapies include advanced behavioral interventions and many novel pharmacological agents for obesity in the pipeline [REF].

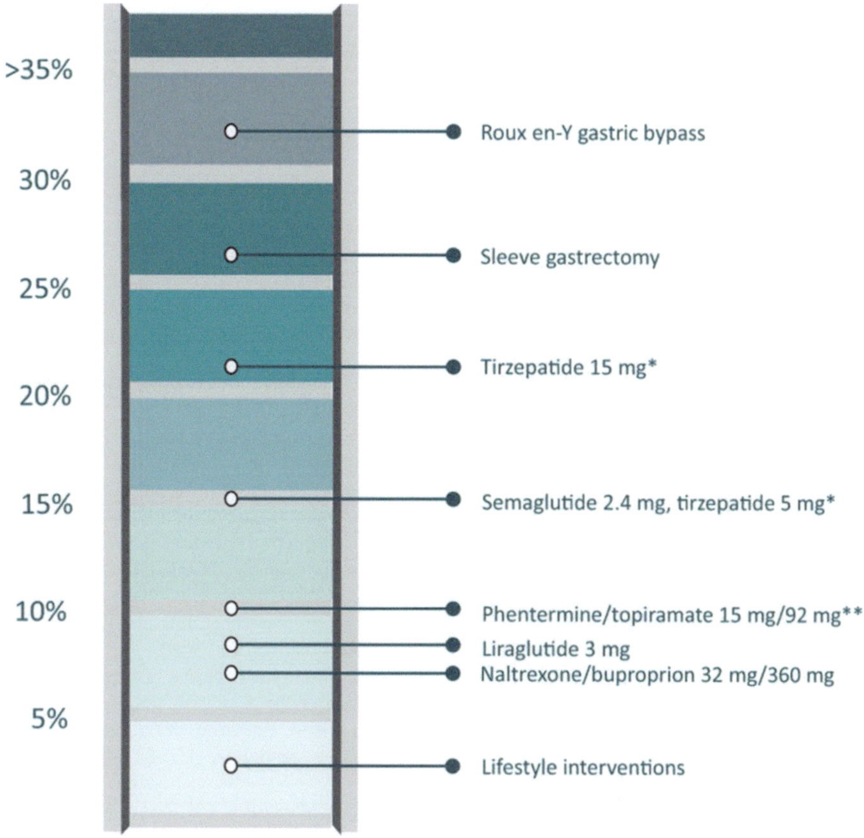

Fig. 4 Lifestyle intervention, Pharmacotherapy and Metabolic surgery show variable effect on BMI% reduction in adults with obesity. (Figure licensed under CC-BY 4.0) Future therapies for obesity Article in Melson [8])

The integration of personalized medicine, based on genetic and metabolic profiling, holds promise for more tailored and effective obesity treatments in the future.

6 Future Challenges

Obesity represents one of the biggest public health challenge of the twenty-first century. Advances in understanding its pathophysiology, decrease stigmatization, redefine diagnostic criteria, and warrants innovative treatments [9]. However, addressing the root causes of obesity requires prevention which needs a coordinated systems approach. Policy makers face significant challenges when addressing this topic. A “whole-of-society” approach involving governments, healthcare systems, industries, and communities is urgently needed to tackle this epidemic effectively.

In conclusion, the management of obesity requires a comprehensive, structured, multidisciplinary approach that combines lifestyle modifications, pharmacotherapy, and surgical interventions. Prevention and care with a deeper understanding of the underlying pathogenicity of obesity and continued advancements in treatment options will be crucial in addressing this global health challenge.

References

1. World Health Organization. Topic Obesity and overweight. https://www.who.int/news-room/fact-sheets/detail/obesity-and-overweight.
2. World Obesity Atlas 2024: No area of the world is unaffected by the consequences of obesity. https://www.worldobesity.org/news/world-obesity-atlas-2024.
3. Steinbeck KS, Lister NB, Gow ML, et al. Treatment of adolescent obesity. Nat Rev Endocrinol. 2018;14:331–44. https://doi.org/10.1038/s41574-018-0002-8.
4. Patton GC, et al. Overweight and obesity between adolescence and young adulthood: a 10-year prospective cohort study. J Adolesc Health. 2011;48:275–80. Treatment of adolescent obesity | Nature Reviews Endocrinology.
5. Centraal bureau voor Statistiek (CBS). https://opendata.cbs.nl/statline/#/CBS/nl/dataset/81565NED/table?ts=1553851467369.
6. World Health Organization (WHO). Obesity and overweight fact sheet. https://www.who.int/news-room/factsheets/detail/obesity-and-overweight. Accessed 15 Nov 2020.
7. Rubino F. et al., Definition and diagnostic criteria of clinical obesity. Lancet Diabetes Endocrinol. 2025; https://doi.org/10.1016/S2213-8587(24)00316-4.
8. Melson E. Future therapies for obesity. Clin Med (London, England). 2023;23(4):337–46. https://doi.org/10.7861/clinmed.2023-01; AND Pediatric guideline: Hampl et al 2023: 10.1542/peds.2022-060640.
9. Angelidi AM, Belanger MJ, Kokkinos A, Koliaki CC, Mantzoros CS. Novel noninvasive approaches to the treatment of obesity: from pharmacotherapy to gene therapy. Endocr Rev. 2022;43(3):507–57. https://doi.org/10.1210/endrev/bnab034. PMID: 35552683; PMCID: PMC9113190. Novel Noninvasive Approaches to the Treatment of Obesity: From Pharmacotherapy to Gene Therapy – PubMed.

Clinical Obesity Disorders

Prader-Willi Syndrome

G. F. Kerkhof and A. F. Juriaans

1 Introduction

In 1956, Andrea Prader, Alexis Labhart and Heinrich Willi, were the first to describe a group of patients with the Prader-Willi phenotype [1]. Diagnostic criteria for PWS were developed, based on clinical findings. In 1976, an abnormal karyotype with a 15/15 Robertsonian translocation, was found in a patient who was clinically diagnosed with PWS [2]. We now know that PWS is caused by the lack of expression of the paternally inherited genes of the PWS critical region, located on chromosome 15q11.2-q13 [3] (Fig. 1).

Currently, the estimated prevalence of PWS is 1 in 10.000-30.000 births and affects both genders equally [4, 5].

2 Aetiology and Pathophysiology

PWS is categorized as a genomic imprinting disorder. Due to the process of genomic imprinting, genes are expressed in a parent-of-origin manner. Some genes are expressed from maternally inherited chromosomes and others from paternally inherited chromosomes [6]. In healthy subjects, the PWS region on the maternally

G. F. Kerkhof (✉)
Pediatric Endocrinology, Department of pediatrics, ErasmusMC Sophia Childrens Hospital, Rotterdam, The Netherlands
e-mail: G.kerkhof@erasmusmc.nl

A. F. Juriaans
Human Development and Health, Human Genetics and Genomics Medicine group, Faculty of Medicine, University of Southampton, Southampton, UK
e-mail: A.F.Juriaans@soton.ac.uk

M. van Haelst, E. van den Akker (eds.), *Clinical Obesity Genetics*,
https://doi.org/10.1007/978-3-032-04095-4_3

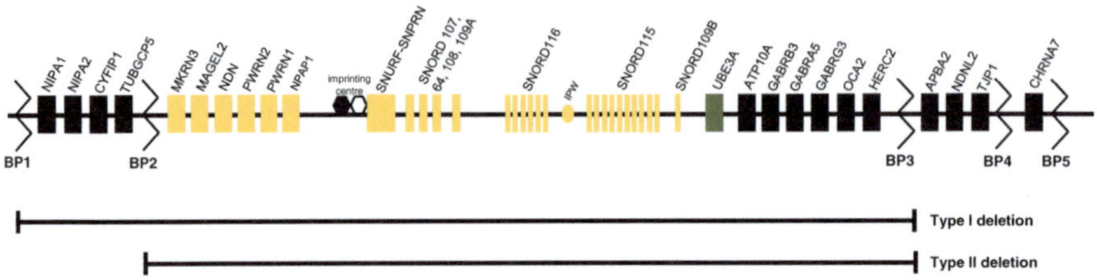

Fig. 1 PWS-region on chromosome 15; yellow: paternally expressed genes; green: maternally expressed genes; black: non-imprinted genes

inherited chromosome 15 is silenced by imprinting. The PWS critical region contains multiple genes and the loss of expression of these genes results in PWS [7] (Fig. 1).

The PWS region spans several genes, namely *MKRN3*, *MAGEL2*, *NDN*, PWRN2, PWRN1, *NPAP1*, *SNURF-SNRPN*, and several non-coding small nucleolar RNA genes; SNORD 107, 64, 108, 109A and B, 116, 115 and IPW [7].

The imprinted domain at 15q11-13 contains two imprinting centres, the PWS Imprinting Centre (PWS-IC), and the Angelman Imprinting Centre (AS-IC). The latter is implicated in the rare neurodevelopmental disorder Angelman syndrome, which is caused by the absence of expression of the *UBE3A* gene. The PWS-IC is maternally methylated and paternally unmethylated and located at the SNURF-SNRPN promotor/exon 1. The AS-IC does not have a parent-specific imprint and is located 31 kB centromeric to the PWS-IC [8]. The PWS-IC and AS-IC cooperate in regulating the epigenetic status and gene expression at the locus [8].

2.1 Molecular Genetics

2.1.1 Deletion (50–75%)

The 15q11.2-q13 region is highly vulnerable to structural rearrangements due to the presence of low-copy repeats (LCRs) in the region [9, 10]. These LCRs also flank the breakpoints of the deletions. A type I deletion extends from breakpoint 1 (BP1) to breakpoint 3 (BP3), and includes imprinted genes in the PWS region as well as four non-imprinted genes. A type II deletions extends from BP2 to BP3 and includes only the imprinted genes in the PWS region. (Fig. 1).

2.1.2 Uniparental Disomy (20–44%)

In patients with UPD(15)mat, the paternal chromosome 15 is missing entirely and both chromosomes are inherited from the mother. There are several mechanisms that can lead to a UPD, (1) gamete complementation; (2) trisomic zygote rescue; (3)

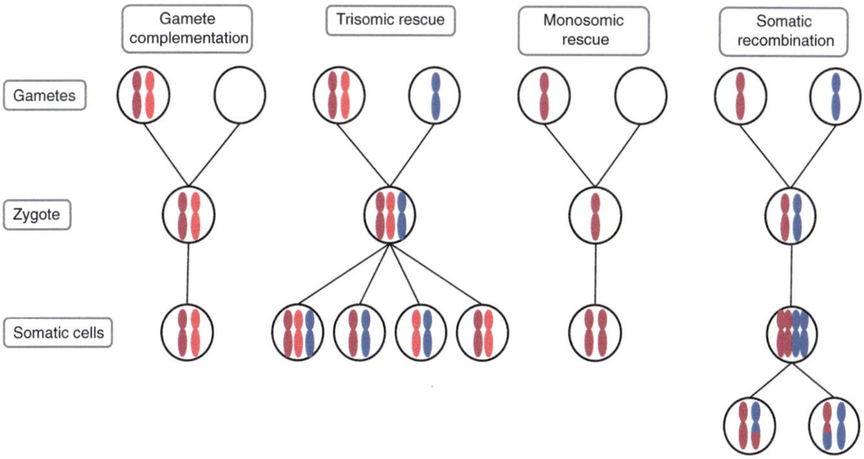

Fig. 2 Different mechanisms causing uniparental disomy, resulting in either heterodisomy, isodisomy or segmental disomy

monosomic rescue; and (4) postzygotic errors, such as somatic recombination. The mechanisms can lead to either a heterodisomy, isodisomy, regions of both iso- and heterodisomy, and/or segmental disomy [11] (Fig. 2).

2.1.3 Imprinting Defect (<5%)

Most imprinting defects result from epigenetic causes (epimutations) without any DNA sequence changes [3] (see Chapter "Methylation Analysis in Diagnostics; the Episignature"). The imprinting defects are thought to be random errors in the imprinting process or in early embryogenesis [12]. A small number of patients with an imprinting defect have a very small deletion in the PWS-IC region.

PWS is usually a *de novo* disorder. However, familial cases can occur in imprinting defects when the deletion is inherited from the unaffected father with a deletion on his maternally inherited chromosome 15 [13] (Fig. 3).

2.2 Genotype-Phenotype Correlation

PWS patients with deletions, specifically atypical deletions (different from the typical type I and type II deletion), have been studied to attempt to gain insight into phenotype-genotype correlations. Several case reports have suggested that disruptions of the SNORD-116 gene cause the primary characteristics of the PWS phenotype [14–19]. Patients with only a small SNURF-SNPRN deletion [20–22] or point mutation [23, 24] can also present with a PWS phenotype. These patients do

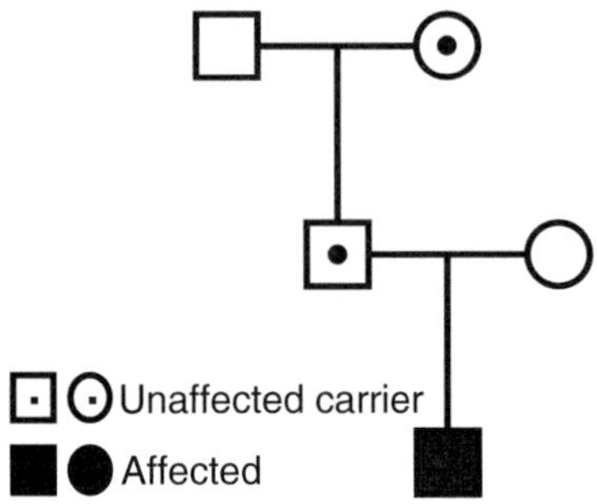

Fig. 3 Example of a family with a pathogenetic variant in the PWS critical region, showing PWS due to paternal transmission of the variant

however usually present with an 'incomplete' phenotype, lacking core symptoms, such as short stature and hypotonia in infancy.

There are no features of the PWS phenotype known to occur exclusively in either one of the genetic subgroups. Particularly, obesity and hyperphagia occurs equally across the genetic subgroups. Some studies have found, however, that some features are more common in patients with either a deletion or UPD(15)mat. Post-term delivery, higher verbal IQ, psychosis and the occurrence of an autism spectrum disorder are more common in patients with a UPD(15)mat [25, 26]. Patients with deletions have a higher occurence of hypopigmentation, sleep disturbances, feeding problems, and speech and language deficits [27].

3 Molecular Diagnosis

Most cases of Prader-Willi syndrome (>99%) can be easily identified by DNA methylation analysis through methylation-specific multiplex ligation-dependent probe amplification (MS-MLPA) (see Chapter "Methylation Analysis in Diagnostics; the Episignature"). With this technique, a maternal-only imprint at the PWS locus will be identified, confirming the clinical diagnosis. It can also assess the approximate size of a deletion and distinguish between a type 1 and 2 deletion [7]. Often, it can also identify mosaicism. However, it can not distinguish UPD(15)mat from an imprinting defect caused by an epimutation.

It is generally advised to perform a SNP-array as well, to determine the exact size of the deletion or to identify a UPD(15)mat due to isodisomy. In patients with an abnormal MS-MLPA of the locus, without a deletion, a SNP-array of both the patient and parents is recommended to identify an epigentic imprinting defect, or a UPD(15)mat due to heterodisomy (Fig. 4).

Alternative diagnostic methods would include multilocus methylation test, which includes detection of other imprinting disorders as well, such as Silver-Russell syndrome and Temple syndrome (see Chapter "Methylation Analysis in Diagnostics; the Episignature").

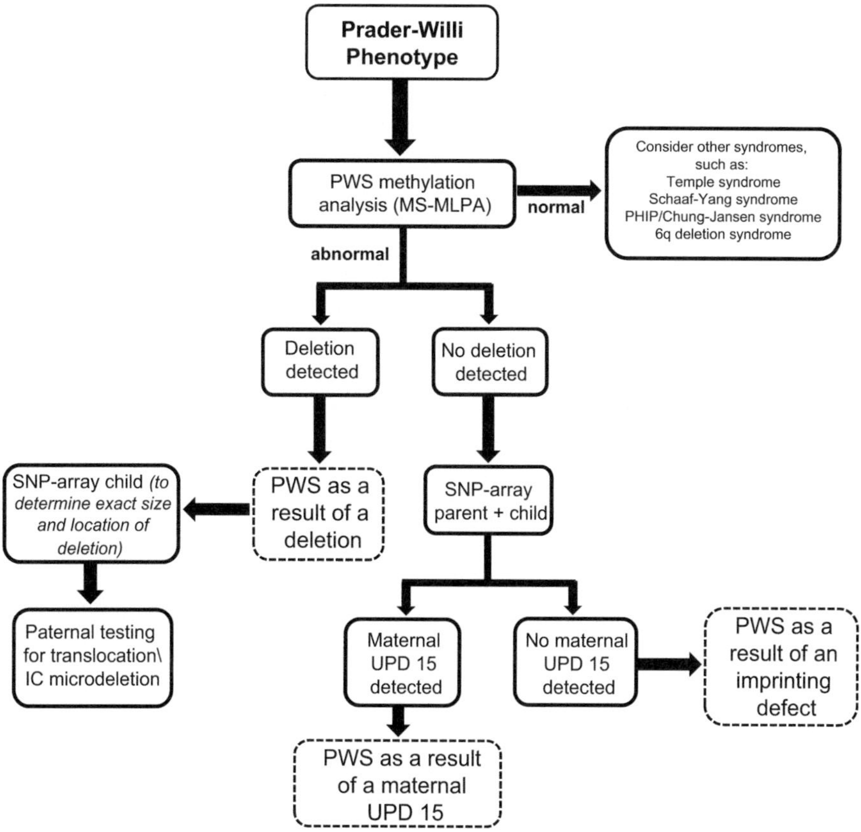

Fig. 4 Molecular analyses in children with a Prader-Willi phenotype

4 Clinical Presentation

Providing that diagnostic testing is available, Prader-Willi syndrome is usually already diagnosed during infancy. Occurrence of hypotonia and subsequent neonatal feeding problems, possibly together with small for gestational age (SGA) birth and cryptorchidism in boys, is often the main reason for targeted PWS diagnostics. Thus, when comparing children with PWS, the clinical presentation during infancy is often comparable. However, when the children become older, the phenotype diverges and leads to a spectrum of clinical features. At the age of approximately 2 years, appetite often increases, leading to hyperphagia later in childhood. During childhood and adulthood, the phenotype of PWS varies significantly between individuals. Taking this into account, we will describe the most common clinical features of PWS, which are mostly caused by hypothalamic dysfunction.

5 Features and Treatment

Many features of Prader-Willi syndrome are related to hypothalamic dysfunction. For example hyperphagia, disturbed temperature regulation and sleeping problems. Also various pituitary endocrine deficiencies can be present.

5.1 *Dysmorphic Features*

Prader-Willi syndrome is characterized by specific facial features. Holm et al. published guidelines in 1993 for clinical diagnosis of PWS and described the "typical facies" of PWS: dolichocephaly (long, narrow skull shape) during infancy, a narrow face with narrow forehead, almond shaped eyes, and a small, downturned mouth with a thin upper lip [28]. Hypopigmentation (fair hair and blue eyes) has been frequently observed in PWS patients with a paternal deletion [29]. Furthermore, patients with PWS often have small hands and feet.

5.2 *Appetite Dysregulation*

Hyperphagia is one of the most distinctive features of PWS, and occurs in 64% of Prader-willi patients [30]. At this moment, hyperphagia in PWS is not fully understood. It is thought to be caused by several mechanisms, such as hypothalamic abnormality, altered orbitofrontal cortex responses, abnormal brain reward system activity, and abnormal levels of ghrelin and oxytocin [31]. The characteristic course of eating behaviour and appetite in PWS has been previously described using different nutritional phases [32]. Starting with a period with failure to thrive after birth because of feeding difficulties, followed by periode with normal growth and without feeding problems. After this, around the age of 18-36 months, children start to gain excessive body weight without a particular interest in food or increase in calorie intake. Thereafter, appetite increases abnormally and turns into a state of hyperphagia [32].

At this moment several studies are being (and have been) performed with regard to hyperphagia treatment. Currently there is no consistent treatment regime, other than behavioural treatment of the individual with PWS, and offering advice to the caregivers on, for example, a structured daily routine.

5.3 *Obesity*

Obesity and its complications are the most common causes of morbidity and mortality in PWS. Obesity is often the consequence of hyperphagia, however other features of PWS, such as hypotonia, behavioural issues and related medication, reduced energy expenditure, and scoliosis can also play a role. Furthermore, body composition is often altered in PWS, with patients having increased adiposity and reduced muscle mass, independent of the presence of obesity. Although growth hormone treatment improves body composition, (abdominal) adiposity remains present. Usually, at time of diagnosis, obesity is not yet present. As PWS is currently often diagnosed during infancy and hyperphagia and subsequent obesity typically occurs at a later age.

Optimal lifestyle intervention and multidisciplinary care including psychological/parental guidance, also with regard to eating behaviour, is essential to prevent obesity-related comorbidities. Early diagnosis of Prader-Willi syndrome leads to appropriate intervention and guidance at a younger age, which causes obesity to develop at a later age [33].

5.4 *Development/Cognitive Impairment*

Patients with PWS usually have a mild intellectual disability with an IQ ranging approximately between 60 and 70 [34]. Part of the patients with PWS has an IQ in the lower-normal range. However, also with a borderline disability or low-normal intelligence, the authors' experience is that patients with PWS often struggle to finish regular education, for example due to their impaired socio-emotional development and/or a disharmonic intelligence profile.

5.5 *Behaviour and Socio-emotional Development*

Patients with PWS often have a similar behavioural profile, including autistic features with cognitive rigidity, behavioural outburst, anxiety, skin-picking and obsessive compulsive behaviour. The challenging behaviour in PWS centers mainly around hyperphagia and early (dietary) intervention. Clear agreements about food in and outside of the home, can be helpful for management of food related behaviours throughout life.

Furthermore, there is an increased risk for psychosis, which usually becomes evident in young adulthood, especially In those who have a UPD(15)mat as the underlying cause of PWS. In case of sudden behavioural changes without a clear substrate, one should be aware of the possibility of psychosis.

5.6 *Neurologic and Neuromuscular Symptoms*

5.6.1 Hypotonia

One of the main features of PWS is neonatal hypotonia. This is one of the most important causes of motor developmental delay. Furthermore, most of the infants have feeding problems requiring tube feeding, because of poor sucking as a result of hypotonia [35]. Usually, physical therapy is already started at a young age to increase muscle mass. Growth hormone treatment also increases muscle mass and is subsequently thought to improve motor development in PWS.

5.6.2 Sleep Disorders

Circadian rhythm abnormalities often result in sleeping problems in PWS, which is thought to be caused by hypothalamic dysfunction. Furthermore, patients with PWS have increased risk for narcolepsy with or without cataplexy [36]. Sleep-disordered breathing is more prevalent in PWS. Including both central- and obstructive sleep apnea, with central sleep apnea mainly being present in infancy. This often results in tiredness during the day, which is already commont in PWS, independent of sleep apnea.

As sleep disorders have a great impact on daily functioning, medical history with regard to sleep and fatigue during the day, should be reviewed frequently and overnight polysomnography (PSG) should be performed if needed, in order to evaluate the presence of hypoventilation and/or central—or obstructive apnoea. Growth hormone treatment is regarded safe, but surveillance for obstructive sleep anoea is important, and adenotonsillectomiy is sometimes indicated before start or during growth hormone treatment [37].

5.6.3 Epilepsy

In Prader-Willi syndrome, seizures occur more often than in children without PWS, mainly during childhood. Epilepsy in PWS is often transient. Some children do need anti-epileptic medication.

5.7 Endocrine Deficiencies

5.7.1 Growth Hormone Deficiency

Some features of subjects with PWS resemble those seen in growth hormone deficiency, and growth hormone treatment partly resolves these issues. Previous studies have shown an increased prevalence of reduced growth hormone response to stimulation tests, as well as low IGF-1 levels and low free IGF-1 levels [38]. However, after reaching final height, the prevalence of growth hormone deficiency is low [39].

Nonetheless, growth hormone treatment is beneficial for children and adults with PWS, as it improves body composition, lineair growth, physical strength and cognitive function. Therefore, treatment with growth hormone is strongly advised to patients with PWS, regardless of presence of growth hormone deficiency. According to expert opinion, prevalence of obesity in PWS has decreased considerably the last decades as a result of growth hormone treatment, in addition to the multidisciplinary care [40] (Fig. 5).

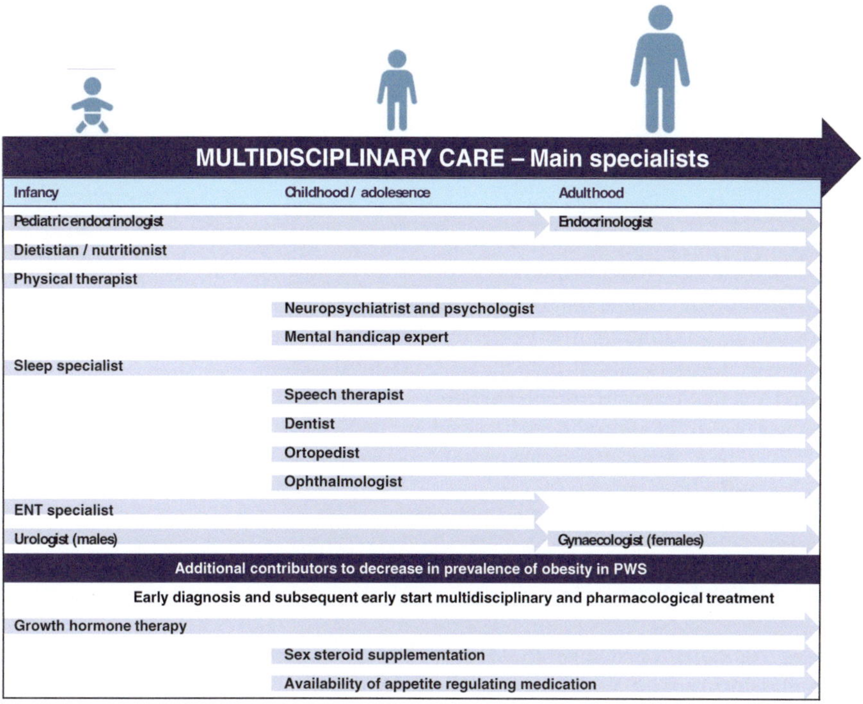

Fig. 5 Multidisciplinary care, early diagnosis [33] and pharmacological treatment lead to decrease in prevalence of obesity in PWS

5.7.2 Pubertal Development and Hypogonadism

Previous research showed that almost all males and a large proportion of females with PWS, have hypogonadism at an adult age [41, 42]. Hypogonadism is therefore one of the main features of PWS. This is already apparent in male infants, who often have cryptorchidism at birth. Furthermore, sexual maturation usually starts at a normal age in boys with PWS, but in most cases it stops in early to mid-puberty [43]. Girls with PWS also have insufficient sexual maturation, although it is clinically les obvious as many cases do have breast development, partly because of the aromatization of androgens in the fat tissue [44, 45]. However, spontaneous menarche and regular periods in females with PWS are rare [44].

Because of stagnation of puberty progression in both boys and girls, they do not reach a sufficient blood level of sex hormones. Sex hormone substitution is highly relevant and important for the overall health and quality of life. It is essential to prevent osteopenia and osteoporosis, lower the risk for cardiovascular diseases and it improves body composition, energy level and general wellbeing [46]. All these aspects are in particular important in patients with PWS, who are already at increased risk for osteoporosis [47] and cardiovascular disease, and almost all have pre-existing hypotonia and fatigue.

In contrast with hypogonadism in later childhood, some children with PWS have precocious puberty and many have premature adrenarche [48].

5.7.3 Hypothyroidism

Central hypothyroidism has been described in patients with PWS. Furthermore, some patients have a mild and transient central hypothyreoidism during early childhood. Thyroid hormone suppletion is not always necessary in these cases as the hypothyreoidism often spontaneously resolves. Growth hormone use is a possible contributor to this finding. Many patients with PWS use growth hormone treatment, and growth hormone might interact with the thyroid hormone axis. Some studies reported low fT4 levels in growth hormone treated children with PWS [49]. Because of the possibility of central hypothyreoidism and additional effects of growth hormone treatment, thyroid function should be monitored in all patients with PWS, with or without growth hormone treatment.

5.7.4 Adrenal Insufficiency

Central Adrenal Insufficiency (CAI) has been described in patients with PWS, in particular during childhood. This could be an explanation for the described increased prevalence of sudden and unexpected deaths, and clinical deterioration in case of mild viral infections in children with PWS. Complete adrenal insufficiency is very rare, also in PWS, and children usually do not need daily treatment with corticosteroids. CAI has been described during acute stress, and data suggests that children with PWS have a delayed stress response, indicating that in some patients stress dosing with corticosteroids is beneficial [50]. Therefore, clinical symptoms should be evaluated and hypothalamic-pituitary-adrenal axis testing and/or corticosteroids stress dosing should be considered in children with PWS, in particular in cases of severe illness or during surgery and anesthesia. In contrast, in adults with PWS, CAI seems to bo very rare [51]. This suggests that there could be a component of delayed maturation of the hypothalamic-pituitary-adrenal axis in PWS.

5.8 Orthopedic Manifestations

The majority of patients with PWS develops scoliosis, which might be even more frequent in patients with a paternal deletion than a mUPD [52]. Repeated imaging is therefore necessary during growth in childhood in order to monitor progression of scoliosis. Physical therapy can be initiated and in more severe cases a corset or surgery can be indicated. Studies have shown that scoliosis in PWS is not related to growth hormone therapy [53, 54].

Also, hip dysplasia occurs more often in patients with PWS. Therefore, there should be a low threshold to perform imaging when hip dysplasia is suspected.

5.8.1 Gastrointestinal

Patients with PWS can have disordered pharyngeal and oesophageal swallowing. Furthermore, gastric emptying is often delayed and vomiting is rare. This, together with hyperphagia, can lead to abdominal distention and other gastro-intestinal problems, which can even be life-threatening [55].

5.8.2 Other Symptoms

Physical illness can be masked in patients with PWS, because of an increased pain threshold, absence of fever (because of temperature dysregulation), and/or inability to vomit due to hypotonia [56]. This is important to consider when examining a patient with PWS.

Patients with PWS can have ophthalmologic manifestations, in particular strabismus, but myopia and hyperopia are also common.

6 Differential Diagnosis

Prader-Willi syndrome is often diagnosed relatively early, because of its symptoms during infancy. However, some conditions show overlap with the features of Prader-Willi syndrome, these conditions are often labelled as 'Prader-Willi-like' or as part of the 'Prader-Willi spectrum' [57]. These patients have, for example developmental delay/intellectual disability, speech problems, overweight/obesity, hypotonia and psychobehavioural problems.

The most common genetic causes of a Prader-Will-like phenotype are: Temple syndrome, Schaaf-Yang syndrome, and PHIP syndrome/Chung-Jansen syndrome [57].

7 Follow-Up Advices

Surveillance of patients consists of a multidisciplinary approach, with particular focus on supporting a healthy and structured lifestyle, with for example involvement of a dietician, psychologist, physiotherapist, endocrinologist, neurologist, geneticist, ENT specialist, ophthalmologist and an ortopedist. (Fig. 5) Growth hormone suppletion is advised, in particular because of beneficial metabolic effects, and substitution of other hormones is prescribed on indication.

8 Family Screening

In the majority of PWS patients the underlying genetic cause developed *de novo* with a recurrence risk of less than 1% [7]. There are, however, underlying mechanisms that involve a significant recurrence risk. For example, if the patient has an imprinting defect, caused by a point mutation, it could be inherited from the unaffected father, which would result in a recurrence risk of 50%. The recurrence risk assessment therefore starts with determining the underlying genetic mechanism of PWS in the patient and should be followed by parental testing to assess the presence of an underlying genetic alteration in the parents, such as a balanced translocation or an imprinting center mutation.

Take Home Message

Prader-Willi syndrome is characterized by distinct dysmorphic features in early life, such as muscular hypotonia and neonatal feeding difficulties often requiring nasal tube feeding. Because of the new genetic techniques that are directly available in the neonatal period, diagnosis is usually genetically confirmed in infancy. And because of the course of the symptoms with hyperphagia not being present during infancy/early childhood, obesity is rarely the main feature in first presentation.

From around the age of 2 onwards, children with PWS often present with increased appetite and in a later stage hyperphagia, neurobehavioral problems and mild to moderate cognitive impairement. Furthermore, hypothalamic dysregulation can result in endocrine deficits, such as growth hormone deficiency, hypothyroidism, hypogonadism, and adrenal insufficiency. Other frequent symptoms are, for example, temperature dysregulation, ear infections, dental problems, gastro-intestinal complaints, scoliosis and strabismus.

Many of the symptoms can be attributed to hypothalamic dysfunction. Growth hormone suppletion is an important part of treatment strategy. Furthermore, multidisciplinary follow-up is essential, with particular focus on supporting a healthy and structured lifestyle. With this treatment strategy, together with availability of early genetic diagnostic techniques and subsequent early diagnosis and start of treatment, progress has been made to improve body composition of patients with PWS.

References

1. Prader A LA WH. Ein Syndrom von Adipositas, Kleinwuchs, Kryptorchismus und Oligophrenie nach myatonieartigem Zustand im Neugeborenenalter. Schweiz Med Wochenschr. 1956;6(1260-1)
2. Hawkey CJ, Smithies A. The Prader-Willi syndrome with a 15/15 translocation. Case report and review of the literature. J Med Genet. 1976;13(2):152–7. https://doi.org/10.1136/jmg.13.2.152.
3. Cassidy SB, Schwartz S, Miller JL, Driscoll DJ. Prader-Willi syndrome. Genet Med. 2012;14(1):10–26. https://doi.org/10.1038/gim.0b013e31822bead0.
4. Akefeldt A. Prader-Will1 syndrome in a Swedish Rural County: epidemiological. Published online; 1991. p. 715–21.
5. Burd L, Vesely B, Martsolf J, Kerbeshian J. Prevalence study of Prader-Willi syndrome in North Dakota. Am J Med Genet. 1990;37(1):97–9. https://doi.org/10.1002/ajmg.1320370122.
6. Reik W, Walter J. Genomic imprinting: parental influence on the genome. Nat Rev Genet. 2001;2(1):21–32. https://doi.org/10.1038/35047554.
7. Cheon CK. Genetics of prader-willi syndrome and prader-will-like syndrome. Ann Pediatr Endocrinol Metab. 2016;21(3):126–35. https://doi.org/10.6065/apem.2016.21.3.126.
8. Horsthemke B, Wagstaff J. Mechanisms of imprinting of the Prader-Willi/Angelman region. Am J Med Genet A. 2008;146(16):2041–52. https://doi.org/10.1002/ajmg.a.32364.
9. Donlon TA, Lalande M, Wyman A, Bruns G, Latt S. Isolation of molecular probes associated with the chromosome 15 instability in the Prader-Willi syndrome. Proc Natl Acad Sci. 1986;83(6):4408–12.
10. Christian SL, Fantes JA, Mewborn SK, Huang B, Ledbetter DH. Large genomic duplicons map to sites of instability in the Prader-Willi/Angelman syndrome chromosome region (15q11-q13). Hum Mol Genet. 1999;8(6):1025–37. https://doi.org/10.1093/hmg/8.6.1025.
11. Robinson WP. Mechanisms leading to uniparental disomy and their clinical consequences. BioEssays. 2000;22(5):452–9. https://doi.org/10.1002/(SICI)1521-1878(200005)22:5<452::AID-BIES7>3.0.CO;2-K.
12. Glenn CC, Driscoll DJ, Yang TP, Nicholls RD. Genomic imprinting: potential function and mechanisms revealed by the Prader-Willi and Angelman syndromes. Mol Hum Reprod. 1997;3(4):321–32. https://doi.org/10.1093/molehr/3.4.321.
13. Buiting K, Groß S, Lich C, Gillessen-Kaesbach G, El-Maarri O, Horsthemke B. Epimutations in Prader-Willi and Angelman syndromes: a molecular study of 136 patients with an imprinting defect. Am J Hum Genet. 2003;72(3):571–7. https://doi.org/10.1086/367926.
14. Duker AL, Ballif BC, Bawle EV, et al. Paternally inherited microdeletion at 15q11.2 confirms a significant role for the SNORD116 C/D box snoRNA cluster in Prader-Willi syndrome. Eur J Hum Genet. 2010;18(11):1196–201. https://doi.org/10.1038/ejhg.2010.102.
15. Sahoo T, Del Gaudio D, German JR, et al. Prader-Willi phenotype caused by paternal deficiency for the HBII-85 C/D box small nucleolar RNA cluster. Nat Genet. 2008;40(6):719–21. https://doi.org/10.1038/ng.158.
16. Tan Q, Potter KJ, Burnett LC, et al. Prader – Willi-Like phenotype caused by an atypical. Genes (Basel). 2020;11(2):1–7. https://doi.org/10.3390/genes11020128.
17. de Smith AJ, Purmann C, Walters RG, et al. A deletion of the HBII-85 class of small nucleolar RNAs (snoRNAs) is associated with hyperphagia, obesity and hypogonadism. Hum Mol Genet. 2009;18(17):3257–65. https://doi.org/10.1093/hmg/ddp263.
18. Bieth E, Eddiry S, Gaston V, et al. Highly restricted deletion of the SNORD116 region is implicated in Prader-Willi syndrome. Eur J Hum Genet. 2015;23(2):252–5. https://doi.org/10.1038/ejhg.2014.103.
19. Hassan M, Butler MG. Prader-Willi syndrome and atypical submicroscopic 15q11-q13 deletions with or without imprinting defects. Eur J Med Genet. 2016;59(11):584–9. https://doi.org/10.1016/j.ejmg.2016.09.017.

20. Kuslich CD, Kobori JA, Mohapatra G, Gregorio-King C, Donlon TA. Prader-Willi syndrome is caused by disruption of the SNRPN gene. Am J Hum Genet. 1999;64(1):70–6. https://doi.org/10.1086/302177.
21. Cao Y, AlHumaidi SS, Faqeih EA, Pitel BA, Lundquist P, Aypar U. A novel deletion of SNURF/SNRPN exon 1 in a patient with Prader-Willi-like phenotype. Eur J Med Genet. 2017;60(8):416–20. https://doi.org/10.1016/j.ejmg.2017.05.003.
22. Grootjen LN, Juriaans AF, Kerkhof GF, Hokken-Koelega ACS. Atypical 15q11.2-q13 deletions and the Prader-Willi phenotype. J Clin Med. 2022;11(15):1–14. https://doi.org/10.3390/jcm11154636.
23. Huang Y, Grand K, Kimonis V, et al. Mosaic de novo SNRPN gene variant associated with Prader-Willi syndrome. J Med Genet. 2021;6:1–4. https://doi.org/10.1136/jmedgenet-2020-107674.
24. Pellikaan K, van Woerden GM, Kleinendorst L, et al. The diagnostic journey of a patient with prader–willi-like syndrome and a unique homozygous snurf-snrpn variant; bio-molecular analysis and review of the literature. Genes (Basel). 2021;12(6) https://doi.org/10.3390/genes12060875.
25. Butler MG, Bittel DC, Kibiryeva N, Talebizadeh Z, Thompson T. Behavioral differences among subjects with Prader-Willi syndrome and type I or type II deletion and maternal Disomy. Pediatrics. 2004;113(3 I):565–73. https://doi.org/10.1542/peds.113.3.565.
26. Yang L, Zhan G-D, Ding J-J, et al. Psychiatric illness and intellectual disability in the Prader-Willi syndrome with different molecular defects – a meta analysis. PLoS One. 2013;8(8):1–11. https://doi.org/10.1371/journal.pone.0072640.
27. Torrado M, Araoz V, Baialardo E, Abraldes K, Mazza C, Krochik G, Ozuna B, Leske V, Caino S, Fano V, Chertkoff L. Clinical-etiologic correlation in children with Prader-Willi syndrome (PWS): an interdisciplinary study. Am J Hum Genet. 2007;143(3):460–8. https://doi.org/10.1002/ajmg.a.
28. Holm A, Cassidy B, Whitman Y, Butler C. Prader-Willi syndrome: consensus diagnostic criteria. Pediatrics. 1993;91(2):398–402.
29. Cassidy SB, Forsythe M, Heeger S, et al. Comparison of phenotype between patients with Prader-Willi syndrome due to deletion 15q and uniparental disomy 15. Am J Med Genet. 1997;68(4):433–40. https://doi.org/10.1002/(SICI)1096-8628(19970211)68:4<433::AID-AJMG12>3.0.CO;2-T.
30. Salvatore M, Torreri P, Grugni G, et al. The Italian registry for patients with Prader–Willi syndrome. Orphanet J Rare Dis. 2023;18(1):1–9. https://doi.org/10.1186/s13023-023-02633-5.
31. Madeo SF, Zagaroli L, Vandelli S, et al. Endocrine features of Prader-Willi syndrome: a narrative review focusing on genotype-phenotype correlation. Front Endocrinol (Lausanne). 2024;15(April):1–23. https://doi.org/10.3389/fendo.2024.1382583.
32. Miller JL, Lynn CH, Driscoll DC, et al. Nutritional phases in Prader-Willi syndrome. Am J Med Genet A. 2011;155(5):1040–9. https://doi.org/10.1002/ajmg.a.33951.
33. Kimonis VE, Tamura R, Gold JA, et al. Early diagnosis in prader–willi syndrome reduces obesity and associated co-morbidities. Genes (Basel). 2019;10(11) https://doi.org/10.3390/genes10110898.
34. Trueba-Timmermans DJ, Grootjen LN, Juriaans AF, et al. Cognitive function during 3 years of growth hormone in previously growth hormone-Treated young adults with Prader-Willi syndrome. Eur J Endocrinol. 2023;189(1):132–9. https://doi.org/10.1093/ejendo/lvad084.
35. Grootjen LN, Uyl NEM, van Beijsterveldt IALP, Damen L, Kerkhof GF, Hokken-Koelega ACS. Prenatal and neonatal characteristics of children with Prader-Willi syndrome. J Clin Med. 2022;11(3) https://doi.org/10.3390/jcm11030679.
36. Duis J. Prader-Willi syndrome: an update. Curr Opin Pulm Med. 2023;29(6):539–42.
37. Itani R, Gillett ES, Perez IA. Sleep consequences of Prader-Willi syndrome. Curr Neurol Neurosci Rep. 2023;23(3):25–32. https://doi.org/10.1007/s11910-023-01254-6.
38. Damen L, Elizabeth MSM, Donze SH, van den Berg SAA, de Graaff LCG, Hokken-Koelega ACS. Free Insulin-like Growth Factor (IGF)-I in children with PWS. J Clin Med. 2022;11(5) https://doi.org/10.3390/jcm11051280.

39. Donze SH, Damen L, van Alfen-van der Velden JAEM, et al. Prevalence of growth hormone (GH) deficiency in previously GH-treated young adults with Prader-Willi syndrome. Clin Endocrinol. 2019;91(1):118–23. https://doi.org/10.1111/cen.13988.
40. Salvatoni A, Nosetti L, Salvatore S, Agosti M. Benefits of multidisciplinary care in Prader-Willi syndrome. Expert Rev Endocrinol Metab. 2021;16(2):63–71.
41. Pellikaan K, Ben BY, Rosenberg AGW, et al. Hypogonadism in adult males with Prader-Willi syndrome—clinical recommendations based on a Dutch cohort study, review of the literature and an international expert panel discussion. J Clin Med. 2021;10(24) https://doi.org/10.3390/jcm10245781.
42. Pellikaan K, Ben BY, Rosenberg AGW, et al. Hypogonadism in women with prader-willi syndrome— clinical recommendations based on a dutch cohort study, review of the literature and an international expert panel discussion. J Clin Med. 2021;10(24) https://doi.org/10.3390/jcm10245781.
43. Siemensma EPC, De Lind Van Wijngaarden RFA, Otten BJ, De Jong FH, Hokken-Koelega ACS. Testicular failure in boys with Prader-Willi syndrome: longitudinal studies of reproductive hormones. J Clin Endocrinol Metab. 2012;97(3):452–9. https://doi.org/10.1210/jc.2011-1954.
44. Noordam C, Höybye C, Eiholzer U. Prader–willi syndrome and hypogonadism: a review article. Int J Mol Sci. 2021;22(5):1–12. https://doi.org/10.3390/ijms22052705.
45. Siemensma EPC, Van Alfen-van Der Velden AAEM, Otten BJ, Laven JSE, Hokken-Koelega ACS. Ovarian function and reproductive hormone levels in girls with prader-willi syndrome: a longitudinal study. J Clin Endocrinol Metab. 2012;97(9):1766–73. https://doi.org/10.1210/jc.2012-1595.
46. Prencipe N, Marinelli L, Varaldo E, et al. Isolated anterior pituitary dysfunction in adulthood. Front Endocrinol (Lausanne). 2023;14(March):1–21. https://doi.org/10.3389/fendo.2023.1100007.
47. Bakker NE, Kuppens RJ, Siemensma EPC, et al. Bone mineral density in children and adolescents with prader-willi syndrome: a longitudinal study during puberty and 9 years of growth hormone treatment. J Clin Endocrinol Metab. 2015;100(4):1609–18. https://doi.org/10.1210/jc.2014-4347.
48. Tauber MHC. Endocrine disorders in Prader-Willi syndrome: a model to understand and treat hypothalamic dysfunction. Lancet Diabetes Endocrinol. 2021;9(4):235–46.
49. Tauber M, Barbeau C, Jouret B, Pienkowski C, Malzac PMA. Auxological and endocrine evolution of 28 children with Prader-Willi syndrome: effect of GH therapy in 14 children. Horm Res. 2000;53(6):297–87.
50. Grootjen LN, Kerkhof GF, Juriaans AF, Trueba-Timmermans DJ, Hokken-Koelega ACS. Acute stress response of the HPA-axis in children with Prader-Willi syndrome: new insights and consequences for clinical practice. Front Endocrinol (Lausanne). 2023;14(May):1–9. https://doi.org/10.3389/fendo.2023.1146680.
51. Rosenberg AGW, Pellikaan K, Poitou C, et al. Central adrenal insufficiency is rare in adults with prader–willi syndrome. J Clin Endocrinol Metab. 2020;105(7):2563–71. https://doi.org/10.1210/clinem/dgaa168.
52. Rosenberg AGW, Wellink CM, Tellez Garcia JM, et al. Health problems in adults with Prader–Willi syndrome of different genetic subtypes: cohort study, meta-analysis and review of the literature. J Clin Med. 2022;11(14):1–27. https://doi.org/10.3390/jcm11144033.
53. Grootjen LN, Rutges JPHJ, Damen L, et al. Effects of 8 years of growth hormone treatment on scoliosis in children with Prader-Willi syndrome. Eur J Endocrinol. 2021;185(1):47–55. https://doi.org/10.1530/EJE-21-0211.
54. Crinò A, Armando M, Crostelli M, et al. High prevalence of scoliosis in a large cohort of patients with Prader-Willi syndrome. J Clin Med. 2022;11(6) https://doi.org/10.3390/jcm11061574.

55. Min M, Ferreira J, Wang C. Food for thought: complications of acute gastric distension in Prader-Willi syndrome. Clin Gastroenterol Hepatol. 2015;13(8):A25–6. https://doi.org/10.1016/j.cgh.2015.03.027.
56. Van Loo L, Vogels A, Rochtus A. Behavioral changes in patients with Prader-Willi syndrome can mask severe physical illness. JCEM Case Rep. 2022;1(1):1–4. https://doi.org/10.1210/jcemcr/luac034.
57. Juriaans AF, Kerkhof GF, Hokken-Koelega ACS. The Spectrum of the Prader–Willi-like Pheno- and genotype: a review of the literature. Endocr Rev. 2021:1–18. https://doi.org/10.1210/endrev/bnab026.

Chung-Jansen Syndrome (*PHIP*-Related Disorder)

Wenneke van Weelden, Lotte Kleinendorst, and Mieke van Haelst

1 Introduction

Chung-Jansen syndrome (CHUJANS), also known as *PHIP*-related disorder is a rare genetic disorder caused by haploinsufficiency of the Pleckstrin Homology domain Interacting Protein (PHIP). The *PHIP* gene is located on chromosome 6q14. The syndrome was first identified in the 2016. Patients mainly present with developmental delay, learning difficulties or intellectual disability, behavioral abnormalities, obesity and typical facial features. In 2022, only 67 patients with CHUJANS have been described in the literature [1]. It is likely that the actual number of patients is higher than currently reported. At our outpatient clinic in the Amsterdam UMC, we have seen about 30 patients with CHUJANS.

W. van Weelden
Department of Human Genetics, Section Clinical Genetics, Amsterdam University Medical Center, Amsterdam, The Netherlands
e-mail: w.vanweelden@amsterdamumc.nl

L. Kleinendorst · M. van Haelst (✉)
Department of Human Genetics, Section Clinical Genetics, Amsterdam University Medical Center, Amsterdam, The Netherlands

Emma Center for Personalized Medicine, Amsterdam UMC, University of Amsterdam, Amsterdam, The Netherlands
e-mail: l.kleinendorst@amsterdamumc.nl; m.vanhaelst@amsterdamumc.nl

M. van Haelst, E. van den Akker (eds.), *Clinical Obesity Genetics*,
https://doi.org/10.1007/978-3-032-04095-4_4

2 Aetiology and Pathophysiology

Heterozygous pathogenic *PHIP* variants cause CHUJANS. The *PHIP* gene encodes through alternative splicing for the PHIP protein and neuronal differentiation-related protein. Their function is linked to neurodevelopment processes. Reported *PHIP* alterations encompass a spectrum of variants, including truncating variants, missense substitutions, splice variants, and larger deletions. There appears to be no clear clustering of variants or specific hotspots for pathogenic variants [2]. Although, many of the reported missense variants are located in the WD40 repeat regions of the *PHIP* gene [3].

CHUJANS has an autosomal dominant inheritance pattern. The variant often occurs *de novo* in the patient, but there are several familial cases known and mosaicism has been described [3].

2.1 Obesity

In cellular experiments, it was shown that *PHIP* regulates proopiomelanocortin (*POMC)* transcription. Rare loss-of-function variants in *PHIP* showed a decrease of POMC transcription. For some variants, the *POMC* transcription was shown to be rescuable by leptin stimulation, suggesting a potential therapeutic target [4].

3 Clinical Presentation

CHUJANS is usually diagnosed in children with developmental delay. Patients can also initially present with obesity when the learning problems are mild. The clinical characteristics are summarized in Table 1. The largest published cohort included 47 patients, with a median age of 10.9 years (youngest 5 months; oldest 43.7 years old) [3].

3.1 Obesity

The prevalence of obesity in CHUJANS differs in the published cohorts, partly dependent on age. Birth weight is usually normal. About half of the patients have initial feeding problems. Overweight or obesity is reported in approximately 60% of the patients (all ages together) [3]. The onset of obesity is before the age of 8 years old in about half of the cases [1], but starts at a later age as well [3]. Obesity appears to be more prominent in older individuals. Hyperphagia without obesity can also be seen in childhood.

Table 1 Some of the clinical characteristics of Chung-Jansen syndrome reported in three larger cohort studies [1, 3, 5]

Feature	Reported frequency (n = 47) [3]	Reported frequency (n = 23) [5]	Reported frequency (n = 23) [1]
Developmental delay	85.1%	100%	95.7%
Overweight/obesity	55.8%	74%	69.6%
Behavioral challenges (such as ADHD, autism, anxiety and depression)	70.2%	78%	87%
Sleep issues	42.6%	18%	26.1%
Constipation	48.9%	8%	34.8%
Gastroesophageal reflux disease	23.4%	4.3%	Unknown
Hypotonia	78.7%	26%	34.8%
Cryptorchidism	39.1%	27.3%	26.1%
Asthma/reactive airway disease	27.7%	Unknown	Unknown
Urinary tract infection	29.8%	4.3%	4.3%
Visual problems	66%	65%	47.8%
Hearing problems	12.8%	Unknown	Unknown
Physical features, e.g.:			
Scoliosis	25.5%	4.3%	Unknown
Clinodactyly (of the 5th finger)	14.9%	64%	30.4%
Syndactyly	14.9%	30%	26.1%

3.2 *Behavior*

Behavioral challenges are a notable and impactful aspect of CHUJANS. The behavioral problems occur in both childhood and adulthood and are diverse. Many patients are diagnosed with autism spectrum disorder or attention deficit hyperactivity disorder. Anxiety occurs in around 50% of the patients and depression in almost 30%. Depression is more common in patients who are overweight or have obesity [3].

3.3 *Hearing and Vision*

Sensory processing problems are reported in many patients with CHUJANS. Visual problems are diverse but mostly relatively mild. The common visual problems are myopia, hyperopia, strabismus, amblyopia, and astigmatism. Frequent ear-nose-throat problems include otitis media and inflamed tonsils and adenoids [3]. Hearing problems (usually conductive hearing loss) already start at a young age and occur in 12.8% of the patients [3].

3.4 Neurological Problems

In the largest cohort study to date, hypotonia is present in the majority (80%) of patients, which is a higher frequency compared to the smaller cohort studies (approximately 30%). Other neurological problems are less frequent but could involve uncoordinated movements, hypertonia, tics or seizures [3].

3.5 Other Characteristics

Approximately 40% of patients experience sleep issues [3]. Constipation (48.9%), gastroesophageal reflux disease (23.4%), asthma/reactive airway disease (27.7%), urinary tract infection (29.8%) and cryptorchidism (39.1%) can occur. Other features have been described in fewer patients: hypothyroidism (2.1%), heart defects (4.3%; e.g. ventricular septal defect) and renal involvement (horseshoe kidney, unilateral kidney, small kidneys) [3, 6].

3.6 Dysmorphic Features

CHUJANS has a distinct associated facial gestalt [7]. The most characteristic facial features are large ears and earlobes, prominent eyebrows, and anteverted nares. A round face, short nose with broad nasal tip, long philtrum, and deep-set eyes is also observed in the majority of cases. Scoliosis is seen in about a quarter of patients [3]. Syndactyly (29%) and clinodactyly of the fifth finger have been reported as well [8].

3.7 Case

A 42-year-old man was referred to the obesity genetics clinic with the suspicion of a genetic obesity disorder. He was born at 36 weeks of gestation after un eventful pregnancy with a birth weight of 2400 grams (p10–p50). There was no history of neonatal feeding problems. His development was delayed: to stimulate motor development, he had received physiotherapy at the age of 10 months, after which his development progressed. He was able to walk at approximately 14 months of age. He learned to read and write, but later than average. He followed special education, where he was diagnosed with Pervasive Developmental Disorder-Not Otherwise Specified. There were no further behavioral problems. He underwent surgery for cryptorchidism. Now, at an adult age, he works as a waiter. His motor skills are not impaired although he is still a bit clumsy. His hearing is impaired (perceptual hearing loss) due to recurrent otitis media infections. He wears glasses (mild myopia) but has no other eye problems. Because of constipation he sometimes uses

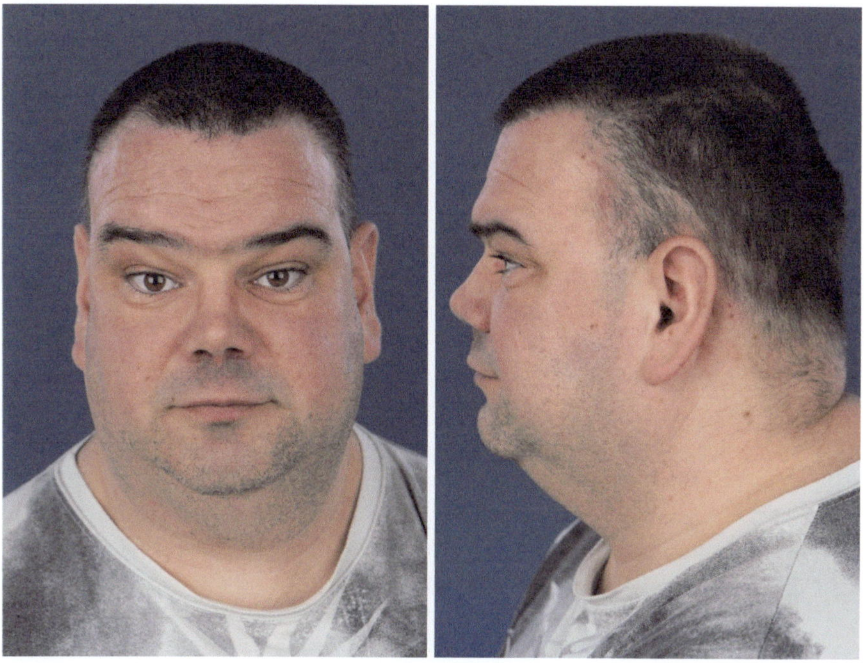

Fig. 1 Photographs of the patient: upslanted palpebral fissure, synophrys, attached earlobes, thin upper lip, dorsocervical fat pad

high-fiber sachets. Until the age of 12 years he was slim, but since then his weight increased and he became obese. He has an increase appetite since childhood and ate the food of his siblings if they did not like it. At the moment he still suffers from hyperphagia; he can continue to eat unless he is stopped. He also sometimes binge-eats without an apparent reason. The increased weight caused comorbidities such as hypertension, dyslipidemia and sleep apnea. There are no people in the family with an intellectual disability or childhood onset obesity.

On physical examination, his height was 180.5 cm (−0.5 SD), weight 110.6 kg, BMI 34 kg/m^2 (+3.3 SD) and head circumference 56,0 cm (−1 SD). Apart from his truncal obesity, he has upslanted palpebral fissure, synophrys, attached earlobes, thin upper lip, dorsocervical fat pad, some breast development (mostly fat tissue) and cubitus valgus of the elbows (Fig. 1).

Genetic testing in the patient showed a heterozygous likely pathogenic *PHIP* variant ((Chr6: NM_017934.7) c.4159_4162del p.(Leu1387Phefs*19)). His mother's DNA was analysed and the *PHIP* variant was not identified. His father is not tested, but it was suspected that he did not have the same variant since he did not have a similar phenotype.

Genotype-Phenotype Correlation

No clear genotype-phenotype correlation is described for CHUJANS. There is intra- and interfamilial phenotypic variability.

4 Clinical and Molecular Diagnosis

The diagnosis CHUJANS can be confirmed by identification of a heterozygous (likely) pathogenic variant in the *PHIP* gene. There are no official diagnostic criteria established for a clinical diagnosis. Patients are often diagnosed via broad genetic tests such as whole exome or genome sequencing or episignature testing. In the Amsterdam UMC a Next-Generation Sequencing (NGS) based obesity gene panel is available which includes the *PHIP* gene. When there is a high suspicion of CHUJANS, one could also order a single-gene analysis of *PHIP*.

4.1 Episignature Testing

Episignature testing for CHUJANS is also offered as a diagnostic test in het laboratory of the Amsterdam UMC. This test can help confirm a high suspicion of CHUJANS in patients where no DNA variant in *PHIP* was found. Episignature analysis can also be helpful to classify variants of unknown significance in the *PHIP* gene. In particular when the methylation pattern fits the suspicion for CHUJANS it can help further interpret these unknown variants and strengthen a clinical diagnosis. CHUJANS has an overlapping episignature with Borjeson-Forssman-Lehmann syndrome (*PHF6* gene) and White-Kernohan syndrome (*DBB1* gene) [9]. Therefore, to definitively confirm CHUJANS a (likely) pathogenic DNA variant in het *PHIP* gene has to be located.

5 Differential Diagnosis

There are many syndromic forms of obesity that share overlapping features with CHUJANS. For many patients, Prader-Willi syndrome is considered as a differential diagnosis [1], but severe neonatal hypotonia is reported less frequently in patients with CHUJANS [1]. Other important diagnoses to consider are Borjeson-Forssman-Lehmann syndrome and White-Kernohan syndrome, as these genetic obesity disorders have similar features as well as overlapping methylation signatures [9]. Cornelia de Lange syndrome also has some overlapping characteristics such as prominent eyebrows. The other striking Cornelia de Lange syndrome features (skeletal anomalies, severe intellectual deficiency) are however lacking in CHUJANS [10].

6 Therapy and Follow-Up Advice

At the moment, there is no specific cure for CHUJANS and no formal guideline for the syndrome exists.

There are also no specific guidelines for obesity treatment in CHUJANS syndrome. Management is done according to standard guidelines for obesity. However, because of the syndromic aspects, patients need a tailored program to support their combined lifestyle intervention by a multidisciplinary team with specific expertise on hyperphagia and intellectual deficit. The effect of untargeted obesity pharmacotherapy is unknown for CHUJANS. Preliminary results of a phase 2 clinical trial with MC4R-agonist Setmelanotide show that over 50% of the patients achieved a BMI reduction greater than 5% [Rhythm Pharmaceuticals Announces Updates on MC4R Pathway Programs at R&D Event | Rhythm Pharmaceuticals, Inc. (rhythmtx.com)].

Doctors should be aware of weight gain when prescribing psychotropic medications such as anti-epileptic or anti-depressive drugs. This is particularly important for people with CHUJANS who are already at a significantly increased risk of developing obesity.

Further management of this syndrome should be tailored to each individual case, although general concepts e.g. for people with intellectual disabilities can be applied. Often speech and/or physical therapy is required. The behavioral problems can require neuropsychological / psychiatric evaluation. Because of visual problems in ~65% of the patients, we recommend ophthalmological surveillance for CHUJANS patients [3].

7 Family Screening

Parents of an index with a (likely) pathogenic variant in *PHIP* are offered testing. Since most cases of CHUJANS are *de novo,* further family screening is often not necessary. The chance of the parents having another child with CHUJANS, when their child has a *de novo* variant, is small, but a bit higher than the population risk due to the change of germline mosaicism (the presence of a pathogenic variant in only the ovaries or testes of a parent). Since CHUJANS is an autosomal dominant condition, affected individuals with a proven molecular diagnosis have a 50% chance of passing the *PHIP* variant on to their children.

Take Home Message

- Chung-Jansen syndrome (CHUJANS) is an autosomal dominant obesity disorder
- It is caused by a heterozygous genetic defect in the *PHIP* gene
- The main characteristics are developmental delay, behavioral problems, obesity and hypotonia
- Facial features include large earlobes and prominent eyebrows
- For obesity treatment, patients need a tailored program for combined lifestyle intervention supported by a multidisciplinary team with specific expertise on hyperphagia and intellectual deficit. The effect of untargeted obesity pharmacotherapy or bariatric surgery is currently unknown.
- An Episignature analysis can further interpret variants of uncertain significance in the *PHIP* gene to confirm a clinical diagnosis

References

1. Kampmeier A, Leitao E, Parenti I, Beygo J, Depienne C, Bramswig NC, et al. PHIP-associated Chung-Jansen syndrome: report of 23 new individuals. Front Cell Dev Biol. 2022;10:1020609.
2. Craddock KE, Okur V, Wilson A, Gerkes EH, Ramsey K, Heeley JM, et al. Clinical and genetic characterization of individuals with predicted deleterious PHIP variants. Cold Spring Harb Mol Case Stud. 2019;5(4):a004200.
3. Sudnawa KK, Calamia S, Geltzeiler A, Chung WK. Clinical phenotypes of individuals with Chung-Jansen syndrome across age groups. Am J Med Genet A. 2024;194(3):e63471.
4. Marenne G, Hendricks AE, Perdikari A, Bounds R, Payne F, Keogh JM, et al. Exome sequencing identifies genes and gene sets contributing to severe childhood obesity, linking PHIP variants to repressed POMC transcription. Cell Metab. 2020;31(6):1107–19 e12.
5. Jansen S, Hoischen A, Coe BP, Carvill GL, Van Esch H, Bosch DGM, et al. A genotype-first approach identifies an intellectual disability-overweight syndrome caused by PHIP haploinsufficiency. Eur J Hum Genet. 2018;26(1):54–63.
6. Kaur H, Panigrahi I. Chung-Jansen syndrome with obesity. Obes Res Clin Pract. 2021;15(3):303–5.
7. van der Donk R, Jansen S, Schuurs-Hoeijmakers JHM, Koolen DA, Goltstein L, Hoischen A, et al. Next-generation phenotyping using computer vision algorithms in rare genomic neurodevelopmental disorders. Genet Med. 2019;21(8):1719–25.
8. Dietrich J, Lovell S, Veatch OJ, Butler MG. PHIP gene variants with protein modeling, interactions, and clinical phenotypes. Am J Med Genet A. 2022;188(2):579–89.
9. Vos N, Haghshenas S, van der Laan L, Russel PKM, Rooney K, Levy MA, et al. The detection of a strong episignature for Chung-Jansen syndrome, partially overlapping with Borjeson-Forssman-Lehmann and white-Kernohan syndromes. Hum Genet. 2024;143(6):761–73.
10. Conti B, Rinaldi B, Rimoldi M, Villa R, Iascone M, Gangi S, et al. Chung-Jansen syndrome can mimic Cornelia de Lange syndrome: another player among chromatinopathies? Am J Med Genet A. 2023;191(6):1586–92.

16p11.2 Deletion Syndrome

Niels Vos, Lotte Kleinendorst, and Mieke van Haelst

1 Introduction

The 16p11.2 chromosomal region is a hotspot of genetic variation. Within this region, both deletions and duplications are regularly seen. They are associated with diverse neurodevelopmental and psychiatric problems. The deletions and duplications also lead to contrasting clinical phenotypes, often referred to as a "mirror phenotype". Deletions of 16p11.2 have been linked to increased frequency of macrocephaly, whereas individuals with the duplication more often have microcephaly. Another striking aspect of this mirror phenotype is the impact on body weight. Individuals with 16p11.2 deletions are more likely to have obesity and associated metabolic concerns, such as insulin resistance. In contrast, individuals with 16p11.2 duplications tend to be underweight.

Recurrent chromosome 16p11.2 deletions are among the most common genetic causes of neurodevelopmental problems and obesity. The most frequently reported recurrent 16p11.2 deletion subtypes are the 'typical' 16p11.2 BP4-BP5 and 'distal'

N. Vos (✉)
Department of Human Genetics, Amsterdam University Medical Center,
Amsterdam, The Netherlands

Amsterdam Reproduction and Development Research Institute, Amsterdam, The Netherlands
e-mail: n.vos12@amsterdamumc.nl

L. Kleinendorst · M. van Haelst
Department of Human Genetics, Amsterdam University Medical Center,
Amsterdam, The Netherlands

Amsterdam Reproduction and Development Research Institute, Amsterdam, The Netherlands

Emma Center for Personalized Medicine, Amsterdam UMC, University of Amsterdam,
Amsterdam, The Netherlands
e-mail: l.kleinendorst@amsterdamumc.nl; m.vanhaelst@amsterdamumc.nl

M. van Haelst, E. van den Akker (eds.), *Clinical Obesity Genetics*,
https://doi.org/10.1007/978-3-032-04095-4_5

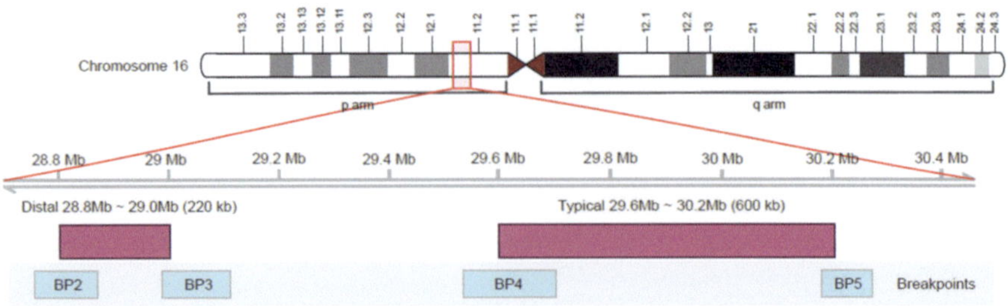

Fig. 1 An overview of chromosome 16. Part of the 16p11.2 region is shown in more detail and the most common deletions of this region, the typical 16p11.2 BP4-BP5 deletion and the distal 16p11.2 BP2-BP3 deletion, are depicted, together with their breakpoints. (Figure adapted from Vos et al. [3])

16p11.2 BP2-BP3 deletions, see Fig. 1, with population prevalence estimates of 1/2000 and 1/4100, respectively [1, 2].

2 Molecular Mechanisms

The chromosome 16p11.2 region consists of low-copy repeats (LCR). Misalignment of these LCRs can lead to non-allelic homologous recombination and so recurrent deletions and duplications can occur [4], Fig. 2.

The 'typical' 16p11.2 deletion (OMIM #611913) affects the breakpoint 4–5 (BP4-BP5) ~29.6–30.2 Mb (size ~600 kb; reference genome GRCh37/hg19) region of chromosome 16 and comprises 25–30 genes. Typical 16p11.2 BP4-BP5 deletions occur *de novo* in ~70–93% of cases [5–7].

The 'distal' 16p11.2 deletion (OMIM #613444) affects the BP2-BP3 ~ 28.8–29 Mb (~220 kb; reference genome GRCh37/hg19) region of chromosome 16 and comprises 9 genes. Distal 16p11.2 BP2-BP3 deletions occur *de novo* in ~33% of cases [2, 5, 8]. Additionally, various typical and distal 16p11.2 region overlapping deletions have been reported [9].

2.1 *SH2B1*

Some genes in these typical and distal 16p11.2 regions have been linked to specific clinical features.

The *SH2B1* gene is particularly noteworthy in the context of genetic obesity. It encodes the SH2B adapter protein 1, which plays a role in the regulation of energy balance and body weight. This gene is implicated in the control of appetite, metabolism, and insulin signaling. SH2B1 serves as an adapter protein that interacts with various signaling molecules involved in metabolic pathways, including those

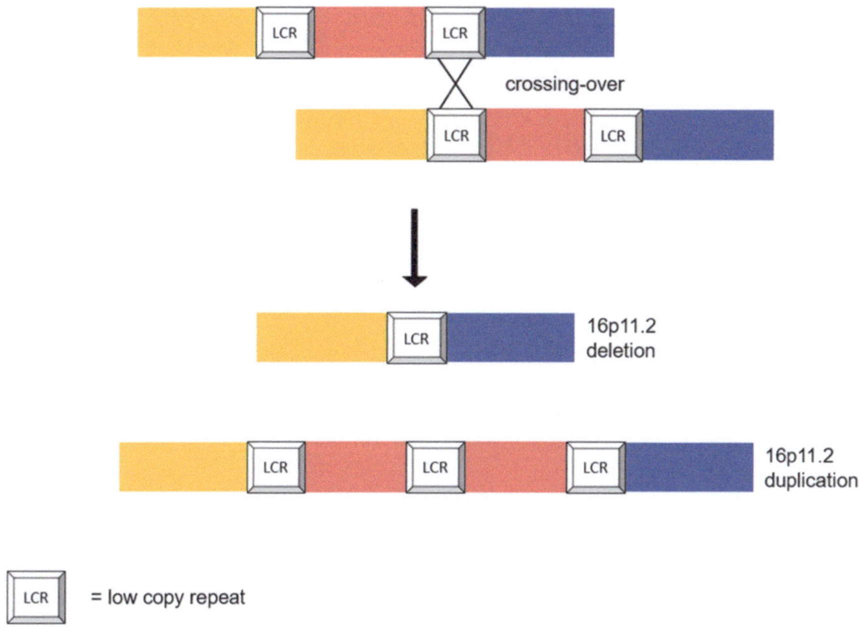

Fig. 2 An illustration of the biological mechanism that can result in 16p11.2 deletions and 16p11.2 duplications. (Credit: Figure made by Lotte Kleinendorst)

triggered by leptin. Patients with single nucleotide variants in *SH2B1* have been shown to present with obesity and severe insulin resistance [10, 11].

3 Clinical Presentation

The amount and severity of clinical features varies between individuals with 16p11.2 deletion, even within the same family. This is important to keep in mind in consultation, especially of young children whose parents might wonder what the developmental and overall clinical outlook is. The observed clinical heterogeneity requires a personalized approach for all individuals with 16p11.2 deletion, see *5.6 Therapy and follow-up*. Most is currently known about the clinical presentation of individuals with a typical 16p11.2 BP4-BP5 deletion.

3.1 *Typical 16p11.2 BP4-BP5 Deletion*

3.1.1 Perinatal Period

The first reported typical 16p11.2 BP4-BP5 deletion case, in 2002, had intra-uterine growth retardation and multiple severe congenital anomalies (cardiovascular, skeletal, genitourinary and ocular), as well as dysmorphic features [12]. Ever since, severe congenital anomalies have rarely been reported and pregnancy is typically uneventful. In comparison to the general population, however, there is an increased rate of congenital anomalies. Vertebral anomalies are most frequent (20%) and can lead to scoliosis later in life [5, 13]. Various congenital cardiac (6%), urogenital (8%) and other malformations have been reported with low frequencies [13]. Neonatal feeding problems (34%) and neonatal hypotonia (12%) are seen in part of individuals with typical 16p11.2 BP4-BP5 deletion in our own cohort [3].

3.1.2 Neurodevelopmental and Psychiatric Features

Developmental milestones are typically delayed. The majority (80–90%) of individuals with typical 16p11.2 BP4-BP5 deletion has a delayed speech and/or language development. Half of individuals with this deletion have motor difficulties [5, 13, 14]. Hypotonia, in combination with hypermobility and clumsiness, likely contribute to this [5, 15].

Large differences in school performance and full-scale IQ (FSIQ) are seen. Overall, a ~26.8 point lower FSIQ compared to familial controls is reported for individuals with typical 16p11.2 BP4-BP5 deletion (average FSIQ ~82.5) [5, 14]. IQ profiles are often disharmonic and verbal IQ is typically lower than non-verbal IQ [14, 16]. Intellectual disability (ID) is reported in 20–30% of individuals with typical 16p11.2 BP4-BP5 deletion [7, 13].

Autistic features are common and approximately 20–25% of individuals with this deletion are officially diagnosed with autism spectrum disorder (ASD). Attention Deficit Hyperactive Disorder (ADHD) is seen in a similar percentage (30%) of cases [7]. Other behavioral and psychiatric symptoms, like anxiety, obsessive compulsive disorder (OCD), tics and mood disorders have also been described, yet less frequently [7]. Currently ongoing large mental health studies will provide more detailed information on development and mental health of cases with typical 16p11.2 BP4-BP5 deletion syndrome.

Epilepsy is reported in 16–24% of cases, of which half are considered benign infantile epilepsy [5] and absence epilepsy is reported in 33% [15]. Even though limited information is available in current literature, individuals with typical 16p11.2 BP4-BP5 deletion seem to have a higher risk of sleep disturbances than the general population [17]. In our own clinical cohort, there is a lower prevalence of epilepsy (10%) and sleep problems are reported in 32% [3].

3.1.3 Weight and Growth

Obesity, often the result of hyperphagia or eating in the absence of hunger, impacts both mental and physical health and is one of the cardinal features of typical 16p11.2 BP4-BP5 deletion syndrome [18, 19]. The combination with the aforementioned neurocognitive problems, can further complicate obesity treatment. Onset of obesity is typically early in childhood. The typical 16p11.2 BP4-BP5 deletion cases' risk of developing obesity is estimated to be 43 times higher than non-carriers [13, 20]. Eventually, approximately 75% of adults with typical 16p11.2 BP4-BP5 deletion develop obesity (45% morbid obesity) [5, 13].

Occipitofrontal circumference (OFC) is generally larger than OFC of non-carrier relatives. Approximately 17% of cases have macrocephaly (OFC standard deviation score; SDS or z-score ≥2) [13, 15]. Final height of individuals with typical 16p11.2 BP4-BP5 deletion is slightly below average [13]. Height SDS is −0.8 SD in our own cohort, consisting of children and adults [3].

3.1.4 Other

Imaging studies have shown a thicker corpus callosum in 16%, cerebellar tonsillar ectopia in ~31% and Chiari I malformations in ~9% of typical 16p11.2 BP4-BP5 deletion cases [21]. Ocular/vision problems have been reported; ptosis, deep-set and downslant of eyes, hypertelorism, strabismus hyperopia and myopia [22, 23]. Even though various dysmorphic features have been described, no specific dysmorphic features stand out as disorder-specific.

3.2 Distal 16p11.2 BP2-BP3 Deletion

3.2.1 Perinatal Period

Less large clinical cohorts of individuals with distal 16p11.2 BP2-BP3 deletions have thus far been published. Non-specific congenital anomalies have been reported in a few cases [24]. In our own clinical cohort of 19 individuals, neonatal feeding difficulties and hypotonia were reported in 5% and 40%, respectively [3].

3.2.2 Neurodevelopmental and Psychiatric Features

The penetrance of distal 16p11.2 BP2-BP3 deletions for neurodevelopmental issues is estimated to be less than that of typical 16p11.2 BP4-BP5 deletions. However, developmental delay is observed in the majority of individuals with distal 16p11.2 BP2-BP3 deletion, according to the Simons Searchlight registry [25] and our own data [3]. In our clinical cohort, motor development was delayed in 87% and speech/

language development in 73% of individuals with distal 16p11.2 BP2-BP3 deletion. FSIQ information in literature and our own cohort is incomplete. Approximately half of individuals with distal 16p11.2 BP2-BP3 deletion in our own cohort had an IQ test (average FSIQ 83) and of those individuals, 40% have ID [3]. ASD is reported in 20–26% and ADHD in 33% [3, 25, 26]. Mental health studies, previously mentioned for individuals with typical 16p11.2 BP4-BP5 deletions are also aiming at clarifying the cognitive functioning and prevalence of mental health disorders in individuals with distal 16p11.2 BP2-BP3 deletions. Approximately 14–16% of individuals have a form of epilepsy [3, 25].

3.2.3 Weight and Growth

The distal 16p11.2 BP2-BP3 deletion is associated with hyperphagia and a strongly increased risk of developing obesity from early childhood and obesity-related comorbidities such as type 2 diabetes [24–26]. In our own cohort, 61% of individuals with distal 16p11.2 BP2-BP3 deletion report hyperphagia and 74% have obesity [3]. On average, individuals with this 16p11.2 deletion had a BMI SDS of 3.2 in our cohort [3]. Macrocephaly is present in ~10% [25] and on average, individuals with this deletion had an increased OFC (OFC SDS 0.9) [3]. Height of individuals with distal 16p11.2 BP2-BP3 deletion is typically normal [3, 27].

4 Diagnosis (Index Case)

The diagnosis is typically established by chromosomal microarray (CMA) analysis. However, other diagnostic techniques with CNV analysis (e.g. Whole Exome Sequencing (WES), Next-Generation Sequencing (NGS) obesity gene panel) are increasingly used in cases with developmental delay, ASD, obesity and/or epilepsy. Future diagnostic advances might additionally lead to this diagnosis (e.g. genome-wide DNA methylation analysis with EpiSign [28, 29]).

5 Flow Chart for Family Screening (Diagnosis in Relatives)

After identification of a pathogenic 16p11.2 deletion in an index patient, relatives can be referred for counseling and targeted chromosome 16p11.2 analysis. Our recommendation is to first perform this analysis in parents of the index, to determine the risk for (future) siblings of the index patient. In case a 16p11.2 occurred *de novo*, risk for (future) siblings of the index patient is low (1–2%) and testing is only recommended if siblings have clear symptoms. If the 16p11.2 deletion is identified in one of the parents, the (future) siblings of the index patient have a 50% chance of having the 16p11.2 deletion as well, see Fig. 3.

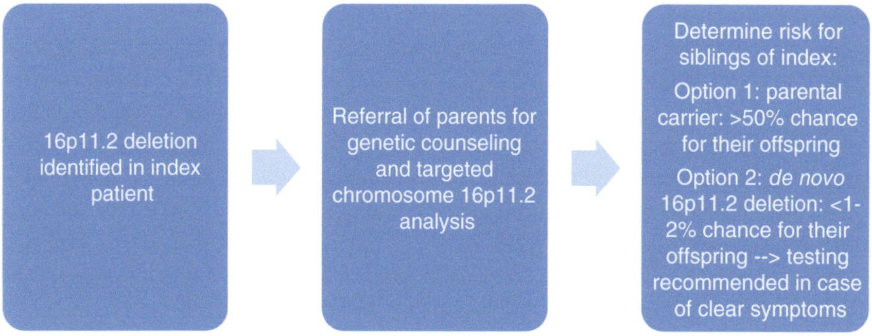

Fig. 3 Flow chart of recommendations for testing of relatives after initial diagnosis of 16p11.2 deletion in index patient

6 Therapy and Follow Up

Currently, no 16p11.2 deletion syndrome guideline exists and a generalized approach is difficult due to the observed clinical heterogeneity. Therapy and follow-up of individuals with 16p11.2 deletion should be tailored to the individual case. Knowledge of this disorder and early detection of associated features can help optimizing guidance and treatment.

These individuals, particularly with typical 16p11.2 BP4-BP5 deletion, are at increased risk of having congenital anomalies. In case a congenital anomaly is suspected (e.g. heart murmur), cardiac, renal, spinal and brain imaging can be considered.

Monitoring of milestones is important for all individuals with 16p11.2 deletion, as speech and/or physical therapy might be required. In case of developmental delay, learning difficulties and/or behavioral problems, a full neuropsychological evaluation is advised and should ideally be repeated prior to or during transitional phases. In case of psychiatric features, a psychiatric evaluation might be required. Caution is required when prescribing psychotropic (and for example anti-epileptic) medication, as these drugs might lead to weight gain and these individuals already have a strongly increased risk of developing obesity. If, however, psychotropic medication is required, extra attention is needed for weight gain, which often accompanies their use. Clinicians can consider starting metformin in an early stage in order to prevent medication induced weight gain [30].

Neurological evaluation can be considered in cases with suspected epilepsy or other neurological features.

Monitoring of weight and growth is recommended due to the increased risk of early onset obesity and potential benefits of early detection and intervention. Individuals with 16p11.2 deletion often require a more specialist and multidisciplinary approach, as obesity is often therapy resistant. Medication trials targeted at specific genetic obesity disorders, in which the efficacy of setmelanotide (an MC4R agonist) is being evaluated, provide hope of an anti-obesity remedy for certain cases with genetic obesity. The *SH2B1* gene, located within the 'distal' 16p11.2 BP2-BP3 region, is considered a component of the leptin-melanocortin pathway, making individuals with a 'distal' 16p11.2 BP2-BP3 deletion eligible for these medication trials. Unfortunately, individuals with 'typical' 16p11.2 BP4-BP5 deletions are currently not included in these studies. Alternative non-targeted pharmacological options are being evaluated and liraglutide, a glucagon-like peptide 1 (GLP-1) analogue was shown to be effective in one case with distal 16p11.2 BP2-BP3 deletion and one case with typical 16p11.2 BP4-BP5 deletion [31]. In case of abnormal growth, endocrine evaluation, including hormonal status and bone age, should be considered to determine whether additional treatment or diagnostics are required. In case of atypical or severe symptoms, additional genetic testing should be considered to search for a potentially underlying second genetic diagnosis.

Current research is aimed at further understanding clinical heterogeneity, by assessing the role of polygenic and epigenetic contribution. Additionally, pharmacogenetic profiles or passports can aid in providing an optimized and personalized treatment for individuals with 16p11.2 deletion syndrome.

7 Summary/Take Home Message

A 16p11.2 deletion, whether 'typical', 'distal' or overlapping, makes an individual susceptible to various neurodevelopmental issues, hyperphagia and childhood onset obesity. Clinical heterogeneity, also within families, requires a personalized and often multidisciplinary approach. Therapeutic anti-obesity options, like currently in medical trials for individuals with a 'distal' 16p11.2 BP2-BP3 deletion and obesity, are needed for individuals with a 'typical' 16p11.2 BP4-BP5 deletion and obesity. Research focusing on further understanding interindividual differences and prediction of clinical trajectories is currently ongoing.

References

1. Männik K, Mägi R, Macé A, Cole B, Guyatt AL, Shihab HA, et al. Copy number variations and cognitive phenotypes in unselected populations. JAMA. 2015;313(20):2044–54.
2. Smajlagić D, Lavrichenko K, Berland S, Helgeland Ø, Knudsen GP, Vaudel M, et al. Population prevalence and inheritance pattern of recurrent CNVs associated with neurodevelopmental disorders in 12,252 newborns and their parents. Eur J Hum Genet. 2021;29(1):205–15.
3. Vos N, Kleinendorst L, van der Laan L, van Uhm J, Jansen PR, van Eeghen AM, et al. Evaluation of 100 Dutch cases with 16p11.2 deletion and duplication syndromes; from clinical manifestations towards personalized treatment options. Eur J Hum Genet. 2024; https://doi.org/10.1038/s41431-024-01601-2.

4. Hastings PJ, Lupski JR, Rosenberg SM, Ira G. Mechanisms of change in gene copy number. Nat Rev Genet. 2009;10(8):551–64.
5. Chung WK, Roberts TP, Sherr EH, Snyder LG, Spiro JE. 16p11.2 deletion syndrome. Curr Opin Genet Dev. 2021;68:49–56.
6. D'Angelo D, Lebon S, Chen Q, Martin-Brevet S, Snyder LG, Hippolyte L, et al. Defining the effect of the 16p11.2 duplication on cognition, behavior, and medical comorbidities. JAMA Psychiatry. 2016;73(1):20–30.
7. Niarchou M, Chawner S, Doherty JL, Maillard AM, Jacquemont S, Chung WK, et al. Psychiatric disorders in children with 16p11.2 deletion and duplication. Transl Psychiatry. 2019;9(1):8.
8. Rosenfeld JA, Coe BP, Eichler EE, Cuckle H, Shaffer LG. Estimates of penetrance for recurrent pathogenic copy-number variations. Genet Med. 2013;15(6):478–81.
9. Sønderby IE, Gústafsson Ó, Doan NT, Hibar DP, Martin-Brevet S, Abdellaoui A, et al. Dose response of the 16p11.2 distal copy number variant on intracranial volume and basal ganglia. Mol Psychiatry. 2020;25(3):584–602.
10. Maures TJ, Kurzer JH, Carter-Su C. SH2B1 (SH2-B) and JAK2: a multifunctional adaptor protein and kinase made for each other. Trends Endocrinol Metab. 2007;18(1):38–45.
11. Doche ME, Bochukova EG, Su HW, Pearce LR, Keogh JM, Henning E, et al. Human SH2B1 mutations are associated with maladaptive behaviors and obesity. J Clin Invest. 2012;122(12):4732–6.
12. Hernando C, Plaja A, Rigola MA, Pérez MM, Vendrell T, Egocue J, Fuster C. Comparative genomic hybridisation shows a partial de novo deletion 16p11.2 in a neonate with multiple congenital malformations. J Med Genet. 2002;39(5):E24.
13. Zufferey F, Sherr EH, Beckmann ND, Hanson E, Maillard AM, Hippolyte L, et al. A 600 kb deletion syndrome at 16p11.2 leads to energy imbalance and neuropsychiatric disorders. J Med Genet. 2012;49(10):660–8.
14. Hanson E, Bernier R, Porche K, Jackson FI, Goin-Kochel RP, Snyder LG, et al. The cognitive and behavioral phenotype of the 16p11.2 deletion in a clinically ascertained population. Biol Psychiatry. 2015;77(9):785–93.
15. Steinman KJ, Spence SJ, Ramocki MB, Proud MB, Kessler SK, Marco EJ, et al. 16p11.2 deletion and duplication: characterizing neurologic phenotypes in a large clinically ascertained cohort. Am J Med Genet A. 2016;170(11):2943–55.
16. Kim SH, Green-Snyder L, Lord C, Bishop S, Steinman KJ, Bernier R, et al. Language characterization in 16p11.2 deletion and duplication syndromes. Am J Med Genet B Neuropsychiatr Genet. 2020;183(6):380–91.
17. Kamara D, De Boeck P, Lecavalier L, Neuhaus E, Beauchaine TP. Characterizing sleep problems in 16p11.2 deletion and duplication. J Autism Dev Disord. 2023;53(4):1462–75.
18. Gill R, Chen Q, D'Angelo D, Chung WK. Eating in the absence of hunger but not loss of control behaviors are associated with 16p11.2 deletions. Obesity (Silver Spring). 2014;22(12):2625–31.
19. Taylor CM, Smith R, Lehman C, Mitchel MW, Singer K, Weaver WC, Chung W. 16p11.2 recurrent deletion. In: Adam MP, Ardinger HH, Pagon RA, Wallace SE, Bean LJH, Mirzaa G, Amemiya A, editors. GeneReviews(®). Seattle: University of Washington; 1993. Copyright © 1993-2021, University of Washington, Seattle. GeneReviews is a registered trademark of the University of Washington, Seattle. All rights reserved.; 1993.
20. Jacquemont S, Reymond A, Zufferey F, Harewood L, Walters RG, Kutalik Z, et al. Mirror extreme BMI phenotypes associated with gene dosage at the chromosome 16p11.2 locus. Nature. 2011;478(7367):97–102.
21. Owen JP, Bukshpun P, Pojman N, Thieu T, Chen Q, Lee J, et al. Brain MR imaging findings and associated outcomes in carriers of the reciprocal copy number variation at 16p11.2. Radiology. 2018;286(1):217–26.
22. Stingl CS, Jackson-Cook C, Couser NL. Ocular findings in the 16p11.2 microdeletion syndrome: a case report and literature review. Case Rep Pediatr. 2020;2020:2031701.

23. Shinawi M, Liu P, Kang SH, Shen J, Belmont JW, Scott DA, et al. Recurrent reciprocal 16p11.2 rearrangements associated with global developmental delay, behavioural problems, dysmorphism, epilepsy, and abnormal head size. J Med Genet. 2010;47(5):332–41.
24. Bachmann-Gagescu R, Mefford HC, Cowan C, Glew GM, Hing AV, Wallace S, et al. Recurrent 200-kb deletions of 16p11.2 that include the SH2B1 gene are associated with developmental delay and obesity. Genet Med. 2010;12(10):641–7.
25. Simons Vip Consortium. Simons Variation in Individuals Project (Simons VIP): a genetics-first approach to studying autism spectrum and related neurodevelopmental disorders. Neuron. 2012;73(6):1063–7.
26. Loviglio MN, Leleu M, Männik K, Passeggeri M, Giannuzzi G, van der Werf I, et al. Chromosomal contacts connect loci associated with autism, BMI and head circumference phenotypes. Mol Psychiatry. 2017;22(6):836–49.
27. Hanssen R, Auwerx C, Jõeloo M, Sadler MC, Henning E, Keogh J, et al. Chromosomal deletions on 16p11.2 encompassing SH2B1 are associated with accelerated metabolic disease. Cell Rep Med. 2023;4(8):101155.
28. Levy MA, McConkey H, Kerkhof J, Barat-Houari M, Bargiacchi S, Biamino E, et al. Novel diagnostic DNA methylation episignatures expand and refine the epigenetic landscapes of Mendelian disorders. HGG Adv. 2022;3(1):100075.
29. Siu MT, Butcher DT, Turinsky AL, Cytrynbaum C, Stavropoulos DJ, Walker S, et al. Functional DNA methylation signatures for autism spectrum disorder genomic risk loci: 16p11.2 deletions and CHD8 variants. Clin Epigenetics. 2019;11(1):103.
30. Fitzgerald I, O'Connell J, Keating D, Hynes C, McWilliams S, Crowley EK. Metformin in the management of antipsychotic-induced weight gain in adults with psychosis: development of the first evidence-based guideline using GRADE methodology. Evid Based Ment Health. 2022;25(1):15–22.
31. Welling MS, de Groot CJ, Kleinendorst L, van der Voorn B, Burgerhart JS, van der Valk ES, et al. Effects of glucagon-like peptide-1 analogue treatment in genetic obesity: a case series. Clin Obes. 2021;11(6):e12481.

Schaaf-Yang Syndrome (*MAGEL2*)

Lotte Kleinendorst and Mieke van Haelst

1 Introduction

Schaaf-Yang syndrome (SYS) is a rare genetic disorder that affects neurodevelopment. It was first described in 2013 and currently over 250 cases have been published [1]. The syndrome is caused by heterozygous pathogenic variants on the paternal allele of the *MAGEL2* gene. This gene is located within the Prader-Willi critical region, chromosome locus 15q11.2, see Fig. 1. Large deletions or methylation defects of this region lead to Prader-Willi syndrome (Chapter "16p11.2 Deletion Syndrome"). There are many clinical similarities between SYS and PWS. In both disorders, the patients typically present with neonatal hypotonia and feeding problems. All patients have developmental delay, which can lead to intellectual disability ranging from mild to severe. An important distinctive feature of SYS is the presence of joint contractures, which can range in severity from mild contractures in the fingers to lethal arthrogryposis multiplex congenita or foetal akinesia.

L. Kleinendorst (✉) · M. van Haelst
Department of Human Genetics, Section Clinical Genetics, Amsterdam University Medical Center, Amsterdam, The Netherlands

Emma Center for Personalized Medicine, Amsterdam University Medical Center, Amsterdam, The Netherlands
e-mail: L.Kleinendorst@amsterdamumc.nl

M. van Haelst, E. van den Akker (eds.), *Clinical Obesity Genetics*,
https://doi.org/10.1007/978-3-032-04095-4_6

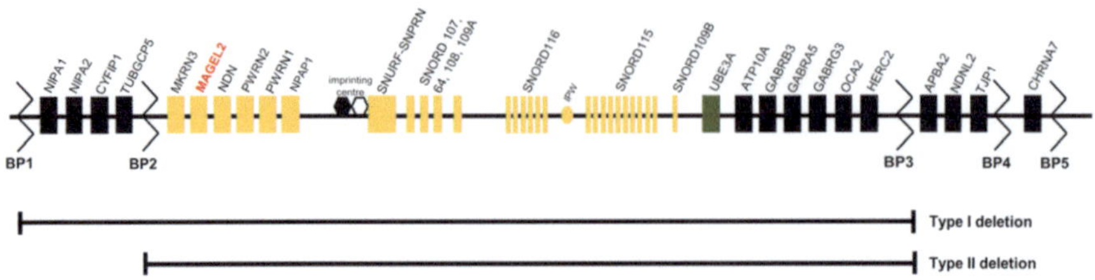

Fig. 1 Prader-Willi critical region (chromosome locus 15q11.2) including the *MAGEL2* gene shown in red

2 Aetiology and Pathophysiology

Schaaf-Yang syndrome is caused by heterozygous (likely) pathogenic variants on the paternal *MAGEL2* allele. Since *MAGEL2* is maternally imprinted, only the paternally derived allele is expressed. Therefore, maternal pathogenic variants will not lead to a phenotype. The penetrance for paternal pathogenic variants is considered to be 100% [1].

2.1 *Obesity*

The *MAGEL2* gene is involved in the food-satiety centre in the hypothalamus. *Magel2* null-mice have obesity and are less active than normal mice. These mice show a progressive loss of leptin sensitivity, probably caused by decreased LepR trafficking to the cell surface in the POMC neurons [2]. This reduced POMC activity would lead to hypoactivation of downstreaming MC4R expressing neurons, causing hyperphagia and obesity. In addition, people with Schaaf-Yang syndrome are likely more prone to obesity due to other factors, such as a lack of physical activity because of the developmental delay. Similarly to Prader-Willi syndrome, the low muscle tone (hypotonia) and low amount of muscle mass (low lean body mass) in people with SYS could also lead to a low resting energy expenditure [3]. The contractures and other skeletal abnormalities such as scoliosis could also cause patients with SYS to perform less exercise.

3 Clinical Presentation

SYS is usually diagnosed in the neonatal period because of generalized hypotonia and feeding problems. The muscular hypotonia is present in all cases, but can be variable in severity. Similar to PWS, almost all new-borns with SYS have feeding problems, with many of them needing nasogastric tube feeding.

Many children with SYS have difficulty breathing at birth and about half need respiratory support. In the majority of cases, pregnancy is without abnormalities, but decreased fetal movement and polyhydramnios can occur [4]. Some patients have very severe joint contractures that can be detected during pregnancy. Most patients have less severe distal joint contractures.

All patients have neurodevelopmental delay and around 75% have autistic behaviour [4]. The severity of intellectual disability differs: there are cases with low-normal intellectual performance, but there are also patients that never acquire speech or walking. Seizures and epilepsy is present in around 30–40% of the patients [1].

Various endocrine problems can be seen in SYS, such as growth hormone deficiency, hypopituitarism, and hypogonadism.

3.1 Dysmorphic Features

The reported dysmorphic features are non-specific and include a prominent forehead, low-set ears, and prognathism with a squared-off chin [5]. Other physical features reported are small hands, short feet, scoliosis, and kyphosis.

3.2 Obesity

In Schaaf-Yang syndrome, obesity and excessive hunger (hyperphagia) tend to appear later in childhood than they do in Prader-Willi syndrome [1, 6]. Because of high variability between the patients, there is no clear age-of-onset for the obesity in SYS. About 40% of people with Schaaf-Yang syndrome experience significant weight gain or obesity [1, 7]. It is important to realize that obesity can be a life-threatening complicating factor for the respiratory problems in SYS [7]. Obesity in SYS is more frequently seen in patients with a mild cognitive impairment compared to those with severe cognitive impairment [6]. One reason why people with SYS may be less prone to obesity in childhood compared to those with PWS could be that SYS patients generally have lower cognitive ability and are often not able to independently obtain food. This may contribute to the development of obesity later in life as cognitive skills improve.

4 Clinical Diagnosis

The diagnosis SYS is established by identification of a (likely) pathogenic variant in the paternally derived *MAGEL2* allele. There are no official criteria for a clinical diagnosis. Neuroimaging can be considered at diagnosis, which can show delayed myelination, abnormalities of the corpus callosum, and an abnormal pituitary gland [4].

5 Differential Diagnosis

The differential diagnosis of SYS is highly dependent on the age of the patient because the neonatal presentation differs from the clinical features later in life.

Differential diagnosis for neonatal presentation (hypotonia and feeding problems)

- Prader-Willi syndrome
- Temple syndrome
- Spinal muscular atrophy
- Arthrogryposis multiplex congenita
- Congenital Myasthenic Syndromes
- Congenital myotonic dystrophy

Differential diagnosis childhood/adulthood presentation (developmental delay, autistic features, short stature, obesity).

Syndromic obesity disorders such as

- Prader-Willi syndrome
- GNAS-inactivating disorders
- Temple syndrome
- Chung-Jansen syndrome

6 Molecular Diagnosis

When Schaaf-Yang syndrome is suspected, one can order either single-gene analysis, a gene panel, or broader diagnostics like exome sequencing or genome sequencing. The majority of the cases can be found with sequencing analysis, as only single cases of small deletions have been described [1, 8].

Virtually all pathogenic variants are truncating variants [4]. After detection of a (likely) pathogenic *MAGEL2* variant, testing for the parental origin is needed by methylation-sensitive sequencing.

7 Genotype-Phenotype Correlation

There are some *MAGEL2* variants with well-described genotype-phenotype correlations. The c.1996delC variant is described in multiple perinatal lethal cases. The c.1966dupC variant is the most common described pathogenic variant, which is found in about half of the SYS cases [1]. Patients with this variant have a severe SYS phenotype with a more profound intellectual disability. Interestingly, this subgroup of patients shows less hyperphagia and less excessive weight gain than patients with SYS caused by other pathogenic variants [9]. There is no specific *MAGEL2* variant reported that clearly gives a more pronounced hyperphagia or obesity phenotype.

8 Management

Currently, there is no specific cure for Schaaf-Yang syndrome, and management is primarily supportive in nature. Early intervention services, such as speech and language therapy and occupational therapy, are important to maximize the functional outcomes and quality of life of SYS patients and their caregivers.

In the neonatal phase, assisted ventilation is often needed. Assessment of the respiratory status is crucial in the follow-up phase. Around 20% of the children will require tracheostomy because of the severe respiratory distress [1]. Periodic polysomnography is needed to assess for apnea, which can be both central and obstructive [4].

Another important symptom in the neonatal phase are the severe feeding problems. Many infants will need nasogastric tube feeding. Prolonged feeding problems can lead to the placement of a gastrostomy tube in a significant part of the patients.

For all patients, the assessment of development and behavioural problems is needed. As autism spectrum disorder is often diagnosed in SYS, we recommend testing when the parents see signs of autism in their child. There are screening questionnaires and checklist especially designed to test for autism in toddlers.

Evaluation of height and weight is very important in SYS because of the possibility of growth hormone deficiency and to monitor the development of overweight and obesity.

When prescribing psychotropic medication or antiepileptic drugs, healthcare professionals should consider the obesogenic effects of these drugs because of the increased risk for obesity in SYS patients.

8.1 Clinical Trials

Studies with rapamycin are proposed and might influence the neurodevelopmental problems in SYS [10].

9 Therapy

Children with SYS and growth retardation can be treated with recombinant human growth hormone. A clear increase in height and a decrease in BMI have been reported. Moreover, the parents of the patients report improved muscle strength and some even improved motor and cognitive development during the treatment [11]. One person with SYS who was receiving growth hormone therapy reported a worsening of their sleep apnea. It is therefore recommended to perform a polysomnography before starting growth hormone therapy [1]. Other than growth hormone therapy, there are currently no specific treatment options for the obesity in SYS, but Magel2-null mice appear to be very responsive to setmelanotide, a melanocortin 4 receptor agonist [12]. Further research will have to show whether setmelanotide also has a clinical effect in SYS patients.

10 Family Screening

In approximately 50% of patients with SYS, the pathogenic *MAGEL2* variant is inherited from an unaffected father. In the other half of the patients, the variant occurred *de novo* on the paternal allele.

Paternal germline mosaicism of a *MAGEL2* variant is also reported [13].

When the father carries the *MAGEL2* variant, the recurrence risk for siblings is 50%.

For other family members, it is important to test the paternal grandmother of the proband for the presence of the *MAGEL2* variant. Paternal aunts of the proband will not have children with SYS if they carry the pathogenic variant, but their sons do have an increased risk of having a child with SYS.

Take Home Message
Schaaf-Yang syndrome is a neurodevelopmental disorder closely related to Prader-Willi syndrome. The obesity and hyperphagia in Schaaf-Yang syndrome generally develop later than in Prader-Willi syndrome and appear to be less severe. Approximately 40% of the reported patients have excessive weight gain or obesity.

References

1. Schaaf CP, Marbach F. Schaaf-Yang Syndrome. In: Adam MP, Everman DB, Mirzaa GM, Pagon RA, Wallace SE, Bean LJH, et al., editors. GeneReviews((R)). Seattle: University of Washington; 1993.
2. Oncul M, Dilsiz P, Ates Oz E, Ates T, Aklan I, Celik E, et al. Impaired melanocortin pathway function in Prader-Willi syndrome gene-Magel2 deficient mice. Hum Mol Genet. 2018;27(18):3129–36.
3. Driscoll DJ, Miller JL, Schwartz S, Cassidy SB. Prader-Willi syndrome. In: Adam MP, Everman DB, Mirzaa GM, Pagon RA, Wallace SE, Bean LJH, et al., editors. GeneReviews((R)). Seattle: University of Washington; 1993.

4. Castilla-Vallmanya L, Centeno-Pla M, Serrano M, Franco-Valls H, Martinez-Cabrera R, Prat-Planas A, et al. Advancing in Schaaf-Yang syndrome pathophysiology: from bedside to subcellular analyses of truncated MAGEL2. J Med Genet. 2023;60(4):406–15.
5. Fountain MD, Aten E, Cho MT, Juusola J, Walkiewicz MA, Ray JW, et al. The phenotypic spectrum of Schaaf-Yang syndrome: 18 new affected individuals from 14 families. Genet Med. 2017;19(1):45–52.
6. Marbach F, Elgizouli M, Rech M, Beygo J, Erger F, Velmans C, et al. The adult phenotype of Schaaf-Yang syndrome. Orphanet J Rare Dis. 2020;15(1):294.
7. Kleinendorst L, Pi Castan G, Caro-Llopis A, Boon EMJ, van Haelst MM. The role of obesity in the fatal outcome of Schaaf-Yang syndrome: early onset morbid obesity in a patient with a MAGEL2 mutation. Am J Med Genet A. 2018;176(11):2456–9.
8. Jobling R, Stavropoulos DJ, Marshall CR, Cytrynbaum C, Axford MM, Londero V, et al. Chitayat-Hall and Schaaf-Yang syndromes:a common aetiology: expanding the phenotype of MAGEL2-related disorders. J Med Genet. 2018;55(5):316–21.
9. McCarthy J, Lupo PJ, Kovar E, Rech M, Bostwick B, Scott D, et al. Schaaf-Yang syndrome overview: report of 78 individuals. Am J Med Genet A. 2018;176(12):2564–74.
10. Crutcher E, Pal R, Naini F, Zhang P, Laugsch M, Kim J, et al. mTOR and autophagy pathways are dysregulated in murine and human models of Schaaf-Yang syndrome. Sci Rep. 2019;9(1):15935.
11. Hebach NR, Caro P, Martin-Giacalone BA, Lupo PJ, Marbach F, Choukair D, Schaaf CP. A retrospective analysis of growth hormone therapy in children with Schaaf-Yang syndrome. Clin Genet. 2021;100(3):298–307.
12. Bischof JM, Van Der Ploeg LH, Colmers WF, Wevrick R. Magel2-null mice are hyper-responsive to setmelanotide, a melanocortin 4 receptor agonist. Br J Pharmacol. 2016;173(17):2614–21.
13. Patak J, Gilfert J, Byler M, Neerukonda V, Thiffault I, Cross L, et al. MAGEL2-related disorders: a study and case series. Clin Genet. 2019;96(6):493–505.

Bardet-Biedl Syndrome

Wenneke van Weelden, Elizabeth Forsythe, and Mieke van Haelst

1 Introduction

Bardet-Biedl syndrome (BBS) is a pleiotropic genetic disorder that affects multiple organ systems such as the eyes, kidneys and central nervous system. It is caused by (likely) pathogenic variants in genes that are important for the structure and/or function of the cilia, and is therefore referred to as a ciliopathy. Cilia are hair-like projections localised to the surface of most cell types, which explains why multiple organ systems are involved in BBS [1]. The main characteristics of BBS are retinal dystrophy, obesity, urogenital anomalies, polydactyly and learning disabilities (see Fig. 1).

Bardet-Biedl syndrome is named after the French physician Georges Bardet who in 1920 described several patients with retinitis pigmentosa, polydactyly and obesity [2], and a Hungarian physician Artur Biedl who 2 years later described siblings with similar characteristics [3] and recognized the overlap with Bardet's patients.

The prevalence of BBS varies between geographical areas, with the highest report of 1:3700 on the Danish Faroe Islands [4], followed by the Canadian island

W. van Weelden
Department of Human Genetics, Section Clinical Genetics, Amsterdam University Medical Center, Amsterdam, The Netherlands
e-mail: w.vanweelden@amsterdamumc.nl

E. Forsythe
Guy's and St Thomas' Hospitals, Great Ormond Street Hospital, London, UK
e-mail: elizabeth.forsythe@ucl.ac.uk

M. van Haelst (✉)
Department of Human Genetics, Section Clinical Genetics, Amsterdam University Medical Center, Amsterdam, The Netherlands

Emma Center for Personalized Medicine, Amsterdam UMC, University of Amsterdam, Amsterdam, The Netherlands
e-mail: m.vanhaelst@amsterdamumc.nl

M. van Haelst, E. van den Akker (eds.), *Clinical Obesity Genetics*, https://doi.org/10.1007/978-3-032-04095-4_7

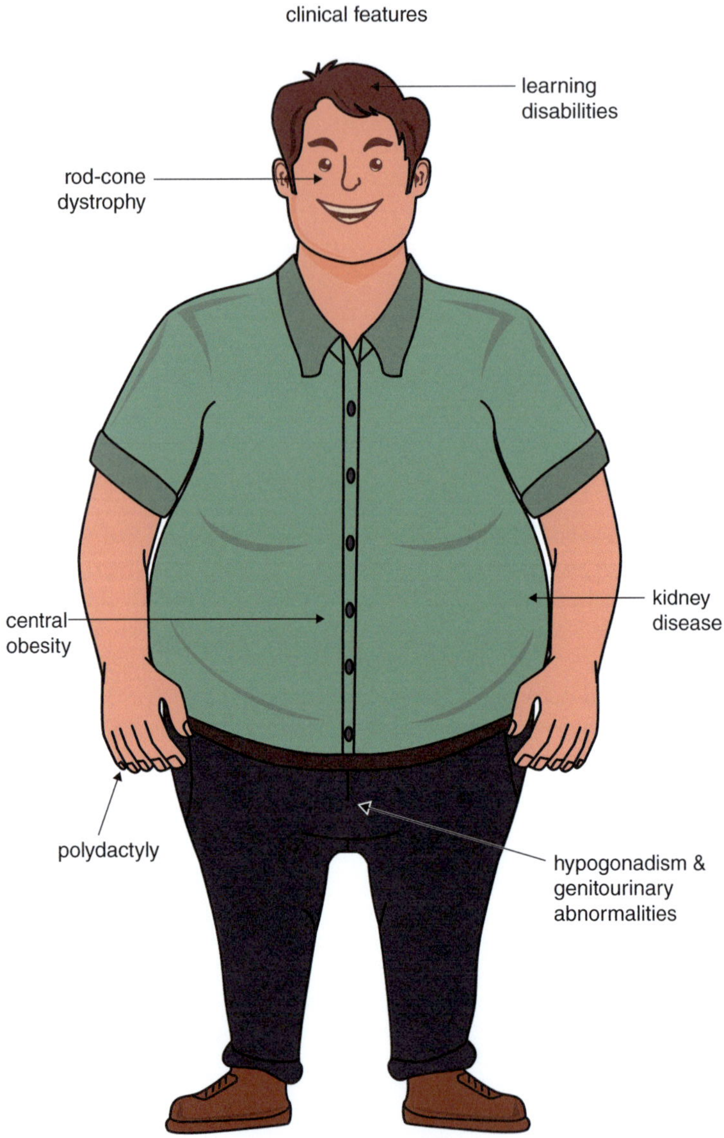

Fig. 1 Diagram of the main characteristics of Bardet-Bield syndrome

Newfoundland with a prevalence of 1:18,000 [5] and La Réunion Island with a prevalence between 1:45,000 and 1:66,000 [6]. In consanguineous populations such as the Bedouin population of Kuwait the prevalence of BBS is also high (1:13,500) [7]. These high prevalences are caused by the geographical isolation and founder effects. In Spain an estimated prevalence of 1:407,000 was described in 2015 [8]. The prevalence in the United Kingdom and North America is estimated to be around

1:100,000 [9]. Epidemiological studies on BBS from Asia and Africa are limited. A nationwide survey in Japan in 2015 identified only seven BBS patients [10], with variants in the *BBS2*, *BBS5* and *BBS7* gene.

2 Aetiology and Pathophysiology

BBS is a ciliopathy. Ciliopathies are divided into two groups: motile and immotile. Immotile cilia are primary cilia and, as the name suggests, lack the ability to move actively but play an important role in cell signaling. In BBS the nonmotile cilia are affected. They are present on most cell types, including the photoreceptors, neurons, renal tubular cells, kinocilia (inner ears) and osteocytes [1].

At least 26 genes are known to be associated with BBS. Eight of them encode highly conserved BBS proteins (BBS1, BBS2, BBS4, BBS5, BBS7, BBS8/TTC8, BBS9, and BBS18/BBIP1) that form an octameric complex called the BBSome, which is important for the function of the cilium. The formation of the BBSome is established by Chaperonin-like BBS proteins (BBS6, BBS10 and BBS12) and small GTPases [11]. The BBSome has ciliary functions as well as intracellular functions such as vesicular trafficking, cell cytoskeleton dynamics, gene expression, and cellular and organelle homeostasis [11]. The pathophysiology of the retinal dystrophy in BBS involves changes in the structure of the photoreceptor, including mislocalization of rhodopsin, and apoptosis [12].

2.1 Obesity

The pathogenicity of the obesity and hyperphagia phenotype in BBS is not completely understood. The BBSome appears to be a regulator of energy balance by influencing the hypothalamic leptin-melanocortin pathway (see Chapter "Non-syndromic Leptin Melanocortin Pathway Disorders"). The BBsome plays a role in localizing the leptin and insulin receptor on the plasma membrane. In mice with a targeted *BBS1* gene deletion, the impaired BBSome in both the proopiomelanocortin (POMC) and agouti-related peptide (AgRP) neurons leads to obesity and hyperphagia [13].

2.2 Inheritance

BBS is inherited in an autosomal recessive manner and is caused by biallelic (likely) pathogenic variants in any of the 26 BBS associated genes. There is significant intra- and interfamilial phenotypic variability. In most cases, both parents of an affected patient are healthy heterozygote carriers. In some cases, uniparental disomy and *de novo* occurrence of one variant has been described [14]. While oligogenic inheritance of BBS was proposed, this has not been substantiated in recent studies [15].

3 Clinical Presentation

Apart from obesity, multiple organ systems such as the eyes, kidneys and central nervous system are affected in BBS. Although the presentation of polydactyly in combination with genital and/or kidney anomales can lead to a pre- or neonatal diagnosis of BBS, the diagnosis is usually established in childhood or early adulthood, coinciding with the onset of the visual deterioration. Common characteristics of BBS are summarized in Table 1.

3.1 Obesity

Obesity is present in up to 89% of patients and usually develops in the first year of life. Birth weight is within normal range in the majority of cases. The highest median BMI z-scores in childhood is seen at the age of two to five [16]. As children progress to adolescence the fat distribution is typically centrally located; also known

Table 1 Common clinical characteristics of Bardet-Biedl syndrome

Feature		Reported frequency [15]
Major	Obesity	89%
	Retinal dystrophy	94%
	Postaxial polydactyly	79%
	Hypogonadism and genitourinary malformations	59%
	Kidney disease and/or malformations	52%
	Cognitive impairment	66%
Minor	Olfactory dysfunction	47–100%
	Dental abnormalities	~50%
	Liver disease	30%
	Type 2 diabetes	15.8%
	Gastrointestinal abnormalities	Up to 30%
	Cardiovascular & other thoraco-abdominal abnormalities	Up to 29%
	Subclinical hypothyroidism	19.4%
	Polycystic ovary syndrome	14.7%
	Epilepsy	9.6%

as truncal obesity [15, 16]. Metabolic syndrome is more prevalent in individuals with BBS compared with matched controls [17].

Obesity can lead to an earlier onset of puberty and therefore patients with BBS can be taller during childhood compared to other children their age. The final height at adulthood is normal [16]. Excessive hunger (hyperphagia) is frequently reported and associated with the obesity [18]. Comorbidities of obesity are common and include type 2 diabetes mellitus, cardiovascular morbidities, non-alcoholic fatty liver disease (NAFLD), sub-clinical hypothyroidism, polycystic ovary syndrome (PCOS) and skin conditions such as striae and acanthosis nigricans.

3.2 *Retinal Dystrophy*

Retinal degeneration is seen in approximately 94% of all BBS patients and is therefore the most prominent characteristic of BBS [15]. There is significant variation in the age of visual deterioration. The lack of retinal dystrophy in the absence of molecular confirmation should prompt the clinician to consider differential diagnoses. Night blindness in the first decade of life is often the initial sign of visual deterioration in patients. After that, peripheral vision will progressively decrease and often patients are registered legally blind between the second and third decade of life. Patients also experience diminution of color discrimination and visual acuity [12]. BBS patients typically have a rod-cone dystrophy with early macular involvement.

3.3 *Cognitive Impairment*

Learning disabilities and developmental delay are present in 66% of the BBS patients [15], equally affecting females and males.

3.4 *Genital Anomalies*

Males with BBS may present with a micropenis, small-testicular volume and/or cryptorchidism (9%) [15]. Females with BBS can have structural genital anomalies such as a hypoplastic uterus, ovaries or fallopian tubes. Relatively few men and women with BBS have been reported in the literature to have biological offspring [15, 19]. This may in part be due to subfertility but for many it may also relate to personal choice and developmental delay.

3.5 Kidney Disease

Kidney disease and/or malformations occur in 52% of the BBS patients [15]. A wide spectrum of structural renal anomalies have been reported including hydronephrosis, vesicoureteral reflux, horseshoe kidney, kidney cysts and ectopic, duplex, or absent kidneys. Less than 10% of patients need a kidney transplantation due to end stage renal failure.

3.6 Skeletal Abnormalities

The most frequent congenital malformation seen in patients with BBS is polydactyly (79%) [15]. The extra digits are typically postaxial. *BBS17* is associated with mesoaxial polydactyly [20]. Brachydactyly is frequently reported. Syndactyly can be present but is less common.

3.7 Facial Dysmorphic Features

The facial dysmorphic features are not very distinct and may also be completely absent. Typical features include brachycephaly, macrocephaly, narrow forehead, deep-set eyes, hypertelorism, downslanted palpebral fissures, a flat midface, flat nasal bridge, long and smooth philtrum, dental crowding or hypodontia, high-arched palate and retrognathia [21]. Figure 2 shows photographs of a patient with BBS illustrating some of the dysmorphic features.

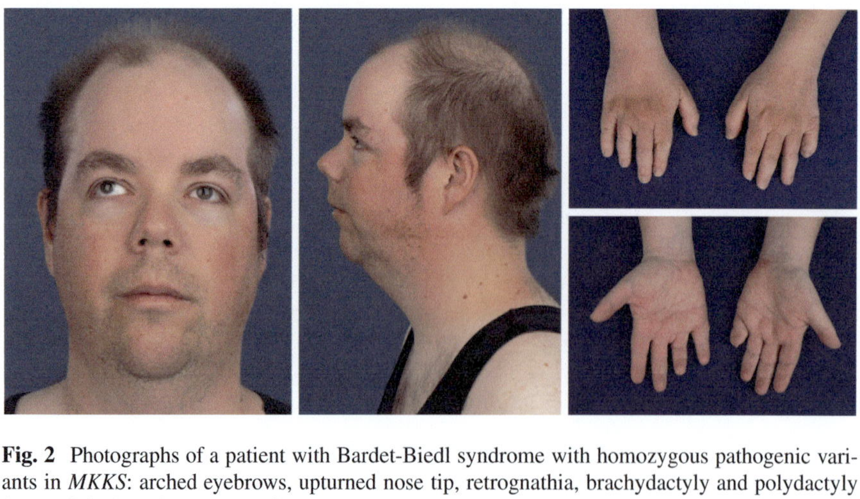

Fig. 2 Photographs of a patient with Bardet-Biedl syndrome with homozygous pathogenic variants in *MKKS*: arched eyebrows, upturned nose tip, retrognathia, brachydactyly and polydactyly (extra digits have been resected)

3.8 *Other Medical Problems*

There are many other physical problems that can be associated with BBS. Examples include: epilepsy, ataxia/poor coordination, anosmia/hyposmia, oral/dental abnormalities, Hirschsprung disease, hearing loss due to recurrent otitits media and laterality defects such as situs inversus [15].

3.8.1 Prenatal Diagnosis

Since whole exome sequencing is increasingly performed during pregnancy and the availability for ultrasounds and fetal MRIs increases, it is likely that BBS will be diagnosed antenatally more often in the future. Typical ultrasound findings include postaxial polydactyly, enlarged and hyperechogenic kidneys or absent or cystic kidneys [22–25]. Urogenital malformations can sometimes also be detected by prenatal ultrasound or after birth.

3.8.2 Genotype-Phenotype Correlation

A meta-analysis of 899 BBS patients analysed genotype-phenotype correlations and indicated that frameshift or splicing *BBS* gene variants are typically associated with a more severe phenotype than those with single amino acid subsitutions or short in-frame deletions [26]. Pathogenic variants in *BBS1*, *BBS2* en *BBS10* were most frequently reported with *BBS1* cases showing a milder phenotype. All pathogenic *BBS* gene variants were associated with a high penetrance of retinal degeneration. Polydactyly is more frequently observed in *BBS2.* Renal anomalies are more frequent in *BBS2, BBS7,* or *BBS9.* Kidney disease is more frequent and manifests itself at a younger age in patients with pathogenic variants in *SDCCAG8* [27]. Interestingly, pathogenic *BBS2* gene variants are considered to lead to a less obese subtype, while cases with pathogenic *BBS4* variants display severse early-onset obesity. However, there was (mostly) no conclusive difference between the different *BBS* genes for the feature obesity [15, 26].

4 Clinical Diagnosis

Revised diagnostic criteria for BBS have been published in 2024 and include the age of the patient, (primary and secondary) clinical criteria and molecular diagnosis (Table 2) [28].

Table 2 Revised diagnostic criteria for BBS [28]

Age	Primary clinical criteria	Secondary clinical criteria	Requirements for BBS diagnosis
In utero	Polydactyly Hyperechogenic kidneys	Hydrometrocolpos Situs inversus	Diagnosis with high level of confidence: Foetus *BBS* genetic testing positive + at least 1 primary criteria Diagnosis with moderate level of confidence: Affected sib *BBS* genetic testing positive + at least 1 primary criteria OR 2 primary +1 secondary criteria Urgent foetus genetic testing is recommended
0–16 years	Polydactyly Early obesity Early onset retinal dystrophy Kidney anomalies/dysfunction	Hydrometrocolpos Micropenis Neurodevelopmental disability Anosmia/hyposmia	Diagnosis with high level of confidence: Child's *BBS* genetic testing positive + at least 1 primary criteria OR If genetic testing is not available for the patient at least 4 primary criteria OR If genetic testing is not available for the patient at least 3 primary criteria + at least 2 secondary criteria Diagnosis with moderate level of confidence: If genetic testing is not available for the patient Affected sib *BBS* genetic testing positive + at least 2 primary criteria

(continued)

Table 2 (continued)

Age	Primary clinical criteria	Secondary clinical criteria	Requirements for BBS diagnosis
≥ 16 years	Polydactyly Obesity Retinal dystrophy Kidney anomalies/dysfunction	Hypogonadism Micropenis Neurodevelopmental disability (NDD) Anosmia/hyposmia	Diagnosis with high level of confidence: *BBS* genetic testing positive Retinal dystrophy + at least 1 other primary criterion OR If genetic testing is not available for the patient Retinal dystrophy + at least 3 other primary criteria OR If genetic testing is not available for the patient Retinal dystrophy + at least 2 other primary criteria + at least 2 secondary criteria Diagnosis with moderate level of confidence: If genetic testing is not available for the patient Affected sib with BBS (proven by genetic testing) + at least 2 primary criteria

5 Differential Diagnosis

The differential diagnosis of BBS varies depending on the phenotype of the patient. Possible differential diagnoses include:

- Alström syndrome
- Joubert syndrome
- Meckel syndrome
- Senior-Løken syndrome
- Laurence-Moon syndrome
- Type 2 Biemond syndrome
- Carpenter syndrome
- Cohen syndrome
- Prader-Willi syndrome

6 Molecular Diagnosis

The diagnosis is established by identification of disease-causing variants in one of the 26 genes known to be associated with BBS (Table 3) [28]. It is likely that more *BBS* genes will be discovered in the future as the identification of novel *BBS* genes has increased in recent years. As an example, in 2010 there were only 14 genes known to be associated with BBS, while now there are 26. *FBN3* is an newly proposed candidate gene [29].

Certain populations have a high prevalence of BBS and some have known founder mutations. A founder splice site variant (c.1091 + 3G > C) in *BBS1* was identified on the Faroe Islands [4]. In Newfoundland and Pakistan variants in the *MKKS/BBS6* gene [5, 30] and in South Africa a specific variant (K243IfsX15) in *BBS10* [31] were more commonly found. In patients with a European/Caucasian

Table 3 Bardet-Biedl syndrome (BBS) associated genes [28]

Gene (BBS type)	Chromosome location	% of all BBS patients [15]
BBS1	11q13.2	23.4%
BBS2	16q13	9.6%
ARL6 (BBS3)	3q11.2	5.1%
BBS4	15q24.1	5.3%
BBS5	2q31.1	3.7%
MKKS (BBS6)	20p12.2	6.3%
BBS7	4q27	4.2%
TTC8 (BBS8)	14q31.3	2.0%
BBS9	7p14.3	3.4%
BBS10	12q21.2	14.5%
TRIM32 (BBS11)	9q33.1	<1%
BBS12	4q27	6.4%
MKS1 (BBS13)	17q22	1.0%
CEP290 (BBS14)	12q21.32	6.3%
WDPCP (BBS15)	2p15	<1%
SDCCAG8 (BBS16)	1q43-q44	4.3%
LZTFL1 (BBS17)	3p21.31	<1%
BBIP1 (BBS18)	10q25.2	<1%
IFT27 (BBS19)	22q12.3	<1%
IFT172 (BBS20)	2p23.3	1%
CFAP418 (BBS21)	8q22.1	1.6%
IFT74 (BBS22)	9p21.2	<1%
CEP19 (BBS23)	3q29	Unknown
SCAPER (BBS24)	15q24.3	Unknown
CEP164 (BBS25)	11q23.3	<1%
SCLT1 (BBS26)	4q28.2	<1%

descent most variants are found in *BBS1* and *BBS10*, while the *BBS3* and *BBS9* gene are affected more often in patients with an Asian descent. In general, most variants are found in de genes affecting the BBSome [1].

When BBS is suspected, a multigene panel can be requested including all the *BBS* genes. If the clinical diagnosis is less certain broader diagnostic testing such as whole exome sequencing or whole genome sequencing may be considered. Broader genetic testing introduces the risk of finding variants of uncertain significance and incidental findings, but makes it possible to find (potential) new *BBS* genes. Recently a likely pathogenic variant in a noncoding region of *BBS10* was indentified [32].

7 Management

There is no cure for BBS. The treatment is aimed at reducing symptoms and preventing complications. Management is personalised and varies between patients based on their phenotype and is often multidisciplinary. Healthcare providers may include the paediatricians, ophthalmologists, nephrologists, endocrinologists, psychologists, dietitians and clinical geneticists. The general practitioner usually has a coordinating and supportive role.

Surveillance in patients with BBS varies between countries. An international consensus statement about the management of BBS [28] describes the importance of early detection of congenital abnormalities. Polydactyly is usually surgically corrected by a plastic surgeon in the first year of life. Since developmental problems and obesity are common, developmental milestones and weight should be monitored from birth. Physiotherapy or speech therapy are often beneficial. Regular ophthalmological examination including ERG and OCT is useful especially whilst residual vision remains. Regular renal examination is advised to monitor for deteriorating renal function, especially in the context of potentially nephrotoxic and/or medication that is excreted via the kidneys [28]. The potential obesogenic effects of some drugs such as some antiepileptics or antidepressants should be considered.

7.1 Management of Obesity

Healthy nutrition and sufficient physical activity are the first steps in the treatment of obesity in patients with BBS. Guidance by a dietician and/or physiotherapist is advisable. The dietician should have experience with hyperphagia, as this can be the underlying cause of the obesity in patients with BBS. Possible learning disabilities and visual impairment must also be taken into account due to the potential impact on mobility. Healthcare providers with a specialist interest in monogenic obesity are usually best placed to provide support.

When lifestyle modifications have not achieved adequate weight management, other treatment options such as medication or bariatric surgery can be considered. The effect of bariatric surgery in people with BBS is not clear. Bariatric procedures may include an adjustable gastric band, sleeve gastrectomy and Roux-en-Y gastric bypass [9]. More recently, the MC4 receptor agonist, setmelanotide, has been approved for BBS in patients aged 2 years and older. Setmelanotide targets the melanocortin 4 receptor pathway and induces weight loss by decreasing appetite. The first study of setmelanotide in patients with BBS was only recently published [33], and long term outcomes are still pending. A short term outcome study identified at least a 10% reduction in bodyweight in 32.3% of the BBS patients after 1 years of setmelanotide use [34]. Frequently reported side effects of setmelanotide are injection site reactions, skin hyperpigmentation and nausea/vomiting. Glucagon-like peptide-1 (GLP-1) receptor agonists can also be prescribed to patients with BBS. The effect of GLP1 receptor agonists specific in patients with BBS has not been studied extensively. It has been suggested that GLP-1 receptor agonists might not be as effective in treating disorders such as BBS that adversely impact the MC4 pathway in the hypothalamus [35].

7.2 Advances in Gene Therapy

A clinical trial for gene therapy targeting retinal dystrophy in patients with disease causing variants in *BBS1* is expected to commence start in the near future. Since gene therapy for some other causes of retinal dystrophy have been proven effective, there is hope this treatment will in the future also be effective for patients with BBS.

8 Genetic Screening of Family Members

BBS is inherited in an autosomal recessive manner. In the majority of cases, both healthy parents of an affected child carry one copy of the pathogenic *BBS* variant. If parents both carry a pathogenic *BBS* variant, the recurrence risk for any future children of having BBS is 25%.

Other family members can have their carrier status tested on request. This may be particularly relevant for family planning. Pre-implantation genetic testing and prenatal genetic testing can be offered to parents who are both carriers of a variant in the same *BBS* gene. On taking a family history it is advisable to note consanguinity and ethnicity.

9 Summary

Take Home Messages

Bardet-Biedl syndrome (BBS) is

- an autosomal recessive ciliopathy
- caused by biallelic disease-causing variants in one of the 26 BBS associated genes
- the main characteristics include retinal dystrophy, obesity, urogenital anomalies, postaxial polydactyly and learning disabilities

Truncal obesity is present in around 89% of patients and usually begins in the first year of life.

Competing Interests The authors Dr. Mieke van Haelst and Dr. Wenneke van Weelden declare that their department, the *Department of Human Genetics at Amsterdam UMC*, receives a sponsorship from Rhythm Pharmaceuticals. However, this chapter was conducted independently, and the content, analysis, and conclusions presented herein were not influenced by the sponsor. No direct funding or input from Rhythm Pharmaceuticals was received for the preparation of this manuscript.

References

1. Priya S, Nampoothiri S, Sen P, Sripriya S. Bardet-Biedl syndrome: genetics, molecular pathophysiology, and disease management. Indian J Ophthalmol. 2016;64(9):620–7.
2. Bardet G. On congenital obesity syndrome with polydactyly and retinitis pigmentosa (a contribution to the study of clinical forms of hypophyseal obesity). 1920. Obes Res. 1995;3(4):387–99.
3. Biedl A. A pair of siblings with adiposo-genital dystrophy. 1922. Obes Res. 1995;3(4):404.
4. Hjortshoj TD, Gronskov K, Brondum-Nielsen K, Rosenberg T. A novel founder BBS1 mutation explains a unique high prevalence of Bardet-Biedl syndrome in The Faroe Islands. Br J Ophthalmol. 2009;93(3):409–13.
5. Moore SJ, Green JS, Fan Y, Bhogal AK, Dicks E, Fernandez BA, et al. Clinical and genetic epidemiology of Bardet-Biedl syndrome in Newfoundland: a 22-year prospective, population-based, cohort study. Am J Med Genet A. 2005;132A(4):352–60.
6. Gouronc A, Zilliox V, Jacquemont ML, Darcel F, Leuvrey AS, Nourisson E, et al. High prevalence of Bardet-Biedl syndrome in La Reunion Island is due to a founder variant in ARL6/BBS3. Clin Genet. 2020;98(2):166–71.
7. Teebi AS. Autosomal recessive disorders among Arabs: an overview from Kuwait. J Med Genet. 1994;31(3):224–33.
8. Castro-Sanchez S, Alvarez-Satta M, Pereiro I, Pineiro-Gallego MT, Valverde D. Algorithm for the molecular analysis of Bardet-Biedl syndrome in Spain. Med Clin (Barc). 2015;145(4):147–52.
9. Tomlinson JW. Bardet-Biedl syndrome: a focus on genetics, mechanisms and metabolic dysfunction. Diabetes Obes Metab. 2024;26(Suppl 2):13–24.
10. Hirano M, Satake W, Ihara K, Tsuge I, Kondo S, Saida K, et al. The first Nationwide survey and genetic analyses of Bardet-Biedl syndrome in Japan. PLoS One. 2015;10(9):e0136317.

11. Tian X, Zhao H, Zhou J. Organization, functions, and mechanisms of the BBSome in development, ciliopathies, and beyond. elife. 2023;12:e87623.
12. Weihbrecht K, Goar WA, Pak T, Garrison JE, DeLuca AP, Stone EM, et al. Keeping an eye on Bardet-Biedl syndrome: a comprehensive review of the role of Bardet-Biedl syndrome genes in the eye. Med Res Arch. 2017;5(9) https://doi.org/10.18103/mra.v5i9.1526.
13. Guo DF, Lin Z, Wu Y, Searby C, Thedens DR, Richerson GB, et al. The BBSome in POMC and AgRP neurons is necessary for body weight regulation and sorting of metabolic receptors. Diabetes. 2019;68(8):1591–603.
14. Gouronc A, Javey E, Leuvrey AS, Nourisson E, Friedmann S, Reichert V, et al. Unexpected inheritance patterns in a large cohort of patients with a suspected ciliopathy. Hum Mutat. 2023;2023:2564200.
15. Forsyth R, Gunay-Aygun M. Bardet-Biedl syndrome overview. In: Adam MP, Feldman J, Mirzaa GM, Pagon RA, Wallace SE, Bean LJH, et al., editors. GeneReviews((R)). Seattle: University of Washington; 1993.
16. Pomeroy J, Krentz AD, Richardson JG, Berg RL, VanWormer JJ, Haws RM. Bardet-Biedl syndrome: weight patterns and genetics in a rare obesity syndrome. Pediatr Obes. 2021;16(2):e12703.
17. Mujahid S, Hunt KF, Cheah YS, Forsythe E, Hazlehurst JM, Sparks K, et al. The endocrine and metabolic characteristics of a large Bardet-Biedl syndrome clinic population. J Clin Endocrinol Metab. 2018;103(5):1834–41.
18. Forsythe E, Mallya UG, Yang M, Huber C, Cala ML, Greatsinger A, et al. Burden of hyperphagia and obesity in Bardet-Biedl syndrome: a multicountry survey. Orphanet J Rare Dis. 2023;18(1):182.
19. Deveault C, Billingsley G, Duncan JL, Bin J, Theal R, Vincent A, et al. BBS genotype-phenotype assessment of a multiethnic patient cohort calls for a revision of the disease definition. Hum Mutat. 2011;32(6):610–9.
20. Schaefer E, Lauer J, Durand M, Pelletier V, Obringer C, Claussmann A, et al. Mesoaxial polydactyly is a major feature in Bardet-Biedl syndrome patients with LZTFL1 (BBS17) mutations. Clin Genet. 2014;85(5):476–81.
21. Forsythe E, Beales PL. Bardet-Biedl syndrome. Eur J Hum Genet. 2013;21(1):8–13.
22. Cassart M, Eurin D, Didier F, Guibaud L, Avni EF. Antenatal renal sonographic anomalies and postnatal follow-up of renal involvement in Bardet-Biedl syndrome. Ultrasound Obstet Gynecol. 2004;24(1):51–4.
23. Dar P, Sachs GS, Carter SM, Ferreira JC, Nitowsky HM, Gross SJ. Prenatal diagnosis of Bardet-Biedl syndrome by targeted second-trimester sonography. Ultrasound Obstet Gynecol. 2001;17(4):354–6.
24. Arora E, Fuks A, Meyer J, Chervenak J. Prenatal diagnosis of Bardet Biedl syndrome: a case report. Radiol Case Rep. 2023;18(1):326–30.
25. Cai M, Lin M, Lin N, Xu L, Huang H. Novel homozygous nonsense mutation associated with Bardet-Biedl syndrome in fetuses with congenital renal malformation. Medicine (Baltimore). 2022;101(32):e30003.
26. Niederlova V, Modrak M, Tsyklauri O, Huranova M, Stepanek O. Meta-analysis of genotype-phenotype associations in Bardet-Biedl syndrome uncovers differences among causative genes. Hum Mutat. 2019;40(11):2068–87.
27. Otto EA, Hurd TW, Airik R, Chaki M, Zhou W, Stoetzel C, et al. Candidate exome capture identifies mutation of SDCCAG8 as the cause of a retinal-renal ciliopathy. Nat Genet. 2010;42(10):840–50.
28. Dollfus H, Lilien MR, Maffei P, Verloes A, Muller J, Bacci GM, et al. Bardet-Biedl syndrome improved diagnosis criteria and management: Inter European Reference Networks consensus statement and recommendations. Eur J Hum Genet. 2024; https://doi.org/10.1038/s41431-024-01634-7.

29. Genovesi ML, Torres B, Goldoni M, Salvo E, Cesario C, Majolo M, et al. Case report: a novel homozygous missense variant of FBN3 supporting it is a new candidate gene causative of a Bardet-Biedl syndrome-like phenotype. Front Genet. 2022;13:924362.
30. Rao AR, Nazir A, Imtiaz S, Paracha SA, Waryah YM, Ujjan ID, et al. Delineating the Spectrum of genetic variants associated with Bardet-Biedl syndrome in consanguineous Pakistani pedigrees. Genes (Basel). 2023;14(2):404.
31. Fieggen K, Milligan C, Henderson B, Esterhuizen AI. Bardet Biedl syndrome in South Africa: a single founder mutation. S Afr Med J. 2016;106(6 Suppl 1):S72–4.
32. Daich Varela M, Bellingham J, Motta F, Jurkute N, Ellingford JM, Quinodoz M, et al. Multidisciplinary team directed analysis of whole genome sequencing reveals pathogenic non-coding variants in molecularly undiagnosed inherited retinal dystrophies. Hum Mol Genet. 2023;32(4):595–607.
33. Haws R, Brady S, Davis E, Fletty K, Yuan G, Gordon G, et al. Effect of setmelanotide, a melanocortin-4 receptor agonist, on obesity in Bardet-Biedl syndrome. Diabetes Obes Metab. 2020;22(11):2133–40.
34. Haqq AM, Chung WK, Dollfus H, Haws RM, Martos-Moreno GA, Poitou C, et al. Efficacy and safety of setmelanotide, a melanocortin-4 receptor agonist, in patients with Bardet-Biedl syndrome and Alstrom syndrome: a multicentre, randomised, double-blind, placebo-controlled, phase 3 trial with an open-label period. Lancet Diabetes Endocrinol. 2022;10(12):859–68.
35. Shoemaker A. Bardet-Biedl syndrome: a clinical overview focusing on diagnosis, outcomes and best-practice management. Diabetes Obes Metab. 2024;26(Suppl 2):25–33.

Pseudohypoparathyroidism and Its Association with Obesity

Erica van den Akker and Mieke van Haelst

1 Introduction

Albright et al. first described pseudohypoparathyroidism (PHP) in 1942 as a novel hormone resistance disorder characterized by hypocalcemia and hyperphosphatemia due to decreased responsiveness to parathyroid hormone (PTH) combined with other features such as neurocognitive, endocrine and growth disorders [4]. PHP was later found to have several subtypes which all share a common defect in the cAMP signaling pathway of G-couples protein receptors. Despite a common cause, there are several subtypes of this disease with important clinical and molecular overlap as well as variation between them (Fig. 1).

PHP is characterized by a wide range of clinical manifestations, including PTH resistance: hypocalcemia, hyperphosphatemia, and elevated PTH levels. PHP can also present as part of Albright's hereditary osteodystrophy (AHO), which is a constellation of skeletal abnormalities which include defects in chondrocyte and osteoblast differentiation, early closure of growth plates, brachydactyly (Fig. 2a, b), adult short stature, and the development of ectopic ossifications (Fig. 3) [11].

E. van den Akker (✉)
Obesity Center CGG, Center of Expertise for Genetic Obesity, Department of Pediatrics, Division of Pediatric Endocrinology, Erasmus University Medical Center-Sophia Children's Hospital, Rotterdam, The Netherlands
e-mail: e.l.t.vandenakker@erasmusmc.nl

M. van Haelst
Department of Human Genetics, Section Clinical Genetics, Amsterdam University Medical Center, Amsterdam, The Netherlands
e-mail: m.vanhaelst@amsterdamumc.nl

M. van Haelst, E. van den Akker (eds.), *Clinical Obesity Genetics*, https://doi.org/10.1007/978-3-032-04095-4_8

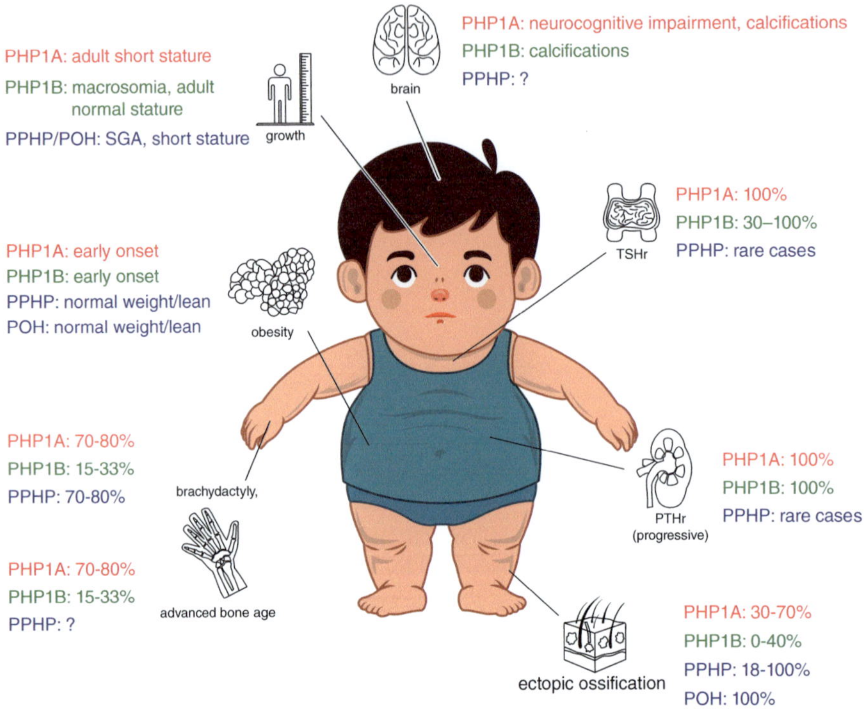

Fig. 1 Main clinical features of PHP related disorders

PHP is classified into several subtypes: PHP type 1A (PHP1A) and PHP type 1B (PHP1B). Pseudohypoparathyroidism type 1 (PHP1) is a rare hereditary disorder characterized by end-organ resistance to the actions of parathyroid hormone (PTH), resulting in a clinical phenotype resembling hypoparathyroidism. Despite the presence of elevated or normal levels of PTH in the blood, affected individuals exhibit hypocalcemia and hyperphosphatemia due to impaired PTH signaling.

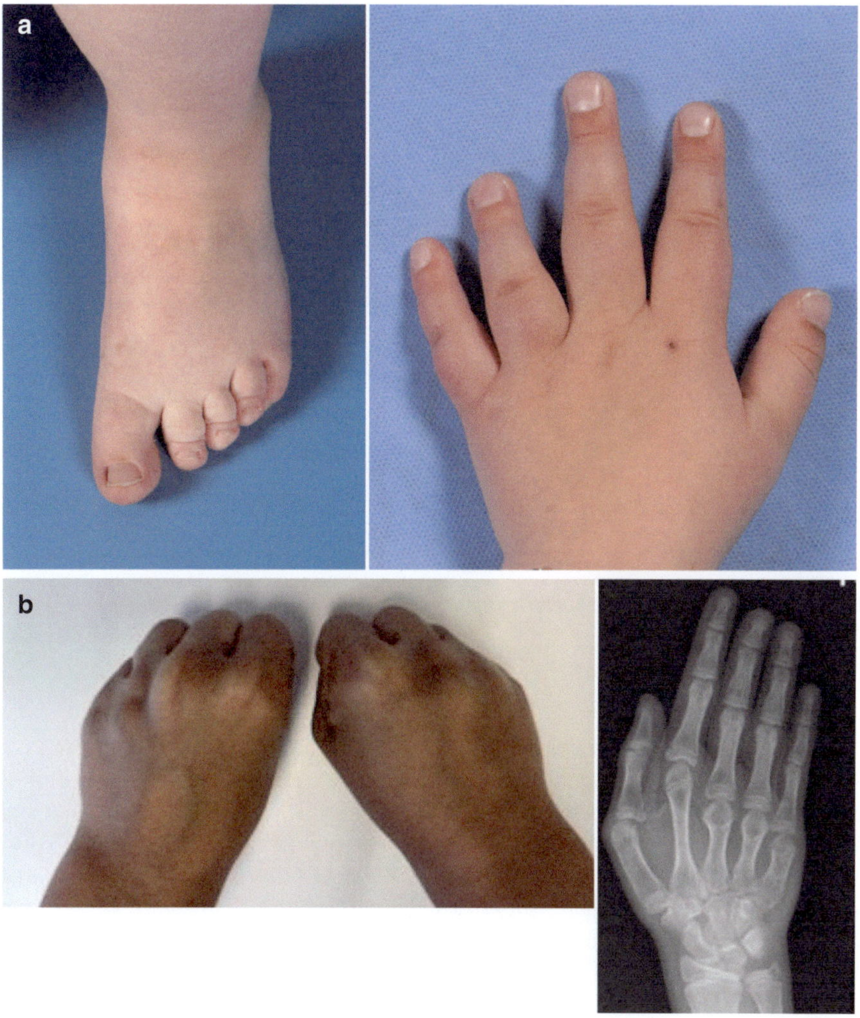

Fig. 2 Brachydacyly. (**a**) Brachydactyly meaning 'short digits, in PHP is typically a shortening of digit III, IV and or V metacarpals or the distal phalanx of digit I due to disturbed bone growth of the metacarpals(hand) or metatarsals (foot). (**b**) Shortening of metacarpal III, IV and V of the right hand and IV and V of the left hand. On physical examination, the knuckles of these digits are absent when making a fist

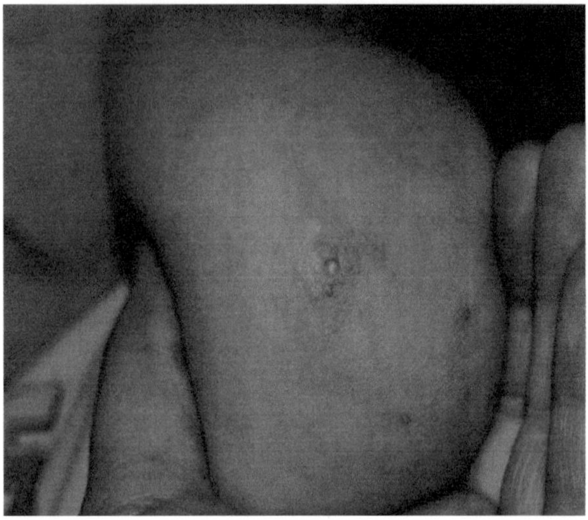

Fig. 3 Ectopic ossification of the skin, located on the elbow. This sign is very specific for PHP

2 Aetiology and Pathophysiology

2.1 PHP Subtypes and Genetic Mechanisms

PHP1A. PHP1A is an autosomal dominant condition characterized by loss-of-function *GNAS* variants on the maternal alelle. *GNAS* encodes the alpha subunit of the stimulatory G protein (Gsα), which is crucial for PTH signaling in bone and kidney. Inactivating *GNAS* mutations reduce intracellular cyclic AMP (cAMP) production, impairing downstream PTH effects. Other G-protein coupled receptors that can show resistance are thyrotropin stimulating hormone (TSH) receptor, growth hormone releasing hormone (GHRH) receptor, and gonadotropin releasing hormone (GnRH) receptor [9]. Other receptors, such as MC4R, β2- and β3-adrenoceptors, and corticotropin-releasing hormone receptor, have been implicated in the pathophysiology of the severe, early-onset obesity that results from (epi)genetic *GNAS* changes [3, 5]. Resting energy expenditure measurements in PHP1a patients have been reported to be lower or equal to controls with obesity [1, 10, 14].

PHP1B is an autosomal dominant disorder caused (methylation) defects or pathogenic variants affecting GNAS regulatory elements rather than the GNAS gene itself.

PHP1B has the receptor resistance phenotype but lacks the skeletal abnormalities (AHO) and is associated with imprinting defects at the *GNAS* locus, leading to reduced Gsα expression from the maternal allele.

PPHP (Pseudo-pseudohypoparathyroidism) is a subtype where only paternally transmitted *GNAS* variants lead to AHO without affecting PTH or serum calcium levels. The unaltered maternal allele preserves renal responsiveness to PTH, resulting in normal calcium homeostasis.

2.2 PHP and Obesity

Several mechanisms contribute to excessive drive for eating (hyperphagia) and fat mass accumulation in PHP. Defects in the Gsα-dependent melanocortin signaling pathway, possibly cause the increased appetite and decreased resting energy expenditure compared to obese controls [1]. In addition, a low sympathetic nervous system activity, decreased lipolysis and GH-releasing hormone resistance in the pituitary can play a role. Dysregulation of GNAS signaling in adipose tissue could impair lipolysis and adipogenesis, promoting fat accumulation. Additionally, altered PTH and calcium signaling may impact adipocyte function and energy homeostasis. Leptin resistance, possibly induced by *GNAS* mutations, could further exacerbate obesity in PHP patients.

2.3 Clinical Presentation

PHP presents with a wide range of clinical manifestations, including PTH resistance: hypocalcemia, hyperphosphatemia, and elevated PTH levels. PTH resistance is progressive and therefore it can present in the first months of life, but can also develop in later years. In addition to these classic endocrine features, PHP is often accompanied by Albright's Hereditary Osteodystrophy (AHO), a constellation of skeletal abnormalities which include defects in chondrocyte and osteoblast differentiation, early closure of growth plates, brachydactyly, adult short stature, and the development of ectopic ossifications. Other symptoms can result from resistance to other hormones such as thyroid-stimulating hormone (TSH) leading to hypothyroidism, gonadotropins leading to hypogonadism, growth-hormone-releasing hormone leading to (partial) growth hormone deficiency [11].

Obesity or overweight is associated with all types of PHP and related disorders, except progressive osseous heteroplasia (POH) which is an ultrarare genetic condition of progressive ectopic ossification and, pseudopseudohypoparathyroidism (PPHP). Patients with PHP1A and 1B often develop early-onset obesity, typically within the first 2 years of life, with an average age of onset of 0,9 years [2]. This may be the initial and sole symptom until a diagnosis is made during adolescence or adulthood.

PHP and related disorders are primarily diagnosed clinically and based on biochemical abnormalities. Diagnosis can be confirmed through genetic testing. Distinguishing between PHP subtypes is crucial, as it determines monitoring strategy.

PHP1a: Individuals with PHP1a typically present with PTH resistance leading to hypocalcemia (in 86.7%), thyroid stimulating hormone (TSH) resistance leading to hypothyroidism or hyperthyroitropinemia (in 75.5%), early onset obesity, developmental delay and a combination of symptoms known as Albright hereditary osteodystrophy (AHO in 87,5%), such as round facies, short stature in adulthood, brachydactyly (especially of III, IV,V metacarpal bones) and subcutaneous ossifications [7]. Children can be born small for gestational age and usually grow within the normal range. However, final height is short due to a (severely) advanced bone age leading to early termination of growth. SGA (prevalence 30%) or growth hormone (GH) deficiency (prevalence 50–60%) can be an indication for the use of recombinant human GH (rhGH) therapy. Recently it was shown that GH treatment may improve final height substantially (+1,9SD) No difference in BMI was found compared to controls [6].

Furthermore individuals with PHP 1a can demonstrate partial resistance gonadotropin releasing hormones: leading hypogonadotropic hypogonadism, delayed puberty or disturbed menstrual cycles. Melanocortin-4 receptor dysfunction leads to hyperphagia and early onset obesity as part of the phenotype. Growth-hormone-releasing hormone resistance leads to (partial) growth hormone deficiency [11].

PHP1B usually presents with PTH resistance without the AHO phenotype, thus with hypo calcemia, hyperphosphatemia, and elevated PTH.

PPHP patients with pseudo-pseudohypoparathyroidism have AHO features despite normal PTH responsiveness. One of the characteristics of PPHP patients is that they are often born small for gestational age.

Patients with POH or osteoma cutis have varying degrees of heterotopic ossifications and brachydactyly. Expert consensus recommendations on diagnosis [11]:

Diagnosis of PHP and Related Disorders Should Be Based on Clinical, Biochemical Characteristics and, in Some Cases, the Family History
Major diagnostic features include PTH resistance and/or ectopic ossifications, early-onset (before 2 years of age) obesity associated with TSH resistance, and/or AHO.

Supporting features include unexplained primary hypothyroidism, hypercalcitoninemia, hypogonadism, growth hormone (GH) deficiency, cognitive impairment, hearing impairment, craniosynostosis and neurosurgical features, and/or CNS calcifications, sleep apnea, ear infections, and being born small for gestational age.

Genetic Testing: Genetic testing plays a pivotal role in confirming the diagnosis of PHP.

2.3.1 Clinical Evaluation

Medical history: asses history of birth (small for gestational age), developmental delays or intellectual disability, epileptic seizures, neonatal thyroid screening result, periods of rapid weight gain, eating behavior and signs of hyperphagia, age of onset obesity, pubertal development, psychosocial evaluation, behavior or learning problems.

Family history: A three-generation family history on hypocalcemia, epilepsy, developmental delay, adult short stature, early onset obesity, hypothyroidism.

Physical examination: asses linear growth, height, weight, BMI, head circumference, (also in both parents) blood pressure, pulse, dysmorphologic examination (including metacarpal length valuation), pubertal status, skin examination for ectopic ossifications and growth chart analysis.

Biochemical and hormonal evaluation: assessment of blood: calcium, phosphorus, PTH, kreatinine, 25OHVitD, 1,25OHVitD, Thyroid function (TSH, FT4), growth factors (in case of growth deceleration), fasting glucose and insulin or oral glucose tolerance test, lipid profile, liver enzymes. Assessment of urine: calcium, phosphorus, creatinine.

Radiologic evaluation asses bone age with an X-ray of the left hand.

On indication neuropsychological assessment of development, behavior and cognition (IQ-test).

3 Differential Diagnosis

The following conditions should be considered in the differential diagnosis and ruled out through clinical evaluation, biochemical tests, and genetic studies.

Primary Hypothyroidism. This can present with growth retardation, obesity and developmental delay, but typically has a stronger decrease of thyroid hormone levels and elevated TSH compared to PHP1a. Nowadays, many countries have a neonatal screening test that pick up congenital primary hypothyroidism very early in life. In children with PHP1a, this screening test can also be abnormal due to TSH resistance. The hyperthyreotropinemia or mild primary hypothyroidism is often transient in the first months of life but can come back at later age. Therefore clinicians should look for signs of PHP in a newborn child with an abnormal neonatal thyroid screening test.

Other forms of syndromal obesity such as:

Prader-Willi (Like) Syndrome (PWS). PWS is characterized by hypotonia and feeding difficulties in infancy, followed by hyperphagia, obesity, and developmental delays in early childhood (after 2 years of age). The onset of hyperphagia and obesity is usually later than in PHP1a. Patients with PWS do not have hypocalcemia or PTH resistance.

Bardet-Biedl Syndrome (BBS). The overlapping features between BBS and PHP1a include early onset obesity, hyperphagia, developmental delay. However BBS specific features are: retinal dystrophy, polydactyly, and renal anomalies.

Other Types of Pseudohypoparathyroidism: including PHP1b, PHP1c, which may have overlapping features but differ in genetic mutations and biochemical profiles.

Multifactorial Obesity. Gsα deficiency is an underappreciated cause of early-onset, severe obesity. Therefore, screening children with unexplained, severe obesity for GNAS defects is recommended [3, 5].

4 Molecular Diagnosis

Molecular Testing is essential for genetic counseling and diagnosis, particularly when clinical features overlap. The primary subtypes of PHP and related disorders arise from either de novo or autosomal dominant inherited inactivating genetic variants or epigenetic alterations at the imprinted GNAS gene. The *GNAS* locus features four distinct differentially methylated regions (DMRs): the paternally methylated region (*GNAS-NESP:*TSS-DMR) and three maternally methylated regions (*GNAS-AS1*:TSS-DMR, GNAS-XL:Ex1-DMR, and GNAS A/B:TSS-DMR).

Genetic Counseling: Crucial for patients with *GNAS* variants, who have a 50% chance of transmitting the molecular defect. Depending on the parental sex, their offspring will develop PPHP, osteoma cutis, or POH (if the transmitting patient is male) or PHP1A (if the transmitting patient is female).

Detection Methods: Single-nucleotide variants can be detected by sequence analysis, Methylation defects can be detected through various methods, such as methylation-sensitive MLPA (MS-MLPA). This test allows simultaneous detection of methylation defects at different GNAS DMRs as well as CNVs, including deletion of the nearby STX16 gene, resulting in loss of methylation in the A/B exon of GNAS. Aberrant methylation without the presence of a deletion is in some cases due to a paternal uniparental disomy, which can be detected using microsatellite typing or SNP array.

5 Therapy

Treatment of PHP includes offering appropriate genetic counselling, screening, treatment of the endocrine deficits, providing supportive to prevent weight gain and complications. A lifelong, coordinated, and multidisciplinary approach is recommended, beginning as early as possible in infancy and continuing through adulthood, with a smooth transition from pediatric to adult care.

Obesity and weight management: To provide supportive care and advice to promote a healthy lifestyle and prevent weight gain should be offered as early as possible. If hyperphagia and obesity are present, provide a multidisciplinary intervention with the approach tailored to the patient needs. Lifestyle modifications, dietary interventions, and tailored exercise regimens should be offered as well as psychologic support and parental coaching. As second step, obesity medication or bariatric surgery can be considered. However, the effectiveness of obesity interventions in PHP-related obesity requires further investigation.

Endocrine treatment: Screen and treat endocrine deficits:

Hypocalcemia or hyperphosphatemia due to PTH resistance. The cornerstone of managing hypocalcemia in PHP involves active vitamin D supplementation. Calcium supplementation until normalisation of calcium. Phosphate binders: If hyperphosphatemia is present, phosphate binders may be prescribed to reduce the absorption of dietary phosphorus, helping to normalize phosphate levels. If a patient is on anti-epileptic drugs, these can often be stopped after normalization of calcium levels.

Hypothyroidism due to TSH resistance is treated with hormone suppletion of thyroxine.

Growth hormone therapy is indicated when growth hormone deficiency is diagnosed. Evidence is lacking that growth hormone treatment is effective to influence final height in the absence of growth hormone deficiency.

Hypogonadism. Hormone replacement therapy (estrogen for females and testosterone for males) is indicated when hypogonadism is present.

6 Follow-Up Advices

Follow-up management aims at early detection of disorders and prevention of complications. The frequency of follow up depends on the subtype diagnosis, endocrine deficits and age. In PHP1A a schedule of monthly follow up in the first year, 3 monthly follow up in infancy and 6–12 month follow up in childhood or adulthood is advised for screening and treatment of endocrine deficits and monitoring of growth, BMI and puberty.

Endocrine Monitoring: Regular monitoring of calcium, phosphate, thyroid function, gonadal hormones, and other relevant endocrine parameters is essential to initiate appropriate treatment on time. If PTH resistance is present, careful monitoring is necessary to avoid complications of hypercalcemia such as nephrocalcinosis. Therefore monitoring of urine calcium excretion and ultrasound of the kidneys is performed with large intervals.

Bone Health: Optimizing bone health is crucial. Physical therapy and weight-bearing exercises can help improve bone density and alleviate musculoskeletal symptoms.

Psychological support and educational programs should be provided early. Skeletal abnormalities can impact physical functioning and self-esteem, influencing patients' psychosocial well-being.

Sleep apnea, a common complication of obesity, is more frequent in patients with PHP1A and may also be present in acrodysostosis. These patients often have round faces, a flattened nasal bridge, and/or maxillary hypoplasia, which, combined with obesity, contribute to sleep and respiratory disturbances. Screening for restless sleep, snoring, inattentiveness, and daytime somnolence is recommended, with polysomnography if symptoms are present.

Metabolic Syndrome. Regular monitoring of blood pressure, lipid profile, and glucose metabolism parameters is recommended within the multidisciplinary follow-up of patients with PHP. Postprandial hyperglycemia and dysglycemia is frequent in children with PHP1A and PHP1B [14]. Decreased insulin sensitivity and type 2 diabetes are common in adult PHP1A patients and may not be solely related to obesity [11]. The lipid profile is generally not profoundly affected in PHP1A patients. Although hypertension has been reported, the incidence of cardiovascular diseases is not increased compared to controls.

Dental checkup. PHP is frequently linked to various dental and oral conditions, including: delayed tooth eruption, hypodontia, enamel hypoplasia, malocclusion, gingival hyperplasia, gingivitis with spontaneous bleeding and pain. Therefore, regular dental check-ups every 6–12 months are advised, especially during childhood.

Registries. Given the lack of strong evidence-based data, particularly for patient management, there is a need for filling data to large international registries such as the initiatives within the European Reference Networks (ERN) EuRREB registry, which recruit data on cohorts of patients to better understand the natural history, and develop novel disease-specific therapies. The ERN centers of expertise can enroll patients after informed consent.

7 Family Screening

The advice for family screening varies per PHP subtype. In case of an autosomal dominant inheritance, family members that show a similar phenotype can be tested for the underlying (epi) genetic cause that was identified, as this can have implication for screening and treatment.

8 Summary

Patients with PHP and related disorders may display a highly heterogeneous and progressive clinical picture over their lifespan, necessitating a lifelong multidisciplinary approach. Each clinical aspect and potential complication should be managed by healthcare professionals with expertise in these disorders, preferably at referral centers. The complex genetic and epigenetic *GNAS* defects underlying these disorders require a specialized approach to establish a correct molecular diagnosis, which can be time-consuming for both patients and their families but is crucial for appropriate management.

Take Home Message

PHP presents with a wide range of clinical manifestations, including PTH resistance: hypocalcemia, hyperphosphatemia, other hormone resistances and osteodystrophy.

The association between PHP and obesity has significant clinical implications. Obesity can exacerbate the metabolic and orthopedic complications already present in PHP patients, leading to reduced quality of life. Therefore, early intervention and management of obesity are crucial.

9 Conclusion

Pseudohypoparathyroidism is a rare genetic disorder with a complex clinical presentation that extends beyond the classic endocrine manifestations. The intriguing association between PHP and obesity sheds light on the intricate interplay between metabolic and endocrine pathways. Further research into the molecular basis of this association may unravel novel therapeutic avenues for managing obesity and improving the overall health of individuals with PHP.

References

1. Abawi O, Koster EC, Welling MS, Boeters SCM, van Rossum EFC, van Haelst MM, van der Voorn B, de Groot CJ, van den Akker ELT. Resting energy expenditure and body composition in children and adolescents with genetic, hypothalamic, medication-induced or multifactorial severe obesity. Front Endocrinol (Lausanne). 2022;13:862817. https://doi.org/10.3389/fendo.2022.862817. PMID: 35898454; PMCID: PMC9309560.
2. Abawi O, Wahab RJ, Kleinendorst L, Blankers LA, Brandsma AE, van Rossum EFC, van der Voorn B, van Haelst MM, Gaillard R, van den Akker ELT. Genetic obesity disorders: body mass index trajectories and age of onset of obesity compared with children with obesity from the general population. J Pediatr. 2023;262:113619. https://doi.org/10.1016/j.jpeds.2023.113619. Epub 2023 Jul 18
3. Abbas A, Hammad AS, Al-Shafai M. The role of genetic and epigenetic GNAS alterations in the development of early-onset obesity. Mutat Res Rev Mutat Res. 2024;793:108487. https://doi.org/10.1016/j.mrrev.2023.108487. Epub 2023 Dec 14
4. Albright F, Burnett CH, Smith PH, Parson W. Pseudo-hypoparathyroidism-an example of 'Seabright-Bantam syndrome': report of three cases. Endocrinology. 1942;30:922.
5. Mendes de Oliveira E, Keogh JM, Talbot F, Henning E, Ahmed R, Perdikari A, Bounds R, Wasiluk N, Ayinampudi V, Barroso I, Mokrosiński J, Jyothish D, Lim S, Gupta S, Kershaw M, Matei C, Partha P, Randell T, McAulay A, Wilson LC, Cheetham T, Crowne EC, Clayton P, Farooqi IS. Obesity-associated GNAS mutations and the Melanocortin pathway. N Engl J Med. 2021;385(17):1581–92. https://doi.org/10.1056/NEJMoa2103329. Epub 2021 Oct 6
6. Ertl DA, de Nanclares GP, Jüppner H, Hanna P, Pagnano A, Pereda A, Rothenbuhler A, Del Sindaco G, Ruiz-Cuevas P, Audrain C, Escribano A, Berkenou J, Gleiss A, Mantovani G, Linglart A. Recombinant growth hormone improves growth and adult height in patients with maternal inactivating GNAS mutations. Eur J Endocrinol. 2023;189(1):123–31. https://doi.org/10.1093/ejendo/lvad085. PMID: 37440712; PMCID: PMC11077274.
7. Jiang S, Yang Y, Song A, Jiang Y, Jiang Y, Li M, Xia W, Nie M, Wang O, Xing X. Genotype-phenotype correlations in pseudohypoparathyroidism type 1a patients: a systemic review. Eur J Endocrinol. 2023;189(5):S103–11. https://doi.org/10.1093/ejendo/lvad142.
8. Germain-Lee EL, Groman J, Crane JL, et al. Growth hormone deficiency in pseudohypoparathyroidism type 1a: another manifestation of multihormone resistance. J Clin Endocrinol Metab. 2003;88:4059–69.
9. Mantovani G, Maghnie M, Weber G, et al. Growth hormone-releasing hormone resistance in pseudohypoparathyroidism type ia: new evidence for imprinting of the Gs alpha gene. J Clin Endocrinol Metab. 2003;88:4070–4.
10. Roizen JD, Danzig J, Groleau V, McCormack S, Casella A, Harrington J, Sochett E, Tershakovec A, Zemel BS, Stallings VA, Levine MA. Resting energy expenditure is decreased

in pseudohypoparathyroidism Type 1A. J Clin Endocrinol Metab. 2016;101(3):880–8. https://doi.org/10.1210/jc.2015-3895. Epub 2015 Dec 28. PMID: 26709970; PMCID: PMC4803160.

11. Mantovani G, Bastepe M, Monk D, de Sanctis L, Thiele S, Ahmed SF, Bufo R, Choplin T, De Filippo G, Devernois G, Eggermann T, Elli FM, Garcia Ramirez A, Germain-Lee EL, Groussin L, Hamdy NAT, Hanna P, Hiort O, Jüppner H, Kamenický P, Knight N, Le Norcy E, Lecumberri B, Levine MA, Mäkitie O, Martin R, Martos-Moreno GÁ, Minagawa M, Murray P, Pereda A, Pignolo R, Rejnmark L, Rodado R, Rothenbuhler A, Saraff V, Shoemaker AH, Shore EM, Silve C, Turan S, Woods P, Zillikens MC, Perez de Nanclares G, Linglart A. Recommendations for diagnosis and treatment of Pseudohypoparathyroidism and related disorders: an updated practical tool for physicians and patients. Horm Res Paediatr. 2020;93(3):182–96. https://doi.org/10.1159/000508985. Epub 2020 Aug 5. PMID: 32756064; PMCID: PMC8140671
12. Linglart A, Menguy C, Couvineau A, et al. Recurrent PRKAR1A mutation in acrodysostosis with hormone resistance. N Engl J Med. 2011;364:2218.
13. Linglart A, Levine MA, Jüppner H. Pseudohypoparathyroidism. Endocrinol Metab Clin N Am. 2018;47:865.
14. Perez KM, Curley KL, Slaughter JC, Shoemaker AH. Glucose homeostasis and energy balance in children with pseudohypoparathyroidism. J Clin Endocrinol Metab. 2018;103(11):4265–74. https://doi.org/10.1210/jc.2018-01067. PMID: 30085125; PMCID: PMC6194807.

Genetic Analysis

Non-syndromic Leptin Melanocortin Pathway Disorders

Lotte Kleinendorst, Ozair Abawi, Erica van den Akker, and Mieke van Haelst

1 Introduction

Body weight is strongly influenced by underlying genetic factors [1, 2]. Twin and family studies have estimated that the heritability of BMI is as high as 40–70% [3]. In most individuals living with obesity, multifactorial obesity, also called common or polygenic obesity, is present. In these individuals, the small effects of hundreds of genetic polymorphisms interact with environmental factors to contribute to their obesity [4]. Currently, over 1000 loci are associated with multifactorial obesity [1], and polygenic risk scores based on large-scale genome-wide association studies can explain around 20% of the variability in BMI on a population level [5]. However, in a minority of individuals with obesity, the obesity phenotype can be explained by disturbances in the leptin-melanocortin pathway, the hypothalamic pathway that regulates body weight, appetite, and energy expenditure [6]. It is estimated that 3–7% of children with obesity who visit a specialized obesity clinic, and up to 3% of adults with obesity [7–10], have an underlying genetic disturbance of the leptin-melanocortin pathway that causes their obesity. These leptin-melanocortin pathway

L. Kleinendorst (✉) · M. van Haelst
Department of Human Genetics, Section Clinical Genetics, Amsterdam University Medical Center, Amsterdam, The Netherlands

Emma Center for Personalized Medicine, Amsterdam UMC, University of Amsterdam, Amsterdam, The Netherlands
e-mail: l.kleinendorst@amsterdamumc.nl; m.vanhaelst@amsterdamumc.nl

O. Abawi · E. van den Akker
Division of Endocrinology, Department of Pediatrics, Erasmus MC-Sophia, University Medical Center Rotterdam, Rotterdam, The Netherlands

Obesity Center CGG, Erasmus MC, University Medical Center Rotterdam, Rotterdam, The Netherlands
e-mail: o.abawi@erasmusmc.nl; e.l.t.vandenakker@erasmusmc.nl

M. van Haelst, E. van den Akker (eds.), *Clinical Obesity Genetics*,
https://doi.org/10.1007/978-3-032-04095-4_9

disorders can be caused by rare defects in a single gene or rare copy number variations (CNVs) involving one or more genes and are typically inherited in a Mendelian pattern (autosomal dominant or recessive) or occur *de novo*. Leptin-melanocortin pathway disorders are generally subdivided into (1) non-syndromic genetic obesity disorders, in which hyperphagia and early-onset severe obesity are the main clinical characteristics, and (2) syndromic genetic obesity disorders, in which the obesity is accompanied by intellectual disability, developmental delay, and/or presence of congenital anomalies or dysmorphic features.

This chapter provides a general overview of the most important clinical, biochemical and genetic features of non-syndromic leptin-melanocortin pathway disorders. The most important individual disorders, namely melanocortin 4 receptor (MC4R) deficiency, leptin (LEP) and leptin receptor (LEPR) deficiency, proopiomelanocortin (POMC) deficiency and proprotein convertase subtilisin/kexin type 1 (PCSK1) deficiency, are described in more detail in the following chapters.

2 Aetiology and Pathophysiology

2.1 Leptin-Melanocortin Pathway

Body weight is tightly regulated by complex systems mainly involving homeostatic neural circuits as well as cognitive-emotional processes that receive information by various hormones and messenger substances [2, 11]. The hypothalamic leptin-melanocortin pathway is the main regulator of homeostatic energy balance, satiety and energy expenditure (Fig. 1). It receives peripheral afferent input from various organs as well as the brainstem and limbic system. These include signals for both short-term and long-term regulation of satiety and weight. The short-term signals mostly derive from the gastrointestinal tract signalling acute changes in hunger and satiety right before and after a meal and include ghrelin produced by the stomach, insulin and amylin by the pancreas, and several hormones produced by the gut, e.g. glucagon-like peptide 1 (GLP-1), cholecystokinin, and peptide YY. Long-term signalling is mostly regulated by the adipose tissue which produces the hormone leptin, the most important indicator of the body's reserve energy stores [12]. Leptin is produced proportional to the amount of adipose tissue present. Upon activation of its receptor, leptin signalling leads to activation of POMC-expressing neurons in the arcuate nucleus of the hypothalamus. This activation leads to the production of POMC, a prohormone that is cleaved by PCSK1 into different hormones, including adrenocorticotropic hormone (ACTH) and α-melanocyte stimulating hormone (MSH). This α-MSH subsequently stimulates the MC4R in the paraventricular nucleus of the hypothalamus. Activation of the MC4R is a critical step which through various downstream signalling pathways ultimately leads to increased satiety and energy expenditure [13]. Disturbances at any level of this leptin-melanocortin pathway lead to decreased MC4R signalling, which results in impaired satiety and decreased energy expenditure.

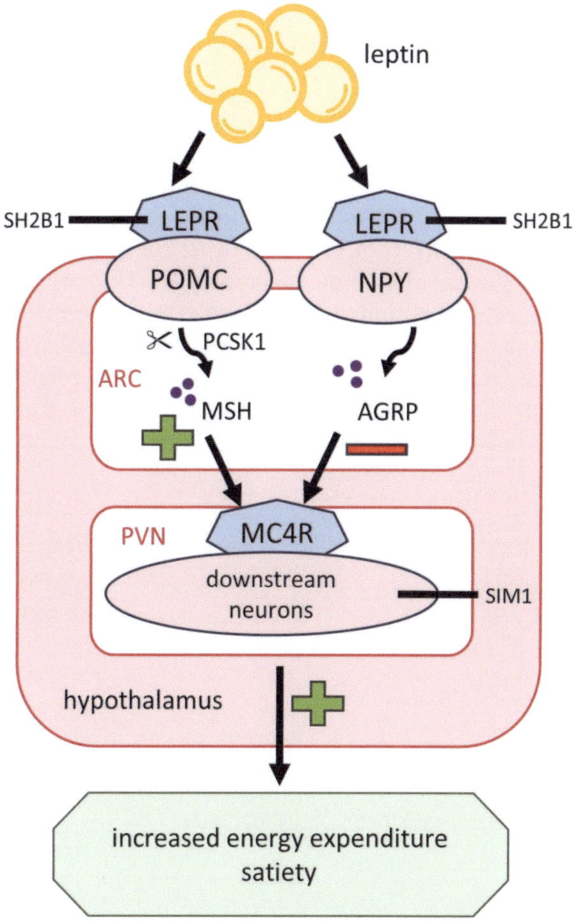

Fig. 1 Schematic overview of the leptin-melanocortin pathway. The adipose tissue produces the hormone leptin. Leptin activates its receptor, after which anorexic pro-opiomelanocortin (POMC) neurons in the arcuate nucleus of the hypothalamus produce the hormone POMC. POMC is subsequently cleaved by proprotein convertase subtilisin/kexin type 1 (PCSK1) into melanocyte stimulating hormone (MSH). This MSH activates downstream melanocortin 4 receptor (MC4R) neurons in the paraventricular nucleus of the hypothalamus resulting in increased energy expenditure and satiety signals. Moreover, leptin decreases the activity of the orexigenic neuropeptide Y (NPY)/ Agouti-related peptide (AgRP) neurons in the arcuate nucleus of the hypothalamus. SH2B1 acts as an adaptor protein at the level of the leptin receptor, enhancing leptin sensitivy. SIM1 is required for the development of PVN neurons that express MC4R. Abbreviations: *AGRP* Agouti-related peptide, *ARC* arcuate nucleus of the hypothalamus, *BDNF* brain-derived neurotrophic factor, *LEPR* leptin receptor, *MC4R* melanocortin 4 receptor, *MSH* melanocyte-stimulating hormone, *NPY* neuropeptide Y, *PCSK1* proprotein convertase subtilisin/kexin type 1, *POMC* pro-opiomelanocortin, *PVN* paraventricular nucleus of the hypothalamus, *SIM1* Single-minded homolog 1. (Credit: Figure made by Lotte Kleinendorst and Ozair Abawi)

2.2 Molecular Genetics

Tables 1a and 1b summarise some of the important genes known to cause non-syndromic obesity disorders that are associated with the leptin-melanocortin pathway, also shown in Fig. 1. In general, patients with biallelic (homozygous or compound heterozygous) variants in *MC4R* have a more severe phenotype than the patients with a single (heterozygous) variant. There is discussion whether heterozygosity for *LEP, LEPR, PCSK1,* or *POMC* confers a genetic obesity disorder or rather an increased risk of having obesity [14–16]. A recent exome sequencing study of 640,000 individuals, showed that heterozygous carriers of loss-of-function variants in *LEP*, *POMC*, *PCSK1*, or *MC4R* have a significantly higher BMI. However, heterozygous carriers of loss-of-function variants in *LEPR* in this study did not have a significantly higher BMI. This suggests that *LEPR* deficiency only results from biallelic pathogenic variants following an autosomal recessive inheritance pattern [17].

Table 1a Overview of most important genes associated with non-syndromic genetic obesity

Gene	Inheritance	OMIM number
LEP	AR Heterozygous LoF variants risk factor	164160
LEPR	AR	601007
MC4R	AR and AD	155541
PCSK1	AR Heterozygous LoF variants risk factor	162150
POMC	AR Heterozygous LoF variants risk factor	176830
SH2B1	AD	608937
SIM1	AD	603128

AD Autosomal dominant, *AR* Autosomal recessive, *LoF* loss-of-function

Table 1b Overview of some of the newly discovered or less studied genes associated with non-syndromic genetic obesity, which are not extensively discussed in this chapter. Clinical features are summarized in Table 2b

Gene	Inheritance	OMIM number
ADCY3	AR	600291
ASIP (*ITCH-ASIP* fusion)	AD	600201
BDNF	AD	113505
DYRK1B	AD	604556
KSR2	AD	610737

AD Autosomal dominant, *AR* Autosomal recessive

3 Clinical Presentation

The key clinical features of all non-syndromic leptin-melanocortin pathway disorders are hyperphagia and early-onset severe obesity. Although there is no uniform definition of hyperphagia, it generally presents as an extreme and insatiable increase in appetite, even when having consumed sufficient amounts of food [18]. Early-onset obesity is defined in current international guidelines as obesity occurring before age 5 years [19, 20]. Depending on the specific genetic obesity disorder, it is estimated that around 80% of patients present with hyperphagia whereas early-onset obesity before the age of 5 years is typically found in 90–95% of pediatric patients [8, 21]. Recently, we proposed that early-onset obesity should be defined as obesity onset before the age of 3.9 years due to the secular trend of increasing obesity worldwide [21]. In adult patients, obesity age of onset is often more difficult to define and occurs later than in pediatric patients [16, 22].

Other features can be present, presented in Tables 2a and 2b.

Table 2a Additional clinical features of the key non-syndromic genetic obesity disorders

Disorder	Clinical features beside obesity
Congenital leptin and leptin receptor deficiency (biallelic)	Increased risk of childhood infections, pituitary hormone disturbances, e.g. growth hormone deficiency (GHD), hypogonadotropic hypogonadism (HH), and central hypothyroidism (CeH) [23, 24]
POMC deficiency (biallelic)	Hyperphagia, red hair, and adrenal insufficiency due to ACTH deficiency [25]
PCSK1 deficiency (biallelic)	Severe neonatal malabsorptive diarrhea, central diabetes insipidus, pituitary hormone disturbances, e.g. GHD, HH, CeH [26]
MC4R deficiency (both mono- and biallelic)	Increased linear growth and increased bone mass, macrocephaly, hyperinsulinemia disproportionate to the degree of obesity [27] Biallelic more severe phenotype than monoallelic
SH2B1 deficiency	Early onset of diabetes with poorer glycaemic control than patients without this deletion, despite higher use of medication. Variable presence of behavioral problems and delayed (speech) development [28]
SIM1 deficiency	Variable presence of learning and behavioral problems. In some cases, a Prader-Willi-like phenotype is described [29]

Table 2b Additional clinical features of some of the newly discovered or less studied genes associated with non-syndromic genetic obesity, which are not extensively discussed in this chapter

Disorder	Clinical features beside obesity
ADCY3 deficiency	Anosmia or hyposmia, type 2 diabetes mellitus [30, 31]
ASIP deficiency	Red hair, hyperinsulinemia [32]. For further information, see paragraph "differential diagnosis" in the chapter on POMC deficiency
BDNF	Behavorial or psychiatric problems [33, 34]
DYRK1B deficiency	Type 2 diabetes mellitus [35]
KSR2 deficiency	Low heart rate, reduced basal metabolic rate, severe insulin resistance [36]

3.1 Clinical Evaluation

A comprehensive clinical evaluation is warranted in all cases with a suspected non-syndromic genetic obesity disorder. This includes:

- Detailed medical history: focusing on eating behaviors, signs of hyperphagia, age of onset of obesity, periods of rapid weight gain, a history of developmental delays or intellectual disability and other associated health issues. A three-generation family history documenting instances of (early-onset) obesity and related metabolic disorders, e.g. diabetes, hypertension, dyslipidemia, and cardiovascular diseases, should be obtained. Comprehensive growth charts analysis can further increase the suspicion of specific genetic obesity disorders and guide genetic testing [21, 37].
- Physical examination: measurement of height (or recumbent length in infants), weight, and head circumference, blood pressure, as well as a thorough dysmorphologic examination. Furthermore, signs of endocrine imbalances should be evaluated, e.g. signs of Cushing syndrome, thyroid or gonadal disfunction, and insulin resistance (acanthosis nigricans). When available, measurement of body composition and energy expenditure can aid in patient-tailored treatment advices, but does not contribute to establishing a diagnosis of a genetic obesity disorder.
- Measurement of parental height, weight, and head circumference.
- Biochemical evaluation: assessment of fasting glucose and insulin, lipid profile, liver enzymes, thyroid function and vitamin D levels is warranted in all patients. If indicated, additional evaluation of adrenal function, growth hormone/IGF-1 axis, gonadal function, white blood cell count and leptin levels are indicated.

4 Clinical Diagnosis

The diagnosis of a non-syndromic genetic obesity disorder is established by identifying (likely) pathogenic (American College of Medical Genetics and Genomics class 4 or 5, see Chapter "General Introduction to Obesity Genetics and Genomics") variants in one of the aforementioned obesity-associated genes (Tables 1a and 1b) in combination with a matching clinical phenotype. There are no formal criteria established for a clinical diagnosis. However, there are patients with a typical phenotype of a non-syndromic genetic obesity disorder without a (presently known) genetic diagnosis, for which future genetic testing might help to pinpoint a diagnosis as new obesity genes and variants in established obesity genes are still regularly discovered [8].

5 Differential Diagnosis

5.1 Multifactorial or Environmental Obesity Including Use of Obesogenic Medication

One of the most difficult problems in the differential diagnosis is to determine whether an environmental cause is the most likely origin of obesity. One should carefully examine the weight course of the patient in relation to lifestyle and environmental factors. Health-care professionals should also ask the patient and/or the parents what they regard as the most likely cause of obesity. A later age-of-onset of obesity and psychosocial problems are more often seen in patients without an underlying genetic cause of obesity [8]. Use of medication can play an important role in multifactorial obesity. Many drugs, such as antidepressants, antipsychotics, and antiepileptics can have an obesogenic effect.

5.2 Polygenic Obesity

Polygenic obesity is a form of obesity influenced by the combined effects of a large amount of genetic variants in numerous genes, each contributing a small amount to an individual's predisposition to gain weight. See Chapter "Genome-Wide Association Studies and Polygenic Risk Prediction in Obesity Research" for extensive information on polygenic obesity.

5.3 Syndromic Obesity

In syndromic obesity, the patient typically also has congenital malformations, organ anomalies, and dysmorphic features. Developmental delay or intellectual disability are often present. Many of these syndromes are discussed elsewhere in this book, with Prader-Willi syndrome as the most well-known syndromic genetic obesity disorder.

5.4 Overgrowth

Genetic obesity syndromes should further be distinguished from overgrowth syndromes such as Beckwith-Wiedemann syndrome [38]. In genetic obesity, the anthropometrics at birth are usually normal. In overgrowth syndromes, patients have macrosomia, tall stature, and a large head circumference. Moreover, patients with an overgrowth syndrome do not typically have the hyperphagia reported in many patients with genetic obesity disorders.

5.5 *Hypothalamic Obesity*

A non-genetic cause of severe obesity with hyperphagia is hypothalamic obesity. This rare type of obesity results from dysfunction or damage to the hypothalamus. When the hypothalamus is damaged, it can lead to abnormal and often uncontrollable weight gain. This condition can be caused by a variety of factors, including tumors, radiation or surgery of the hypothalamic area [39]. A well-known cause of hypothalamic obesity occurs after the surgical removal of a craniopharyngioma. In addition to weight gain and hyperphagia, other symptoms may be present, depending on the underlying cause of the hypothalamic dysfunction. These can include severe fatigue, pituitary hormone deficiencies, growth problems, disturbances in the regulation of body temperature and decreased energy expenditure.

5.6 *Endocrine*

Hypothyroidism and Cushing syndrome should be considered as potential medical causes of obesity.

In adults with obesity, overt hypothyroidism is present in 14% of the patients [40]. Therefore, it is recommended that thyroid function is tested in all adult patients with obesity [41]. In children with obesity, the prevalence of hypothyroidism is unknown, but should be considered in children with decelerating height velocity (endocrine cross) [19, 20]. In adults with obesity, hypercortisolism is present in only 0.9% of patients [40], therefore, testing for Cushing syndrome in patients with obesity is recommended only in patients with additional signs of endogenous hypercortisolism [41]. In children, Cushing syndrome is extremely rare and presents with rapid weight gain coinciding with decelerating height velocity (endocrine cross) [42].

6 Molecular Diagnosis

When patients are suspected of a non-syndromic genetic obesity disorder, analysis of known obesity genes is indicated. These obesity gene panels usually consist of the genes involved in the leptin-melanocortin pathway. For more extensive testing, one could consider whole exome sequencing or whole genome sequencing, although this increases the risk of incidental findings or carrierships that do not explain the phenotype. In cases where it is unclear whether there could also be syndromic component, SNP-array can also be considered, for example to identify the 16p11.2 deletion. Some gene panels incorporate CNV analysis to identify obesity-associated CNVs.

7 Therapy

An individualized tailored treatment plan should be made for every patient with obesity that is appropriate for age, culturally sensitive, and family-centered. The cornerstone treatment is a combined lifestyle intervention (CLI) that focuses on physical activity and dietary advice as well as psychosocial and behavioral interventions. This however rarely suffices in genetic obesity disorders [43], and additional pharmacologic treatment, or in specific cases bariatric surgery might be needed. Several drugs are available in general for obesity without an identified underlying cause. However, data on treatment outcomes in patients with non-syndromic genetic obesity disorders are confined to case reports and case series describing positive results with GLP-1 agonist treatment, naltrexone/bupropion, and central stimulants including methylphenidate and dextroamphetamine [44, 45].

Additionally, targeted drug therapy is available for biallelic POMC, PCSK1, and LEPR deficiency, i.e. MC4R agonist therapy, as well as LEP deficiency, i.e. recombinant leptin therapy. Furthermore, treatment and follow-up of patients with non-syndromic genetic obesity disorders affecting the leptin-melanocortin pathway should include genetic and reproductive counselling and organ system surveillance in specific syndromes (e.g. adrenal insufficiency in POMC deficiency; thyroid, puberty and growth screening in LEP and LEPR deficiency). Moreover, tailored advice pertaining outcomes of bariatric surgery outcomes in genetic obesity should be provided (see Chapter "Metabolic Bariatric Surgery") [46, 47].

8 Follow-up Advices

Management of genetic obesity disorders often requires multidisciplinary, long-term care and varies depending on the specific disorder. There is no uniform surveillance plan for all patients with leptin-melanocortin pathway disorders. Follow-up recommendations that could be considered are:

- Monitoring of adherence to healthy lifestyle
- Monitoring of height, weight, and puberty
- Biochemical evaluation including endocrine evaluation for hormonal disturbances and screening for comorbidities (thyroid function, gonadal hormones, signs of hepatic steatosis, lipid profile). Monitor glucose levels and insulin sensitivity as an increased rate of type 2 is described for some disorders, such as *SH2B1* haploinsufficiency [28]
- Evaluation of treatment of syndrome-associated hormonal deficiencies (e.g. growth hormone therapy in LEPR deficiency, hydrocortisone to treat adrenal insufficiency in POMC deficiency)
- Measurement of body composition and of resting energy expenditure to guide tailored dietary advice

- Cardiovascular assessment: according to severity of the obesity and presence of comorbidities. As of yet, no specific screening strategies are available for genetic obesity disorders

9 Family Screening

The advice for family screening varies per disorder within the leptin-melanocortin pathway.

In case of an autosomal dominant disorder, family members that show a similar phenotype can be tested for the pathogenic variant that was identified in the family, as this can have implication for the follow-up and treatment of obesity. In case of a recessive disorder, it is important to determine the recurrence risk for future siblings of the proband.

10 Summary

Non-syndromic leptin-melanocortin pathway disorders are the most well-known group of monogenic obesity disorders. They typically present with severe obesity with early-onset and marked hyperphagia, generally lacking intellectual disability, neuropsychiatric problems, or congenital anomalies. The inheritance pattern can be autosomal dominant or recessive. The most prevalent condition is heterozygous melanocortin-4 receptor (MC4R) deficiency. Many of the recessive forms of the leptin-melanocortin pathway disorders exhibit associated hormonal imbalances, impacting hormones like adrenocorticotropic hormone (ACTH) and growth hormone. Treatment development is advancing, especially with the recent approval for the use of a specific MC4R agonist.

Take Home Message

The leptin-melanocortin pathway is crucial for the regulation of satiety and body weight. Pathogenic variants in genes involved in this pathway typically lead to a phenotype of hyperphagia and consequently early-onset severe obesity.

References

1. Loos RJF, Yeo GSH. The genetics of obesity: from discovery to biology. Nat Rev Genet. 2022;23(2):120–33.
2. Berthoud HR, Morrison CD, Münzberg H. The obesity epidemic in the face of homeostatic body weight regulation: what went wrong and how can it be fixed? Physiol Behav. 2020;222:112959.
3. Elks CE, den Hoed M, Zhao JH, Sharp SJ, Wareham NJ, Loos RJ, Ong KK. Variability in the heritability of body mass index: a systematic review and meta-regression. Front Endocrinol (Lausanne). 2012;3:29.
4. Loos RJF, Janssens A. Predicting polygenic obesity using genetic information. Cell Metab. 2017;25(3):535–43.
5. Jansen PR, Vos N, van Uhm J, Dekkers IA, van der Meer R, Mannens M, van Haelst MM. The utility of obesity polygenic risk scores from research to clinical practice: a review. Obes Rev. 2024;25(11):e13810.
6. Farooqi IS, O'Rahilly S. The genetics of obesity in humans. 2000.
7. Kleinendorst L, Massink MPG, Cooiman MI, Savas M, van der Baan-Slootweg OH, Roelants RJ, et al. Genetic obesity: next-generation sequencing results of 1230 patients with obesity. J Med Genet. 2018;55(9):578–86.
8. Kleinendorst L, Abawi O, van der Voorn B, Jongejan M, Brandsma AE, Visser JA, et al. Identifying underlying medical causes of pediatric obesity: results of a systematic diagnostic approach in a pediatric obesity center. PLoS One. 2020;15(5):e0232990.
9. Renard E, Thevenard-Berger A, Meyre D. Medical semiology of patients with monogenic obesity: a systematic review. Obes Rev. 2024;25(10):e13797.
10. Serra-Juhé C, Martos-Moreno G, Bou de Pieri F, Flores R, Chowen JA, Pérez-Jurado LA, Argente J. Heterozygous rare genetic variants in non-syndromic early-onset obesity. Int J Obes. 2020;44(4):830–41.
11. Angelidi AM, Belanger MJ, Kokkinos A, Koliaki CC, Mantzoros CS. Novel noninvasive approaches to the treatment of obesity: from pharmacotherapy to gene therapy. Endocr Rev. 2022;43(3):507–57.
12. Pan WW, Myers MG Jr. Leptin and the maintenance of elevated body weight. Nat Rev Neurosci. 2018;19(2):95–105.
13. Krashes MJ, Lowell BB, Garfield AS. Melanocortin-4 receptor-regulated energy homeostasis. Nat Neurosci. 2016;19(2):206–19.
14. Folon L, Baron M, Toussaint B, Vaillant E, Boissel M, Scherrer V, et al. Contribution of heterozygous PCSK1 variants to obesity and implications for precision medicine: a case-control study. Lancet Diabetes Endocrinol. 2023;11(3):182–90.
15. Le Collen L, Delemer B, Poitou C, Vaxillaire M, Toussaint B, Dechaume A, et al. Heterozygous pathogenic variants in POMC are not responsible for monogenic obesity: implication for MC4R agonist use. Genet Med. 2023;25(7):100857.
16. Courbage S, Poitou C, Le Beyec-Le Bihan J, Karsenty A, Lemale J, Pelloux V, et al. Implication of heterozygous variants in genes of the leptin-Melanocortin pathway in severe obesity. J Clin Endocrinol Metab. 2021;106(10):2991–3006.
17. Akbari P, Gilani A, Sosina O, Kosmicki JA, Khrimian L, Fang YY, et al. Sequencing of 640,000 exomes identifies GPR75 variants associated with protection from obesity. Science. 2021;373(6550)
18. Heymsfield SB, Avena NM, Baier L, Brantley P, Bray GA, Burnett LC, et al. Hyperphagia: current concepts and future directions proceedings of the 2nd international conference on hyperphagia. Obesity (Silver Spring). 2014;22(Suppl 1):S1–S17.
19. Hampl SE, Hassink SG, Skinner AC, Armstrong SC, Barlow SE, Bolling CF, et al. Clinical practice guideline for the evaluation and treatment of children and adolescents with obesity. Pediatrics. 2023;151(2)

20. Styne DM, Arslanian SA, Connor EL, Farooqi IS, Murad MH, Silverstein JH, Yanovski JA. Pediatric obesity-assessment, treatment, and prevention: an Endocrine Society Clinical Practice Guideline. J Clin Endocrinol Metab. 2017;102(3):709–57.
21. Abawi O, Wahab RJ, Kleinendorst L, Blankers LA, Brandsma AE, van Rossum EFC, et al. Genetic obesity disorders: body mass index trajectories and age of onset of obesity compared with children with obesity from the general population. J Pediatr. 2023;262:113619.
22. Welling MS, Mohseni M, Meeusen REH, de Groot CJ, Boon MR, Kleinendorst L, et al. Clinical phenotypes of adults with monogenic and syndromic genetic obesity. Obesity (Silver Spring). 2024;32(7):1257–67.
23. Farooqi IS, Wangensteen T, Collins S, Kimber W, Matarese G, Keogh JM, et al. Clinical and molecular genetic spectrum of congenital deficiency of the leptin receptor. N Engl J Med. 2007;356(3):237–47.
24. Besci Ö, Fırat SN, Özen S, Çetinkaya S, Akın L, Kör Y, et al. A National Multicenter Study of leptin and leptin receptor deficiency and systematic review. J Clin Endocrinol Metab. 2023;108(9):2371–88.
25. Gregoric N, Groselj U, Bratina N, Debeljak M, Zerjav Tansek M, Suput Omladic J, et al. Two cases with an early presented proopiomelanocortin deficiency-a long-term follow-up and systematic literature review. Front Endocrinol (Lausanne). 2021;12:689387.
26. Pépin L, Colin E, Tessarech M, Rouleau S, Bouhours-Nouet N, Bonneau D, Coutant R. A new case of PCSK1 pathogenic variant with congenital proprotein convertase 1/3 deficiency and literature review. J Clin Endocrinol Metab. 2019;104(4):985–93.
27. Farooqi IS, Keogh JM, Yeo GS, Lank EJ, Cheetham T, O'Rahilly S. Clinical spectrum of obesity and mutations in the melanocortin 4 receptor gene. N Engl J Med. 2003;348(12):1085–95.
28. Hanssen R, Auwerx C, Jõeloo M, Sadler MC, Estonian Biobank Research T, Henning E, et al. Chromosomal deletions on 16p11.2 encompassing SH2B1 are associated with accelerated metabolic disease. Cell Rep Med. 2023;4(8):101155.
29. Bonnefond A, Raimondo A, Stutzmann F, Ghoussaini M, Ramachandrappa S, Bersten DC, et al. Loss-of-function mutations in SIM1 contribute to obesity and Prader-Willi-like features. J Clin Invest. 2013;123(7):3037–41.
30. Saeed S, Bonnefond A, Tamanini F, Mirza MU, Manzoor J, Janjua QM, et al. Loss-of-function mutations in ADCY3 cause monogenic severe obesity. Nat Genet. 2018;50(2):175–9.
31. Özcabı B, Durmaz A, Aykut A, Önal H, Özen S. A rare case of monogenic obesity due to a novel variant in the ADCY3 gene: challenges in follow-up and treatment. J Clin Res Pediatr Endocrinol. 2023;17:337–44.
32. Kempf E, Landgraf K, Stein R, Hanschkow M, Hilbert A, Abou Jamra R, et al. Aberrant expression of agouti signaling protein (ASIP) as a cause of monogenic severe childhood obesity. Nat Metab. 2022;4(12):1697–712.
33. Gray J, Yeo GS, Cox JJ, Morton J, Adlam AL, Keogh JM, et al. Hyperphagia, severe obesity, impaired cognitive function, and hyperactivity associated with functional loss of one copy of the brain-derived neurotrophic factor (BDNF) gene. Diabetes. 2006;55(12):3366–71.
34. Friedel S, Horro FF, Wermter AK, Geller F, Dempfle A, Reichwald K, et al. Mutation screen of the brain derived neurotrophic factor gene (BDNF): identification of several genetic variants and association studies in patients with obesity, eating disorders, and attention-deficit/hyperactivity disorder. Am J Med Genet B Neuropsychiatr Genet. 2005;132B(1):96–9.
35. Folon L, Baron M, Scherrer V, Toussaint B, Vaillant E, Loiselle H, et al. Pathogenic, total loss-of-function DYRK1B variants cause monogenic obesity associated with type 2 diabetes. Diabetes Care. 2024;47(3):444–51.
36. Pearce LR, Atanassova N, Banton MC, Bottomley B, van der Klaauw AA, Revelli JP, et al. KSR2 mutations are associated with obesity, insulin resistance, and impaired cellular fuel oxidation. Cell. 2013;155(4):765–77.
37. Wabitsch M, Farooqi S, Flück CE, Bratina N, Mallya UG, Stewart M, et al. Natural history of obesity due to POMC, PCSK1, and LEPR deficiency and the impact of Setmelanotide. J Endocr Soc 2022;6(6):bvac057.

38. Klein SD, Nisbet A, Kalish JM. Overgrowth syndromes, diagnosis and management. Curr Opin Pediatr. 2023;35(6):620–30.
39. Müller HL, Tauber M, Lawson EA, Özyurt J, Bison B, Martinez-Barbera JP, et al. Hypothalamic syndrome. Nat Rev Dis Primers. 2022;8(1):24.
40. van Hulsteijn LT, Pasquali R, Casanueva F, Haluzik M, Ledoux S, Monteiro MP, et al. Prevalence of endocrine disorders in obese patients: systematic review and meta-analysis. Eur J Endocrinol. 2020;182(1):11–21.
41. Pasquali R, Casanueva F, Haluzik M, van Hulsteijn L, Ledoux S, Monteiro MP, et al. European Society of Endocrinology Clinical Practice Guideline: endocrine work-up in obesity. Eur J Endocrinol. 2020;182(1):G1–G32.
42. Stratakis CA. Cushing syndrome in pediatrics. Endocrinol Metab Clin N Am. 2012;41(4):793–803.
43. Kleinendorst L, van Haelst MM, van den Akker ELT. Young girl with severe early-onset obesity and hyperphagia. BMJ Case Rep. 2017;2017
44. Welling MS, de Groot CJ, Mohseni M, Meeusen REH, Boon MR, van Haelst MM, et al. Treatment with liraglutide or naltrexone-bupropion in patients with genetic obesity: a real-world study. EClinicalMedicine. 2024;74:102709.
45. Brandt S, von Schnurbein J, Lennerz B, Kohlsdorf K, Vollbach H, Denzer C, et al. Methylphenidate in children with monogenic obesity due to LEPR or MC4R deficiency improves feeling of satiety and reduces BMI-SDS-A case series. Pediatr Obes. 2020;15(1):e12577.
46. Cooiman MI, Alsters SIM, Duquesnoy M, Hazebroek EJ, Meijers-Heijboer HJ, Chahal H, et al. Long-term weight outcome after bariatric surgery in patients with melanocortin-4 receptor gene variants: a case-control study of 105 patients. Obes Surg. 2022;32(3):837–44.
47. Poitou C, Puder L, Dubern B, Krabusch P, Genser L, Wiegand S, et al. Long-term outcomes of bariatric surgery in patients with bi-allelic mutations in the POMC, LEPR, and MC4R genes. Surg Obes Relat Dis. 2021;17(8):1449–56.

Leptin and Leptin Receptor Deficiency

Lotte Kleinendorst and Ozair Abawi

1 Introduction

Leptin deficiency and leptin receptor deficiency are two distinct genetic disorders, both discovered in the mid-1990s, that have significantly advanced our understanding of appetite regulation and energy balance. Leptin deficiency results in the absence or insufficient levels of the hormone leptin, leading to severe hyperphagia and early-onset obesity. The deficiency of the leptin receptor disrupts the body's ability to respond to leptin signals, resulting in similar, less severe, clinical features.

Leptin deficiency is ultra rare, with an estimated global prevalence of 1 in 4.4 million people [1].

Leptin receptor deficiency is less rare, it has a predicted prevalence in Europe of 1 in 750,000 people [2]. The prevalence of these disorders is higher in consanguineous populations as they have an autosomal recessive inheritance pattern. Carriers of a monoallelic pathogenic loss-of-function variant in *LEP* have an increased risk of developing obesity, whereas carriers of a heterozygous *LEPR* pathogenic loss-of-function variant do not have a significantly higher BMI [3].

L. Kleinendorst (✉)
Department of Human Genetics, Section Clinical Genetics, Amsterdam University Medical Center, Amsterdam, The Netherlands

Emma Center for Personalized Medicine, Amsterdam UMC, University of Amsterdam, Amsterdam, The Netherlands
e-mail: l.kleinendorst@amsterdamumc.nl

O. Abawi
Division of Endocrinology, Department of Pediatrics, Erasmus MC-Sophia, University Medical Center Rotterdam, Rotterdam, The Netherlands

Obesity Center CGG, Erasmus MC, University Medical Center Rotterdam, Rotterdam, The Netherlands
e-mail: o.abawi@erasmusmc.nl

M. van Haelst, E. van den Akker (eds.), *Clinical Obesity Genetics*,
https://doi.org/10.1007/978-3-032-04095-4_10

2 Aetiology and Pathophysiology

2.1 *Leptin-Melanocortin Pathway*

Leptin, a hormone produced by white adipose tissue, plays a key role in the regulation of appetite, metabolism, and energy balance. Its production is correlated to the number of adipocytes present and functions as the most important indicator of the body's reserve energy stores [4]. The hypothalamic leptin-melanocortin pathway integrates the leptin signal, as well as other peripheral afferent input from various organs as well as other brain areas, and is the main regulator of homeostatic energy balance, satiety and energy expenditure (see Chapter "Non-syndromic Leptin Melanocortin Pathway Disorders"). Hypothalamic leptin signalling leads to the production of POMC, a precursor hormone that is cleaved into different hormones, including α-melanocyte stimulating hormone (MSH). This α-MSH subsequently activates the MC4R, which through various downstream signalling pathways ultimately leads to increased satiety and energy expenditure [5, 6]. Leptin signalling is also involved in the expression of thyrotropin releasing hormone (TRH) in the paraventricular nucleus of the hypothalmus, thereby regulating thyroid function [7]. Furthermore, leptin is a permissive factor for the initiation of pubertal development [8], stimulates growth hormone secretion via effects at the hypothalamic and pituitary level [9], and has several important immune functions [10]. Disruptions of leptin signalling can have diverse causes, e.g. through absent or insufficient levels of leptin [11], leptin isoforms functioning as antagonists of the leptin receptor [12], or defective leptin receptors [13]. These disruptions lead to a phenotype characterised by hyperphagia and severe, early-onset obesity which can be accompanied by thyroid, gonadal and immune dysfunction, as well as decreased linear growth. It is hypothesized that leptin resistance explains why leptin values in people with obesity are elevated without leading to increased satiety and decreased food intake, but the exact molecular mechanisms are yet to be elucidated [14].

2.1.1 Molecular Genetics

Both in the *LEP* and *LEPR* gene, pathogenic variants can include frameshift, nonsense, missense, or splice variants. For LEPR deficiency, it is suggested that there might be a genotype–phenotype correlation reflecting residual leptin receptor function, but this is not proven yet [2].

SNPs or common variants in *LEP* and *LEPR* associated with an increase in BMI have been described, but these effects on body weight are small [15]. It is suggested that there might also be protective SNPs in *LEP* and *LEPR* that could reduce the obesity risk. There is also a case report published about a mother and son with underweight who both had a rare heterozygous missense variant in *LEP* [16]. The mother and son had reduced appetite and BMI, combined with delayed puberty.

LEP and LEPR deficiencies show complete penetrance, meaning that all individuals with biallelic pathogenic variants (autosomal recessive inheritance) will develop the disorder. However, the expressivity can vary, particularly with regards to the presence of the hormonal disturbances and immune issues. Within families, the presence and type of pituitary hormone deficiency seems to be comparable between family members. However, interfamilial variability has been reported: five unrelated subjects from Reunion Island who were homozygous for the same exon 6–8 deletion in *LEPR*, did not present with a similar phenotype (1 with central hypothyroidism, 3 with growth hormone deficiency, 3 with hypogonadism) [17].

3 Clinical Presentation

The first reported cases with leptin and leptin receptor deficiency were published in the 1990s.

In 1997, two cousins from a highly consanguineous Pakistani family with severe, early-onset obesity were found to have a homozygous pathogenic *LEP* variant. The cousins had very low leptin levels, close to the detection limits [18]. A year later, in 1998, three sisters from a consanguineous Algerian family with comparable severe early-onset obesity were discovered to have LEPR deficiency based on a homozygous *LEPR* defect [19]. These sisters also did not undergo spontaneous puberty development, and they had hypothyroidism and mild growth delay because of decreased growth hormone secretion. These first patients highlight the key clinical features of leptin and leptin receptor deficiency, which highly overlap. Consanguinity is present in about 90% of cases, as fitting with the autosomal recessive inheritance [20]. Besides hyperphagia and severe-early onset obesity, patients with LEP and LEPR deficiency can also have pituitary hormone deficiencies, i.e. central hypothyroidism, hypogonadotropic hypogonadism, or growth hormone deficiency [2, 20]. Hyperphagia can be described as an extreme and insatiable increase in appetite, even when having consumed sufficient amounts of food [21]. Hyperphagia is known to negatively impact quality of life [22]. The age of onset of obesity is usually within the first 2 years of life [20, 23]. The pituitary hormone deficiencies were present in 34% of patients with LEPR deficiency [2]. In patients with LEP deficiency, hypothyroidism is described in 17% and hypogonadism in up to 83% of patients [20]. The clinical phenotype, including obesity severity and age of onset of obesity, seems to be a bit more pronounced in patients with LEP deficiency than LEPR deficiency [20].

People with leptin deficiency can be more prone to infections, mostly pulmonary or upper-airway infections. It is reported that they have a lower circulating CD4+ T cell count, impaired proliferation of T cells and less cytokine release [24]. When treated with recombinant leptin, these measurements improve. In patients with leptin receptor deficiency, lymphocyte counts showed a modest decrease in CD4+ T-cell count and a compensatory higher B-cell count, and frequent infections are described in ~50% of published patients [2, 13]. A retrospective study reported a high mortality rate in children with LEP deficiency (26%) or LEPR deficiency (9%), mainly due to severe pulmonary and gastrointestinal infections [25]. It should be noted that this study was performed in Pakistan, and it is unknown whether this increased mortality due to infections is also present in other countries or populations [2]. Resting energy expenditure is comparable to age-, sex- and weight matched controls [26, 27]. In patients with leptin deficiency, recombinant leptin therapy does not increase energy expenditure, but it prevents the reduction in energy expenditure that is associated with weight loss [11, 28].

4 Differential Diagnosis

Other non-syndromic genetic obesity disorders, for example MC4R deficiency, should be considered when there is early-onset severe obesity. Furthermore, consider multifactorial or environmental obesity including use of obesogenic medication, polygenic obesity, syndromic obesity, overgrowth disorders, hypothalamic obesity, and endocrine obesity. For more details regarding the differential diagnosis, see the differential diagnosis paragraph in Chapter "Non-syndromic Leptin Melanocortin Pathway Disorders".

4.1 Endocrinopathies

The diverse endocrinopathies that can be seen in LEP and LEPR deficiency all have their own differential diagnoses, which fall beyond the scope of this book. The combination of pituitary hormone deficiencies and early-onset severe obesity makes a defect in the leptin-melanocortin pathway most likely. POMC deficiency and PCSK1 deficiency can also present with (some of) these endocrinopathies, see Chapters "MC4R Deficiency" and "PCSK1 Deficiency".

5 Molecular Diagnosis

The molecular diagnosis of leptin and leptin receptor deficiency can be made by sequencing of the *LEP* and *LEPR* gene. Because of the genetic heterogeneity of genetic obesity disorders, especially when the child is young and there are no other features than early-onset obesity and hyperphagia, larger gene panels might be more effective. LEP and LEPR deficiency result from biallelic (homozygous or compound heterozygous) pathogenic variants following an autosomal recessive inheritance pattern. Monoallelic loss-of-function *LEP* variants are likely risk factors for obesity, but monoallelic *LEPR* variants do not appear to increase BMI [3].

6 Therapy

In general, an individualized tailored treatment plan should be made for every patient with non-syndromic genetic obesity, including LEP and LEPR deficiency, that is appropriate for age, culturally sensitive, and family-centered. The cornerstone treatment is a combined lifestyle intervention (CLI) that focuses on physical activity and dietary advice as well as psychosocial and behavioral interventions. This however does not treat the hyperphagia and therefore rarely suffices in LEP and LEPR deficiency [22], and additional pharmacologic treatment, or in specific cases bariatric surgery might be needed. Both for LEP and LEPR deficiency, target treatment is available in the form of recombinant leptin therapy and MC4R agonist therapy, respectively.

6.1 Targeted Therapy for Leptin Deficiency

The treatment for leptin deficiency primarily revolves around leptin replacement therapy. Synthetic recombinant leptin, such as metreleptin, is administered through subcutaneous injections to restore physiological leptin levels. Leptin replacement therapy has demonstrated notable efficacy in improving appetite regulation, metabolic control, reversal of endocrine and immunological disturbances, and body weight management in patients with leptin deficiency [26, 29, 30]. Leptin substitution treatment also shows improvement in psychological traits such as mood and behaviour [31]. In patients with severe obesity, but without biallelic pathogenic variants in *LEP,* leptin levels are increased and leptin treatment does not result in weight loss. This is attributed to central leptin resistance [26]. Anti-metreleptin antibodies have been described in many patients treated with recombinant leptin, some of which, but not all, can have neutralizing activity resulting in inhibition of endogenous leptin action and loss of treatment efficacy [26]. Therefore, it is recommended to test for the presence of these neutralizing antibodies in cases with loss of drug efficacy or severe infections [26].

To our knowledge, there are no published reports on effects of other commonly used anti-obesity medications, such as GLP-1 agonist treatment, naltrexone/bupropione, phentermine, or central stimulants such as methylphenidate or dexamphetamine in patients with LEP deficiency. Moreover, there are no published reports on the effect of bariatric surgery in patients with LEP deficiency, although mice with leptin deficiency (ob/ob mice) show weight regain over the pre-surgery level [32]. Targeted gene therapy using CRISPR has been shown to restore the production and physiological functions of leptin in ob/ob mice and might provide a future therapeutic option [33].

6.2 Targeted Therapy for Leptin Receptor Deficiency

Setmelanotide, a MC4R agonist, is available as treatment for several leptin-melanocortin pathway deficiencies including leptin receptor deficiency. This is currently administered through subcutaneous injections. In a phase 3 trial with 11 patients with LEPR deficiency, 1 year treatment with setmelanotide resulted in an average weight loss of −12.5%, as well as improvements in satiety and hunger feelings and metabolic parameters [34]. The most important side effects are injection side reactions, gastro-intestinal side effects, which usually resolve over time, and skin hyperpigmentation [34, 35]. Qualitative studies also show that treatment with setmelanotide improves quality of life in patients with LEPR deficiency through reduction of the hyperphagia [22, 36]. Neutralizing anti-drug antibodies have not yet been reported.

To our knowledge, no reports have been published on effects of GLP-1 agonist treatment, naltrexone/bupropione or phentermine in patients with LEPR deficiency. There is one study on methylphenidate in children with LEPR deficiency, leading to improved BMI trajectories and decreased appetite [37]. There have been incidental reports of bariatric surgery in LEPR deficiency showing initial weight loss followed by substantial weight gain [38, 39]. It is unknown if there is a preferred type of bariatric surgery for patients with LEPR deficiency. Adenoviral gene therapy has been shown to restore leptin receptor signalling in the arcuate nucleus of the hypothalamus of leptin receptor-deficient mice and might become available as future treatment option [40].

7 Follow-Up Advices

Follow-up of LEP and LEPR deficiency requires multidisciplinary long-term care. There is no uniform follow-up or screening recommendation. Follow-up advices that could be considered are:

- Repeat visits to monitor adherence to healthy lifestyle
- Monitoring of height, weight, and puberty
- Monitoring of associated endocrine deficiencies and evaluation of treatment (growth hormone/IGF1 axis, thyroid function, gonadal hormones)
- Biochemical evaluation including endocrine evaluation for comorbidities (signs of hepatic steatosis, lipid profile, glucose levels, insulin sensitivity). When measuring leptin levels, one should be aware of the possibility of bioinactive leptin
- Upon clinical indication, measurement and follow-up of immune function including CD4+ T cell count
- Measurement of body composition and of resting energy expenditure to guide tailored dietary advice
- Cardiovascular assessment: according to severity of the obesity and presence of comorbidities.

8 Family Screening

Leptin and leptin receptor deficiency follow an autosomal recessive inheritance pattern. The siblings of an affected child have 25% chance of being affected if both parents are carrier. Carriership of a heterozygous pathogenic variant in *LEP* might increase obesity risk. Prenatal diagnostics can be considered in families with known leptin (receptor) deficiency.

9 Summary

LEP (leptin) and LEPR (leptin receptor) deficiencies are genetic disorders that disrupt the leptin-melanocortin pathway, which is crucial for regulating appetite, and energy balance. These ultra rare disorders are most seen in consanguineous populations. They have an autosomal recessive inheritance pattern and are caused by biallelic pathogenic variants in either the *LEP* gene or the *LEPR* gene. The clinical characteristics are severe early-onset obesity caused by hyperphagia and diverse hormonal deficiencies (hypothyroidism, hypogonadotropic hypogonadism, growth hormone deficiency). In the case of LEP deficiency, leptin replacement therapy (such as with recombinant leptin) has shown success in reducing hunger and achieving weight loss. LEPR deficiency can be treated with an MC4R agonist, which also leads to a decrease in hunger and weight loss.

References

1. NORD—National Organization for Rare Disorders. Congenital leptin deficiency; 2024. Available from: https://rarediseases.org/rare-diseases/congenital-leptin-deficiency/#complete-report.
2. Kleinendorst L, Abawi O, van der Kamp HJ, Alders M, Meijers-Heijboer HEJ, van Rossum EFC, et al. Leptin receptor deficiency: a systematic literature review and prevalence estimation based on population genetics. Eur J Endocrinol. 2020;182(1):47–56.
3. Akbari P, Gilani A, Sosina O, Kosmicki JA, Khrimian L, Fang YY, et al. Sequencing of 640,000 exomes identifies GPR75 variants associated with protection from obesity. Science. 2021;373(6550)
4. Pan WW, Myers MG Jr. Leptin and the maintenance of elevated body weight. Nat Rev Neurosci. 2018;19(2):95–105.
5. Krashes MJ, Lowell BB, Garfield AS. Melanocortin-4 receptor-regulated energy homeostasis. Nat Neurosci. 2016;19(2):206–19.
6. Yeo GSH, Chao DHM, Siegert AM, Koerperich ZM, Ericson MD, Simonds SE, et al. The melanocortin pathway and energy homeostasis: from discovery to obesity therapy. Mol Metab. 2021;48:101206.
7. Flier JS, Harris M, Hollenberg AN. Leptin, nutrition, and the thyroid: the why, the wherefore, and the wiring. J Clin Invest. 2000;105(7):859–61.

8. Reinehr T, Roth CL. Is there a causal relationship between obesity and puberty? Lancet Child Adolesc Health. 2019;3(1):44–54.
9. Saleri R, Giustina A, Tamanini C, Valle D, Burattin A, Wehrenberg WB, Baratta M. Leptin stimulates growth hormone secretion via a direct pituitary effect combined with a decreased somatostatin tone in a median eminence-pituitary perifusion study. Neuroendocrinology. 2004;79(4):221–8.
10. Farooqi IS, O'Rahilly S. 20 years of leptin: human disorders of leptin action. J Endocrinol. 2014;223(1):T63–70.
11. Farooqi IS, Jebb SA, Langmack G, Lawrence E, Cheetham CH, Prentice AM, et al. Effects of recombinant leptin therapy in a child with congenital leptin deficiency. N Engl J Med. 1999;341(12):879–84.
12. Funcke JB, Moepps B, Roos J, von Schnurbein J, Verstraete K, Fröhlich-Reiterer E, et al. Rare antagonistic leptin variants and severe, early-onset obesity. N Engl J Med. 2023;388(24):2253–61.
13. Farooqi IS, Wangensteen T, Collins S, Kimber W, Matarese G, Keogh JM, et al. Clinical and molecular genetic spectrum of congenital deficiency of the leptin receptor. N Engl J Med. 2007;356(3):237–47.
14. Cui H, López M, Rahmouni K. The cellular and molecular bases of leptin and ghrelin resistance in obesity. Nat Rev Endocrinol. 2017;13(6):338–51.
15. Cadena-López RO, Hernández-Rodríguez LV, Aguilar-Galarza A, García-Muñoz W, Haddad-Talancón L, Anzures-Cortes ML, et al. Association between SNPs in leptin pathway genes and anthropometric, biochemical, and dietary markers related to obesity. Genes (Basel). 2022;13(6)
16. Murray PG, Read A, Banerjee I, Whatmore AJ, Pritchard LE, Davies RA, et al. Reduced appetite and body mass index with delayed puberty in a mother and son: association with a rare novel sequence variant in the leptin gene. Eur J Endocrinol. 2011;164(4):521–7.
17. Huvenne H, Le Beyec J, Pépin D, Alili R, Kherchiche PP, Jeannic E, et al. Seven novel deleterious LEPR mutations found in early-onset obesity: a ΔExon6-8 shared by subjects from Reunion Island, France, suggests a founder effect. J Clin Endocrinol Metab. 2015;100(5):E757–66.
18. Montague CT, Farooqi IS, Whitehead JP, Soos MA, Rau H, Wareham NJ, et al. Congenital leptin deficiency is associated with severe early-onset obesity in humans. Nature. 1997;387(6636):903–8.
19. Clément K, Vaisse C, Lahlou N, Cabrol S, Pelloux V, Cassuto D, et al. A mutation in the human leptin receptor gene causes obesity and pituitary dysfunction. Nature. 1998;392(6674):398–401.
20. Besci Ö, Fırat SN, Özen S, Çetinkaya S, Akın L, Kör Y, et al. A national multicenter study of leptin and leptin receptor deficiency and systematic review. J Clin Endocrinol Metab. 2023;108(9):2371–88.
21. Heymsfield SB, Avena NM, Baier L, Brantley P, Bray GA, Burnett LC, et al. Hyperphagia: current concepts and future directions proceedings of the 2nd international conference on hyperphagia. Obesity (Silver Spring). 2014;22 Suppl 1(0 1):S1–S17.
22. Wabitsch M, Fehnel S, Mallya UG, Sluga-O'Callaghan M, Richardson D, Price M, Kühnen P. Understanding the patient experience of hunger and improved quality of life with setmelanotide treatment in POMC and LEPR deficiencies. Adv Ther. 2022;39(4):1772–83.
23. Abawi O, Wahab RJ, Kleinendorst L, Blankers LA, Brandsma AE, van Rossum EFC, et al. Genetic obesity disorders: body mass index trajectories and age of onset of obesity compared with children with obesity from the general population. J Pediatr. 2023;262:113619.
24. Farooqi IS, Matarese G, Lord GM, Keogh JM, Lawrence E, Agwu C, et al. Beneficial effects of leptin on obesity, T cell hyporesponsiveness, and neuroendocrine/metabolic dysfunction of human congenital leptin deficiency. J Clin Invest. 2002;110(8):1093–103.
25. Saeed S, Khanam R, Janjua QM, Manzoor J, Ning L, Hanook S, et al. High morbidity and mortality in children with untreated congenital deficiency of leptin or its receptor. Cell Rep Med. 2023;4(9):101187.
26. Paz-Filho G, Mastronardi CA, Licinio J. Leptin treatment: facts and expectations. Metabolism. 2015;64(1):146–56.

27. Abawi O, Koster EC, Welling MS, Boeters SCM, van Rossum EFC, van Haelst MM, et al. Resting energy expenditure and body composition in children and adolescents with genetic, hypothalamic, medication-induced or multifactorial severe obesity. Front Endocrinol (Lausanne). 2022;13:862817.
28. Galgani JE, Greenway FL, Caglayan S, Wong ML, Licinio J, Ravussin E. Leptin replacement prevents weight loss-induced metabolic adaptation in congenital leptin-deficient patients. J Clin Endocrinol Metab. 2010;95(2):851–5.
29. von Schnurbein J, Moss A, Nagel SA, Muehleder H, Debatin KM, Farooqi IS, Wabitsch M. Leptin substitution results in the induction of menstrual cycles in an adolescent with leptin deficiency and hypogonadotropic hypogonadism. Horm Res Paediatr. 2012;77(2):127–33.
30. Paz-Filho G, Mastronardi C, Delibasi T, Wong ML, Licinio J. Congenital leptin deficiency: diagnosis and effects of leptin replacement therapy. Arq Bras Endocrinol Metabol. 2010;54(8):690–7.
31. von Schnurbein J, Remy M, Brandt S, Manzoor J, Kohlsdorf K, Mahmood S, et al. Positive effect of leptin substitution on mood and behaviour in patients with congenital leptin deficiency. Pediatr Obes. 2023;18(8):e13057.
32. Hao Z, Münzberg H, Rezai-Zadeh K, Keenan M, Coulon D, Lu H, et al. Leptin deficient ob/ob mice and diet-induced obese mice responded differently to Roux-en-Y bypass surgery. Int J Obes. 2015;39(5):798–805.
33. Zhu L, Yang X, Li J, Jia X, Bai X, Zhao Y, et al. Leptin gene-targeted editing in ob/ob mouse adipose tissue based on the CRISPR/Cas9 system. J Genet Genomics. 2021;48(2):134–46.
34. Clément K, van den Akker E, Argente J, Bahm A, Chung WK, Connors H, et al. Efficacy and safety of setmelanotide, an MC4R agonist, in individuals with severe obesity due to LEPR or POMC deficiency: single-arm, open-label, multicentre, phase 3 trials. Lancet Diabetes Endocrinol. 2020;8(12):960–70.
35. Kanti V, Puder L, Jahnke I, Krabusch PM, Kottner J, Vogt A, et al. A melanocortin-4 receptor agonist induces skin and hair pigmentation in patients with monogenic mutations in the leptin-melanocortin pathway. Skin Pharmacol Physiol. 2021;34(6):307–16.
36. Welling MS, Kleinendorst L, van Haelst MM, van den Akker ELT. The narrative of a patient with leptin receptor deficiency: personalized medicine for a rare genetic obesity disorder. Obes Facts. 2023;16(5):514–8.
37. Brandt S, von Schnurbein J, Lennerz B, Kohlsdorf K, Vollbach H, Denzer C, et al. Methylphenidate in children with monogenic obesity due to LEPR or MC4R deficiency improves feeling of satiety and reduces BMI-SDS-A case series. Pediatr Obes. 2020;15(1):e12577.
38. Poitou C, Puder L, Dubern B, Krabusch P, Genser L, Wiegand S, et al. Long-term outcomes of bariatric surgery in patients with bi-allelic mutations in the POMC, LEPR, and MC4R genes. Surg Obes Relat Dis. 2021;17(8):1449–56.
39. Zorn S, von Schnurbein J, Kohlsdorf K, Denzer C, Wabitsch M. Diagnostic and therapeutic odyssey of two patients with compound heterozygous leptin receptor deficiency. Mol Cell Pediatr. 2020;7(1):15.
40. Morton GJ, Niswender KD, Rhodes CJ, Myers MG Jr, Blevins JE, Baskin DG, Schwartz MW. Arcuate nucleus-specific leptin receptor gene therapy attenuates the obesity phenotype of Koletsky (fa(k)/fa(k)) rats. Endocrinology. 2003;144(5):2016–24.

POMC Deficiency

Ozair Abawi and Lotte Kleinendorst

1 Introduction

Proopiomelanocortin (POMC) deficiency is a rare autosomal recessive disorder characterized by impaired processing of the POMC protein, which leads to dysfunctional production of various biologically active peptides involved in the hypothalamic leptin-melanocortin pathway. The main clinical features of the disorder are early-onset obesity, adrenal insufficiency, red hair (mostly apparent in white patients), and a lack of skin pigmentation.

In 1998, biallelic (homozygous or compound heterozygous) variants in the *POMC* gene were first identified in two unrelated patients who had severe obesity and adrenal dysfunction. Their distinct features included red hair and a pale skin color [1]. The inheritance pattern of POMC deficiency is autosomal recessive. We currently estimate the prevalence of POMC deficiency to be 1 in 1.9 million people, based on carrier frequency data from the Genome Aggregation Database (gnomAD) [2, 3]. The prevalence of this disorder is higher in consanguineous populations. Heterozygous loss-of-function variants in *POMC* lead to a slightly higher BMI [4].

O. Abawi (✉)
Division of Endocrinology, Department of Pediatrics, Erasmus MC-Sophia, University Medical Center Rotterdam, Rotterdam, The Netherlands

Obesity Center CGG, Erasmus MC, University Medical Center Rotterdam, Rotterdam, The Netherlands
e-mail: o.abawi@erasmusmc.nl

L. Kleinendorst
Department of Human Genetics, Section Clinical Genetics, Amsterdam University Medical Center, Amsterdam, The Netherlands

Emma Center for Personalized Medicine, Amsterdam UMC, University of Amsterdam, Amsterdam, The Netherlands
e-mail: l.kleinendorst@amsterdamumc.nl

M. van Haelst, E. van den Akker (eds.), *Clinical Obesity Genetics*,
https://doi.org/10.1007/978-3-032-04095-4_11

2 Aetiology and Pathophysiology

2.1 Leptin-Melanocortin Pathway

POMC is a key protein in the leptin-melanocortin pathway that is strongly expressed in the arcuate nucleus of the hypothalamus and pituitary gland [5]. It plays a crucial role in the regulation of several physiological processes, including metabolism and response to stress. The hypothalamic leptin-melanocortin pathway is the main regulator of homeostatic energy balance, satiety, and energy expenditure (see Chapter "Non-syndromic Leptin Melanocortin Pathway Disorders"). Leptin signalling through the leptin receptor leads to the production of POMC-expressing neurons. This leads to the production of POMC in the arcuate nucleus of the hypothalamus, which is subsequently cleaved into different hormones such as adrenocorticotropic hormone (ACTH), alpha-melanocyte-stimulating hormone (α-MSH), β-MSH, and γ-MSH [5]. These hormones are involved in several physiologic processes including skin pigmentation, adrenal cortisol production, and, through the MC4R receptor in the paraventricular nucleus of the hypothalamus, satiety and energy expenditure. Biallelic (homozygous or compound heterozygous) defects of the *POMC* gene disrupt the normal post-translational processing of POMC, impairing the formation of bioactive peptides such as ACTH, α-MSH, β-MSH, and γ-MSH, and subsequent downstream signalling. The deficiencies in the ligands and subsequent lack of activation of the melanocortin receptors lead to the different aspects of the phenotype. Lack of MC1R activation leads to the red hair pigmentation and pale skin. Lack of MC2R activation leads to the central adrenal insufficiency. Lack of activation of the MC4R leads to the hyperphagia and severe obesity phenotype.

2.2 Molecular Genetics

Complete POMC deficiency is caused by biallelic loss-of-function *POMC* variants. Several pathogenic variants in *POMC* have been described, including missense variants. Depending on the location of the variant in the *POMC* gene, different functions of the gene can be affected. For example, there were two sisters reported with a homozygous *POMC* variant who only showed obesity, hyperphagia and hypocortisolism, but no red hair of pale skin. Their specific *POMC* defect did not impair the activity of MC1R by β-MSH, leading to normal pigmentation [6].

A recent exome sequencing study showed that heterozygous carriers of *POMC* loss-of-function variants have a significantly higher BMI [7]. There is likely reduced penetrance and variable expressivity for patients who carry a heterozygous loss-of-function variant in POMC. Biallelic POMC deficiency shows complete penetrance.

3 Clinical Presentation

The first reported cases with molecularly confirmed POMC deficiency were published in 1998 [1]. Both patients presented with obesity, red hair pigmentation and pale skin, and ACTH deficiency. Interestingly, an earlier-born sibling of the first patient had died in infancy and was found to have adrenal insufficiency in the post-mortem examination [1]. This first report highlights the key clinical features of POMC deficiency and shows the importance of recognizing the disease, enabling timely glucocorticoid replacement therapy. The commonest presenting sign, in 72% of patients, is neonatal hypoglycemia with or without convulsions, prompting additional laboratory tests leading to the diagnosis of adrenal insufficiency [8]. The clinical presentation in the first years of life is often characterized by hyperphagia, severe obesity, and adrenal insufficiency due to the lack of melanocortin signalling. Hyperphagia is characterized by an extreme and insatiable increase in appetite, even when having consumed sufficient amounts of food [9], which negatively impacts quality of life [10]. The age of onset of obesity is usually within the first two years of life [11, 12]. Additional endocrine disturbances can be present, such as central hypothyroidism, hypogonadotropic hypogonadism, type 1 diabetes and growth hormone deficiency [8]. A pitfall can be that not all patients exhibit the typical pale skin and red hair. Depending on their ethnicity and exact genetic variant, about 55% of patients have red hair, 30% have reddish-brown hair and 25% have brown or dark hair [8]. The first two patients with POMC were reported to have a lower resting energy expenditure (REE) than predicted [1], but this has not subsequently been reported [13].

4 Differential Diagnosis

Other non-syndromic genetic obesity disorders, for example LEP and LEPR deficiency, should be considered when there is early-onset severe obesity. Furthermore, consider multifactorial or environmental obesity including use of obesogenic medication, polygenic obesity, syndromic obesity, overgrowth disorders, hypothalamic obesity, and endocrine obesity. For more details regarding the differential diagnosis, see the differential diagnosis paragraph in Chapter "Non-syndromic Leptin Melanocortin Pathway Disorders".

The most important key symptoms for the differential diagnosis of POMC deficiency are red hair or hypopigmentation and central adrenal insufficiency. A comprehensive overview of the differential diagnoses associated with these symptoms falls beyond the scope of this book. Non-exhaustive examples of important diagnoses to consider are given below.

4.1 Red Hair and Obesity

- Melanocortin-1 receptor: MC1R is one of the most important regulators of human skin and hair color. Red hair can be an indication of biallelic inherited POMC deficiency but can also coincidentally occur with obesity.
- Ectopic ASIP expression: In 2022, a novel genetic obesity disorder typically associated with red hair was published [14]. It is caused by a specific genetic rearrangement where the *ASIP* gene is placed under control of the promoter of the *ITCH* gene, which results in ectopic ASIP expression. This causes red hair because ASIP functions as an antagonist at MC1R in the skin and hair. As ASIP also works as an antagonist on MC4R, patients will develop hyperphagia and obesity.

4.2 Central Adrenal Insufficiency and Obesity

- PCSK1 deficiency: overlapping phenotype of obesity and adrenal failure [15]. See Chapter "PCSK1 deficiency" on the further clinical features of this disorder (severe diarrhoea in the first year of life, other endocrinopathies).
- *TBX19:* This gene is involved in the gene transcription of *POMC*. Patients with biallelic pathogenic variants in *TBX19* present with congenital isolated adreno-corticotropic hormone deficiency [16].
- As part of a multiple pituitary hormone deficiency. For example, *PROP1, HESX1* [17].

5 Molecular Diagnosis

POMC deficiency is caused by biallelic defects of the *POMC* gene. Both pathogenic truncating and missense variants are described. Over the years, there has been a debate about a potential dominant inheritance pattern, where it was thought that heterozygous pathogenic *POMC* variants could lead to obesity with hyperphagia. A recent study assessed this association in 190,000 exomes from the UK Biobank [4]. They found that these heterozygous pathogenic variants did not significantly elevate the risk of obesity, but that they did increase BMI. Therefore, heterozygous *POMC* variants could still be considered as a risk factor for obesity, but not as a typical genetic obesity disorder.

6 Therapy

In general, an individualized tailored treatment plan should be made for every patient with non-syndromic genetic obesity, including POMC deficiency, that is appropriate for age, culturally sensitive, and family-centered. Because of the pale skin, one could consider advising to be cautious with sun exposure.

The cornerstone obesity treatment is a combined lifestyle intervention (CLI) that focuses on physical activity and dietary advice as well as psychosocial and behavioral interventions. This however rarely suffices in POMC deficiency [18], and additional pharmacologic treatment, or in specific cases bariatric surgery might be needed. Setmelanotide, an MC4R agonist, is available as treatment for several leptin-melanocortin pathway deficiencies including POMC deficiency. This is currently administered through subcutaneous injections. In a phase 3 trial with 9 patients with POMC deficiency and 11 patients with LEPR deficiency, 1 year treatment with setmelanotide resulted in an average weight loss of −25.6%, which was more than double the effect size seen in the patients with LEPR deficiency. Moreover, improvements in satiety and hunger feelings and metabolic parameters were clearly seen [19]. The most important side effects are injection side reactions, gastrointestinal side effects, which usually resolve over time, and skin hyperpigmentation [19, 20]. During setmelanotide treatment, red hair and blue eye color can also change to brown [8]. Qualitative studies also show that treatment with setmelanotide improves quality of life in patients with POMC deficiency through reduction of the hyperphagia [10]. Neutralizing anti-drug antibodies have not yet been reported.

To our knowledge, no reports have been published on effects of GLP-1 agonist treatment, naltrexone/bupropione, phentermine, or central stimulants such as methylphenidate and dexamphetamine in patients with POMC deficiency. There have been incidental reports of bariatric surgery in homozygous POMC deficiency showing initial weight loss followed by substantial weight gain [21] and heterozygous *POMC* variants showing similar weight loss as patients without a heterozygous *POMC* variant [22]. It is not known whether the type of bariatric surgery can influence weight loss in patients with POMC deficiency. To our knowledge, no gene therapy possibilities restoring POMC function *in vivo* have yet been reported.

7 Follow-up Advices

Follow-up of POMC deficiency requires multidisciplinary long-term care. There is no uniform follow-up or screening recommendation.

Follow-up advices that could be considered are:

- Monitoring of height, weight, and puberty

- Monitoring of associated endocrine deficiencies and evaluation of treatment. People with POMC deficiency are generally treated with oral hydrocortisone or another glucocorticoid to treat adrenal insufficiency.
- Biochemical evaluation including endocrine evaluation for hormonal disturbances and screening for comorbidities (thyroid function, gonadal hormones, signs of hepatic steatosis, lipid profile, glucose levels, insulin sensitivity)
- Measurement of body composition and of resting energy expenditure to guide tailored dietary advice
- Cardiovascular assessment: according to severity of the obesity and presence of comorbidities.

8 Family Screening

Since POMC deficiency is associated with autosomal recessive inheritance, siblings of an affected child have 25% chance of being affected if both parents are moleculary confirmed carrier. After the genetic diagnosis of a child with *POMC* deficiency, prenatal diagnostics are available to assess whether the future child of the same parents is at risk for *POMC* deficiency. If the future child is affected, glucocorticoid therapy can be started shortly after birth.

9 Summary

- POMC deficiency is a rare genetic obesity disorder with an autosomal recessive inheritance pattern. It is caused by pathogenic biallelic (homozygous or compound heterozygous) *POMC* variants
- Key clinical characteristics are hyperphagia and early-onset obesity, hypopigmentation (leading to red hair or pale skin in around 50% of the cases), and adrenal insufficiency.
- Growth hormone deficiency and central hypothyroidism can also be part of the disorder.
- Heterozygous (monoallelic) carriers of pathogenic loss-of-function *POMC* variants are at risk to develop a higher BMI, but they do not have the other phenotypic features of POMC deficiency.
- Hyperphagia and obesity caused by biallelic POMC deficiency can be treated with MC4R agonist setmelanotide. Setmelanotide does not work for the adrenal insufficiency, therefore these patients should be treated with oral glucocorticoids.

References

1. Krude H, Biebermann H, Luck W, Horn R, Brabant G, Grüters A. Severe early-onset obesity, adrenal insufficiency and red hair pigmentation caused by POMC mutations in humans. Nat Genet. 1998;19(2):155–7.
2. Karczewski KJ, Francioli LC, Tiao G, Cummings BB, Alföldi J, Wang Q, et al. The mutational constraint spectrum quantified from variation in 141,456 humans. Nature. 2020;581(7809):434–43.
3. Baxter S, Grant R, Lee J, Watts N, Chan Zuckerberg Initiative Rare as One Network, O'Donnell-Luria A, Rehm H. GeniE, the Genetic Prevalence Estimator: Broad Institute; 2024 [updated 06/04/2024. Available from: https://genie.broadinstitute.org/.
4. Le Collen L, Delemer B, Poitou C, Vaxillaire M, Toussaint B, Dechaume A, et al. Heterozygous pathogenic variants in POMC are not responsible for monogenic obesity: implication for MC4R agonist use. Genet Med. 2023;25(7):100857.
5. Harno E, Gali Ramamoorthy T, Coll AP, White A. POMC: the physiological power of hormone processing. Physiol Rev. 2018;98(4):2381–430.
6. van der Valk ES, Kleinendorst L, Delhanty PJD, van der Voorn B, Visser JA, van Haelst MM, et al. Obesity and hyperphagia with increased defective ACTH: a novel POMC variant. J Clin Endocrinol Metab. 2022;107(9):e3699–e704.
7. Akbari P, Gilani A, Sosina O, Kosmicki JA, Khrimian L, Fang YY, et al. Sequencing of 640,000 exomes identifies GPR75 variants associated with protection from obesity. Science. 2021;373(6550)
8. Gregoric N, Groselj U, Bratina N, Debeljak M, Zerjav Tansek M, Suput Omladic J, et al. Two cases with an early presented proopiomelanocortin deficiency-a long-term follow-up and systematic literature review. Front Endocrinol (Lausanne). 2021;12:689387.
9. Heymsfield SB, Avena NM, Baier L, Brantley P, Bray GA, Burnett LC, et al. Hyperphagia: current concepts and future directions proceedings of the 2nd international conference on hyperphagia. Obesity (Silver Spring). 2014;22(Suppl 1):S1–S17.
10. Wabitsch M, Fehnel S, Mallya UG, Sluga-O'Callaghan M, Richardson D, Price M, Kühnen P. Understanding the patient experience of hunger and improved quality of life with setmelanotide treatment in POMC and LEPR deficiencies. Adv Ther. 2022;39(4):1772–83.
11. Abawi O, Wahab RJ, Kleinendorst L, Blankers LA, Brandsma AE, van Rossum EFC, et al. Genetic obesity disorders: body mass index trajectories and age of onset of obesity compared with children with obesity from the general population. J Pediatr. 2023;262:113619.
12. Besci Ö, Fırat SN, Özen S, Çetinkaya S, Akın L, Kör Y, et al. A National Multicenter Study of leptin and leptin receptor deficiency and systematic review. J Clin Endocrinol Metab. 2023;108(9):2371–88.
13. Abawi O, Koster EC, Welling MS, Boeters SCM, van Rossum EFC, van Haelst MM, et al. Resting energy expenditure and body composition in children and adolescents with genetic, hypothalamic, medication-induced or multifactorial severe obesity. Front Endocrinol (Lausanne). 2022;13:862817.
14. Kempf E, Landgraf K, Stein R, Hanschkow M, Hilbert A, Abou Jamra R, et al. Aberrant expression of agouti signaling protein (ASIP) as a cause of monogenic severe childhood obesity. Nat Metab. 2022;4(12):1697–712.
15. Pépin L, Colin E, Tessarech M, Rouleau S, Bouhours-Nouet N, Bonneau D, Coutant R. A new case of PCSK1 pathogenic variant with congenital proprotein convertase 1/3 deficiency and literature review. J Clin Endocrinol Metab. 2019;104(4):985–93.
16. Kardelen Al AD, Poyrazoğlu Ş, Aslanger A, Yeşil G, Ceylaner S, Baş F, Darendeliler F. A rare cause of adrenal insufficiency—isolated ACTH deficiency due to TBX19 mutation: long-term follow-up of two cases and review of the literature. Horm Res Paediatr. 2019;92(6):395–403.
17. Avbelj Stefanija M, Kotnik P, Bratanič N, Žerjav Tanšek M, Bertok S, Bratina N, et al. Novel mutations in HESX1 and PROP1 genes in combined pituitary hormone deficiency. Horm Res Paediatr. 2015;84(3):153–8.

18. Wabitsch M, Farooqi S, Flück CE, Bratina N, Mallya UG, Stewart M, et al. Natural history of obesity due to POMC, PCSK1, and LEPR deficiency and the impact of setmelanotide. J Endocr Soc. 2022;6(6):bvac057.
19. Clément K, van den Akker E, Argente J, Bahm A, Chung WK, Connors H, et al. Efficacy and safety of setmelanotide, an MC4R agonist, in individuals with severe obesity due to LEPR or POMC deficiency: single-arm, open-label, multicentre, phase 3 trials. Lancet Diabetes Endocrinol. 2020;8(12):960–70.
20. Kanti V, Puder L, Jahnke I, Krabusch PM, Kottner J, Vogt A, et al. A melanocortin-4 receptor agonist induces skin and hair pigmentation in patients with monogenic mutations in the leptin-melanocortin pathway. Skin Pharmacol Physiol. 2021;34(6):307–16.
21. Poitou C, Puder L, Dubern B, Krabusch P, Genser L, Wiegand S, et al. Long-term outcomes of bariatric surgery in patients with bi-allelic mutations in the POMC, LEPR, and MC4R genes. Surg Obes Relat Dis. 2021;17(8):1449–56.
22. Cooiman MI, Kleinendorst L, Aarts EO, Janssen IMC, van Amstel HKP, Blakemore AI, et al. Genetic obesity and bariatric surgery outcome in 1014 patients with morbid obesity. Obes Surg. 2020;30(2):470–7.

MC4R Deficiency

Ozair Abawi and Lotte Kleinendorst

1 Introduction

Melanocortin-4 receptor deficiency (MC4R deficiency) is the most common genetic disease that influences appetite regulation and energy balance [1]. The clinical phenotype of MC4R deficiency can be seen as a spectrum, from moderate obesity to severe early-onset forms with hyperphagia, often accompanied by metabolic disturbances and increased linear growth (Fig. 1). The *MC4R* gene codes for a G-protein coupled receptor that is a key element of the hypothalamic leptin-melanocortin pathway, which regulates satiety and energy expenditure [2]. MC4R deficiency can be inherited through both recessive and dominant patterns, with the recessive form representing the severe side of the spectrum. There are typically no other endocrinopathies associated with MC4R deficiency, in contrast to LEP, LEPR or POMC deficiency. The disorder was first described in 1998 as the earliest known genetic form of obesity with autosomal dominant inheritance [3]. Currently, there are large patient cohorts described and the prevalence in the general population is estimated at around 1 in 500–2000. In cohorts of adults with obesity, the prevalence of MC4R

O. Abawi (✉)
Division of Endocrinology, Department of Pediatrics, Erasmus MC-Sophia, University Medical Center Rotterdam, Rotterdam, The Netherlands

Obesity Center CGG, Erasmus MC, University Medical Center Rotterdam, Rotterdam, The Netherlands
e-mail: o.abawi@erasmusmc.nl

L. Kleinendorst
Department of Human Genetics, Section Clinical Genetics, Amsterdam UMC location University of Amsterdam, Amsterdam, The Netherlands

Emma Center for Personalized Medicine, Amsterdam UMC, University of Amsterdam, Amsterdam, The Netherlands
e-mail: l.kleinendorst@amsterdamumc.nl

M. van Haelst, E. van den Akker (eds.), *Clinical Obesity Genetics*,
https://doi.org/10.1007/978-3-032-04095-4_12

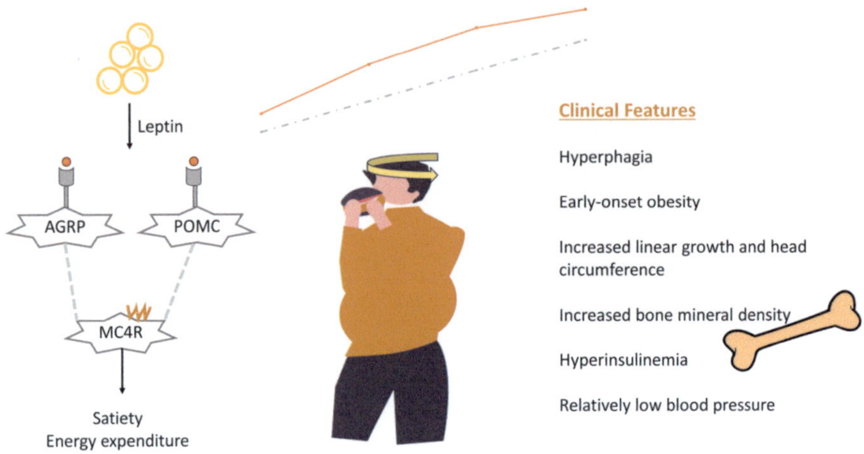

Fig. 1 Graphical abstract of the molecular mechanisms and clinical features of MC4R deficiency. (Credit: Figure made by Lotte Kleinendorst and Ozair Abawi)

deficiency has been estimated at around 1% [4, 5]. In our Dutch center of expertise for genetic obesity, in the pediatric cohort, we found a prevalence of 3.2% [6]. A Spanish early-onset obesity cohort showed a prevalence of 1.5% [7].

2 Aetiology and Pathophysiology

2.1 Leptin-Melanocortin Pathway

The hypothalamic leptin-melanocortin pathway is the main regulator of homeostatic energy balance, satiety and energy expenditure (see Chapter "Non-syndromic Leptin Melanocortin Pathway Disorders"). It receives peripheral afferent input from various organs as well as other brain areas. The adipose tissue is involved in long-term signalling of satiety and energy expenditure by producing the hormone leptin, the most important indicator of the body's reserve energy stores [8]. Hypothalamic leptin signalling leads to the production of POMC, a prohormone that is cleaved into different hormones, including α-melanocyte stimulating hormone (MSH). This α-MSH subsequently activates the MC4R, which through various downstream signalling pathways ultimately leads to increased satiety and energy expenditure [2, 9]. Stimulation of the MC4R expressed on sympathetic preganglionic cholinergic neurons also leads to increased sympathetic tone, which mediates its effects on heart rate, blood pressure and glucose homeostasis [9]. Furthermore, MC4R signalling influences gastric emptying [10].

2.2 Molecular Genetics

The *MC4R* gene encodes for the MC4R receptor. Variants with complete loss-of-function (for example caused by a frameshift) and missense variants have been described as pathogenic. The website www.mc4r.org.uk shows an overview of the current data about the pathogenicity of the rare variants and the specific cellular mechanisms that are affected by the variant [5]. The MC4R signal is mainly conveyed through activation of the Gsα protein, however, recent studies show evidence for biased signalling through other intracellular pathways, e.g. intracellular calcium signalling, receptor trafficking and β-arrestin recruitment [11, 12]. The variants do not appear to cluster at a specific locus in the gene. There are also gain-of-function variants described in the *MC4R* gene. Interestingly, these gain-of-function variants are associated with a lower BMI and less obesity in the UK biobank cohort [13].

2.3 Common Variants

Besides rare *MC4R* variants, large genome-wide association studies (GWAS) have identified several common single nucleotide polymorphisms (SNPs) near the *MC4R* gene that are associated with increased BMI and fat mass [14]. These SNPs are highly prevalent in the general population and they have only a small impact on obesity risk, unlike rare *MC4R* mutations that can cause severe obesity.

2.4 Variable Expressivity and Reduced Penetrance

The severity of obesity caused by rare *MC4R* mutations can vary greatly due to different genetic and environmental factors. It is known that polygenic susceptibility influences the impact of pathogenic *MC4R* variants on BMI [15]. In some families, these influences can also decrease the impact of the mutation. This means that not everyone with the *MC4R* variant will have the same degree of obesity, and in some cases, they might not develop obesity at all. These phenomena are called variable expressivity and reduced penetrance, where variable expressivity refers to variability of the phenotypic features, and reduced penetrance refers to individuals who have the genetic defect but do not show the phenotype.

3 Clinical Presentation

The key clinical features of MC4R deficiency are hyperphagia and early-onset obesity [11, 16]. Hyperphagia is characterized by an extreme and insatiable increase in appetite, even when having consumed sufficient amounts of food [17]. The age of onset of obesity can be variable but is typically before the age of 4–5 years [18]. Patients with biallelic MC4R deficiency have a more severe phenotype with typically more hyperphagia and an earlier age of onset of obesity, often before the age of 2 years [18]. In a UK birth cohort, the mean difference in anthropometrics between carriers and non-carriers of MC4R LoF variants increased throughout childhood [19]. The largest difference was seen at age 18 years, where carriers of MC4R LoF variants weighed on average 17.8 kg more (BMI +4.8 kg/m^2).

Other features of MC4R deficiency include increased linear growth and head circumference, hyperinsulinemia disproportionate to the severity of the obesity, and increased bone mineral density and bone mineral content [11, 20]. The largest difference in height between carriers of MC4R LoF variants and non-carriers is found at age 12 years (on average + 6.5 cm) [19]. Furthermore, carriers of *MC4R* variants have relatively lower blood pressure compared to controls with obesity [21]. Although decreased resting energy expenditure in MC4R deficiency has been reported in individual cases, it is not present more often than in control patients with obesity [22].

3.1 Clinical Evaluation

A comprehensive clinical evaluation is warranted in all cases with suspected or established MC4R deficiency. This includes:

- Detailed medical history: focusing on eating behaviors, signs of hyperphagia, age of onset of obesity, periods of rapid weight gain, and other associated health issues. A three-generation family history documenting consanguinity, instances of (early-onset) obesity, increased linear growth and head circumference and related metabolic disorders, e.g. diabetes, hypertension, dyslipidemia, and cardiovascular diseases, should be obtained. Comprehensive growth charts analysis can further increase the suspicion of MC4R deficiency [18].
- Physical examination: measurement of height (or recumbent length in infants), weight, and head circumference, blood pressure and heart rate. Furthermore, physical signs of insulin resistance (acanthosis nigricans) should be evaluated. When available, measurement of body composition and energy expenditure can aid in patient-tailored treatment advices.
- Measurement of parental height, weight, and head circumference.
- Biochemical evaluation: assessment of fasting glucose and insulin, lipid profile, liver enzymes, thyroid function and vitamin D levels is warranted in all patients.

4 Differential Diagnosis

Other non-syndromic genetic obesity disorders such as LEPR deficiency should be considered when there is a suspicion of MC4R deficiency. Furthermore, consider multifactorial or environmental obesity including use of obesogenic medication, polygenic obesity, syndromic obesity, overgrowth disorders, hypothalamic obesity, and endocrine obesity. For more details regarding the differential diagnosis, see the differential diagnosis paragraph in Chapter "Non-syndromic Leptin Melanocortin Pathway Disorders".

5 Molecular Diagnosis

Sanger sequencing for *MC4R* is a relatively easy and affordable test to identify pathogenic variants in *MC4R*. Because of the genetic heterogeneity of genetic obesity disorders, using a larger obesity gene panel might be a more effective strategy. For more information on the genetic testing, see Chapter "Non-syndromic Leptin Melanocortin Pathway Disorders".

6 Therapy

In general, an individualized tailored treatment plan should be made for every patient with non-syndromic genetic obesity, including MC4R deficiency, that is appropriate for age, culturally sensitive, and family-centered. The cornerstone treatment is a combined lifestyle intervention (CLI) that focuses on physical activity and dietary advice as well as psychosocial and behavioral interventions. This however rarely suffices in MC4R deficiency [23], and additional pharmacologic treatment and/or in specific cases bariatric surgery might be needed. Several case series show short-term positive results of GLP-1 agonist treatment in adults with heterozygous MC4R deficiency [23–25], with an average weight loss of −5% (ranging from −2% to −13%) after 4 months of treatment [25]. For children with MC4R deficiency, only case reports are published to date, with one reporting −11% weight loss after one year of treatment with semaglutide in heterozygous MC4R deficiency [26], and one reporting stabilisation of BMI percentile after 1 year of treatment with liraglutide in homozygous MC4R deficiency [27].

Other treatment options include naltrexone-buproprione and phentermine in adults with heterozygous MC4R deficiency showing modest weight loss [25, 28, 29] and methylphenidate in children with MC4R deficiency showing improved BMI trajectories and decreased appetite [30]. Treatment with setmelanotide, an MC4R agonist (currently approved for treatment of biallelic POMC, PCSK1 and LEPR deficiency) led to a slight reduction of body weight (−2.6% over placebo) in a small phase 1 trial of adults with heterozygous MC4R deficiency, but it is not established as a treatment option as of yet [31]. Bariatric surgery in MC4R deficiency is efficacious in the short term, but more variable in the long term [32, 33]. Furthermore, the type of bariatric surgery can influence weight loss in patients with MC4R deficiency, with Roux-en-Y gastric bypass showing larger effects than sleeve gastrectomy [34]. Mean total body weight loss after 2 years was 33.7% for MC4R heterozygotes who underwent Roux-en-Y gastric bypass; for the sleeve gastrectomy in MC4R heterozygotes total body weight loss after 2 years was 21.5% [34]. Targeted gene therapy using CRISPR has already been shown to revert the obesity phenotype in heterozygous Mc4r deficient mice and might become available as future treatment option [35].

7 Follow-up Advices

There is no uniform follow-up plan for all patients with MC4R deficiency, but management often requires multidisciplinary, long-term care. Some follow-up recommendations that could be considered are:

- Repeat visits to monitor adherence to healthy lifestyle
- Monitoring of height, weight, head circumference, and puberty
- Biochemical evaluation including endocrine evaluation for hormonal disturbances (e.g. thyroid function, hypogonadism) and screening for comorbidities (signs of hepatic steatosis, lipid profile, glucose levels, insulin sensitivity)
- Measurement of body composition and of resting energy expenditure to guide tailored dietary advice
- Cardiovascular assessment: according to severity of the obesity and presence of comorbidities

8 Family Screening

MC4R deficiency is associated with both dominant and recessive inheritance of obesity. Siblings can be tested when they have an obesity phenotype. Because of the known variable expressivity and reduced penetrance of the disorder, it is possible that family members with the genetic defect have a different phenotype than the index patient.

9 Summary

Melanocortin-4 receptor deficiency (MC4R deficiency) is the most common genetic obesity disorder that influences appetite regulation and energy balance, with an estimated prevalence of around 1% of people with obesity. The inheritance pattern can be autosomal dominant or autosomal recessive. The main clinical features are hyperphagia and early-onset obesity. Patients can also have increased linear growth and a large head circumference. Treatment options include GLP-1 receptor agonists, naltrexone-buproprione, phentermine, methylphenidate, and tailored advices regarding bariatric surgery types and outcomes.

References

1. Farooqi IS, O'Rahilly S. The genetics of obesity in humans. 2000.
2. Krashes MJ, Lowell BB, Garfield AS. Melanocortin-4 receptor-regulated energy homeostasis. Nat Neurosci. 2016;19(2):206–19.
3. Yeo GS, Farooqi IS, Aminian S, Halsall DJ, Stanhope RG, O'Rahilly S. A frameshift mutation in MC4R associated with dominantly inherited human obesity. Nat Genet. 1998;20(2):111–2.
4. Orphanet. Obesity due to melanocortin 4 receptor deficiency: Orphanet; 2024 [updated 10–14]. Available from: https://www.orpha.net/en/disease/detail/71529
5. University of Cambridge Metabolic Research Laboratories. MC4R Gene: MC4R Ltd; 2024. Available from: https://www.mc4r.org.uk/
6. Kleinendorst L, Abawi O, van der Voorn B, Jongejan M, Brandsma AE, Visser JA, et al. Identifying underlying medical causes of pediatric obesity: results of a systematic diagnostic approach in a pediatric obesity center. PLoS One. 2020;15(5):e0232990.
7. Serra-Juhé C, Martos-Moreno G, Bou de Pieri F, Flores R, Chowen JA, Pérez-Jurado LA, Argente J. Heterozygous rare genetic variants in non-syndromic early-onset obesity. Int J Obes. 2020;44(4):830–41.
8. Pan WW, Myers MG Jr. Leptin and the maintenance of elevated body weight. Nat Rev Neurosci. 2018;19(2):95–105.
9. Yeo GSH, Chao DHM, Siegert AM, Koerperich ZM, Ericson MD, Simonds SE, et al. The melanocortin pathway and energy homeostasis: from discovery to obesity therapy. Mol Metab. 2021;48:101206.
10. Seelig E, Henning E, Keogh JM, Gillett D, Shin E, Buscombe J, et al. Obesity due to melanocortin 4 receptor (MC4R) deficiency is associated with delayed gastric emptying. Clin Endocrinol. 2022;96(2):270–5.
11. Kühnen P, Krude H, Biebermann H. Melanocortin-4 receptor signalling: importance for weight regulation and obesity treatment. Trends Mol Med. 2019;25(2):136–48.
12. Ju SH, Cho GB, Sohn JW. Understanding melanocortin-4 receptor control of neuronal circuits: toward novel therapeutics for obesity syndrome. Pharmacol Res. 2018;129:10–9.
13. Lotta LA, Mokrosiński J, Mendes de Oliveira E, Li C, Sharp SJ, Luan J, et al. Human gain-of-function MC4R variants show signaling bias and protect against obesity. Cell. 2019;177(3):597–607 e9.
14. Loos RJ, Lindgren CM, Li S, Wheeler E, Zhao JH, Prokopenko I, et al. Common variants near MC4R are associated with fat mass, weight and risk of obesity. Nat Genet. 2008;40(6):768–75.
15. Chami N, Preuss M, Walker RW, Moscati A, Loos RJF. The role of polygenic susceptibility to obesity among carriers of pathogenic mutations in MC4R in the UK biobank population. PLoS Med. 2020;17(7):e1003196.

16. Farooqi IS, Keogh JM, Yeo GS, Lank EJ, Cheetham T, O'Rahilly S. Clinical spectrum of obesity and mutations in the melanocortin 4 receptor gene. N Engl J Med. 2003;348(12):1085–95.
17. Heymsfield SB, Avena NM, Baier L, Brantley P, Bray GA, Burnett LC, et al. Hyperphagia: current concepts and future directions proceedings of the 2nd international conference on hyperphagia. Obesity (Silver Spring). 2014;22(Suppl 1):S1–S17.
18. Abawi O, Wahab RJ, Kleinendorst L, Blankers LA, Brandsma AE, van Rossum EFC, et al. Genetic obesity disorders: body mass index trajectories and age of onset of obesity compared with children with obesity from the general population. J Pediatr. 2023;262:113619.
19. Wade KH, Lam BYH, Melvin A, Pan W, Corbin LJ, Hughes DA, et al. Loss-of-function mutations in the melanocortin 4 receptor in a UK birth cohort. Nat Med. 2021;27(6):1088–96.
20. Martinelli CE, Keogh JM, Greenfield JR, Henning E, van der Klaauw AA, Blackwood A, et al. Obesity due to melanocortin 4 receptor (MC4R) deficiency is associated with increased linear growth and final height, fasting hyperinsulinemia, and incompletely suppressed growth hormone secretion. J Clin Endocrinol Metab. 2011;96(1):E181–8.
21. Greenfield JR, Miller JW, Keogh JM, Henning E, Satterwhite JH, Cameron GS, et al. Modulation of blood pressure by central melanocortinergic pathways. N Engl J Med. 2009;360(1):44–52.
22. Abawi O, Koster EC, Welling MS, Boeters SCM, van Rossum EFC, van Haelst MM, et al. Resting energy expenditure and body composition in children and adolescents with genetic, hypothalamic, medication-induced or multifactorial severe obesity. Front Endocrinol (Lausanne). 2022;13:862817.
23. Iepsen EW, Zhang J, Thomsen HS, Hansen EL, Hollensted M, Madsbad S, et al. Patients with obesity caused by melanocortin-4 receptor mutations can be treated with a glucagon-like peptide-1 receptor agonist. Cell Metab. 2018;28(1):23–32 e3.
24. Iepsen EW, Have CT, Veedfald S, Madsbad S, Holst JJ, Grarup N, et al. GLP-1 receptor agonist treatment in morbid obesity and type 2 diabetes due to pathogenic homozygous melanocortin-4 receptor mutation: a case report. Cell Rep Med. 2020;1(1):100006.
25. Welling MS, de Groot CJ, Mohseni M, Meeusen REH, Boon MR, van Haelst MM, et al. Treatment with liraglutide or naltrexone-bupropion in patients with genetic obesity: a real-world study. EClinicalMedicine. 2024;74:102709.
26. Gokul PR, Apperley L, Parkinson J, Clark K, Lund K, Owens M, Senniappan S. Semaglutide, a long-acting GLP-1 analogue, for the management of early onset obesity due to MC4R defect—a case report. Horm Res Paediatr. 2024;
27. Zaitoon H, Lubetzky R, Amir AZ, Moran-Lev H, Sagi L, Yacobi-Bach M, et al. Glucagon-like peptide-1 analog therapy in rare genetic diseases: monogenic obesity, monogenic diabetes, and spinal muscular atrophy. Acta Diabetol. 2023;60(8):1099–108.
28. Welling MS, Mohseni M, van der Valk ES, van Hagen JM, Burgerhart JS, van Haelst MM, van Rossum EFC. Successful naltrexone-bupropion treatment after several treatment failures in a patient with severe monogenic obesity. iScience. 2023;26(3):106199.
29. Salazar-Valencia IG, Villamil-Ramírez H, Barajas-Olmos F, Guevara-Cruz M, Macias-Kauffer LR, García-Ortiz H, et al. Effect of the melanocortin 4-receptor Ile269Asn mutation on weight loss response to dietary, phentermine and Bariatric Surgery Interventions. Genes (Basel). 2022;13(12)
30. Brandt S, von Schnurbein J, Lennerz B, Kohlsdorf K, Vollbach H, Denzer C, et al. Methylphenidate in children with monogenic obesity due to LEPR or MC4R deficiency improves feeling of satiety and reduces BMI-SDS-A case series. Pediatr Obes. 2020;15(1):e12577.
31. Collet TH, Dubern B, Mokrosinski J, Connors H, Keogh JM, Mendes de Oliveira E, et al. Evaluation of a melanocortin-4 receptor (MC4R) agonist (Setmelanotide) in MC4R deficiency. Mol Metab. 2017;6(10):1321–9.
32. Fojas EGF, Radha SK, Ali T, Nadler EP, Lessan N. Weight and glycemic control outcomes of bariatric surgery and pharmacotherapy in patients with melanocortin-4 receptor deficiency. Front Endocrinol (Lausanne). 2021;12:792354.

33. Poitou C, Puder L, Dubern B, Krabusch P, Genser L, Wiegand S, et al. Long-term outcomes of bariatric surgery in patients with bi-allelic mutations in the POMC, LEPR, and MC4R genes. Surg Obes Relat Dis. 2021;17(8):1449–56.
34. Cooiman MI, Alsters SIM, Duquesnoy M, Hazebroek EJ, Meijers-Heijboer HJ, Chahal H, et al. Long-term weight outcome after bariatric surgery in patients with melanocortin-4 receptor gene variants: a case-control study of 105 patients. Obes Surg. 2022;32(3):837–44.
35. Matharu N, Rattanasopha S, Tamura S, Maliskova L, Wang Y, Bernard A, et al. CRISPR-mediated activation of a promoter or enhancer rescues obesity caused by haploinsufficiency. Science. 2019;363(6424)

PCSK1 Deficiency

Lotte Kleinendorst and Ozair Abawi

1 Introduction

Proprotein convertase subtilisin/kexin type 1 (PCSK1) deficiency is a very rare genetic disorder that affects the function of the enzyme proprotein convertase 1 (also known as prohormone convertase 3 or PC1/3). This hormone is critical for the processing of various precursor proteins, including prohormones and neuropeptides in the hypothalamic leptin-melanocortin pathway [1]. Because of the diverse roles of PCSK1, the patients do not only have hyperphagia and severe obesity, but also suffer from severe gastrointestinal problems in childhood and diverse complete or partial hormonal deficiencies including growth hormone deficiency, hypocortisolism, hypothyroidism, arginine vasopressine (AVP) deficiency, low levels of sex hormones or diabetes mellitus [1, 2].

The first patient diagnosed with PCSK1 deficiency was published in 1997 [3]. She had compound heterozygous pathogenic variants in *PCSK1*, which led to a phenotype of severe early-onset obesity and impaired glucose tolerance with postprandial hypoglycemia. She also had adrenal insufficiency and hypogonadotropic

L. Kleinendorst (✉)
Department of Human Genetics, Section Clinical Genetics, Amsterdam University Medical Center, Amsterdam, The Netherlands

Emma Center for Personalized Medicine, Amsterdam University Medical Center, Amsterdam, The Netherlands
e-mail: L.kleinendorst@amsterdamumc.nl

O. Abawi
Division of Endocrinology, Department of Pediatrics, Erasmus MC-Sophia, University Medical Center Rotterdam, Rotterdam, The Netherlands

Obesity Center CGG, Erasmus MC, University Medical Center Rotterdam, Rotterdam, The Netherlands
e-mail: o.abawi@erasmusmc.nl

M. van Haelst, E. van den Akker (eds.), *Clinical Obesity Genetics*,
https://doi.org/10.1007/978-3-032-04095-4_13

hypogonadism. After the publication of three more cases, which had a phenotype of severe intestinal malabsorption, the medical history of the first published case was reviewed and it was found that she had also suffered from frequent diarrhea in the first decade of her life [1].

PCSK1 deficiency is an autosomal recessive disorder. Many of the currently described patients are from highly consanguineous populations. There is a suggestion of a higher prevalence in males versus females, but it is unclear what causes this difference [4]. Carriership of a single loss-of-function variant (monoallelic/heterozygous) in *PCSK1* could also lead to an increased risk of obesity [5]. We currently estimate the prevalence of PCSK1 deficiency to be 1 in 3.8 million, based on carrier frequency data from the Genome Aggregation Database (gnomAD) [6, 7].

2 Aetiology and Pathophysiology

2.1 Leptin-Melanocortin Pathway

PCSK1 is an enzyme involved in the proteolytic cleavage and activation of various precursor molecules, in particular proopiomelanocortin (POMC) and proinsulin (Fig. 1). These precursor molecules are crucial for the production of various hormones, neuropeptides, and other bioactive substances. In the leptin-melanocortin pathway, it is particularly important in the conversion of pro-opiomelanocortin (POMC), after stimulation of POMC-neurons by leptin signaling, into ACTH, alpha-melanocyte-stimulating hormone (α-MSH), β-MSH, and γ-MSH [8]. Alpha-MSH is a key agonist for the melanocortin 4 receptor (MC4R) involved in regulating appetite and energy expenditure. Deficiencies in PCSK1 can lead to impaired cleavage of POMC, resulting in reduced levels of α-MSH and, consequently, decreased MC4R activation. This subsequently leads to hyperphagia and early-onset obesity [1, 8].

The *PCSK1* gene is also expressed broadly in other areas of the hypothalamus such as the supraoptic nucleus (SON) and peripheral tissues such as the adrenal medulla, pituitary gland, thyroid gland, endocrine pancreas and small intestine [1], where it is involved in many metabolic processes beyond the leptin-melanocortin pathway. Therefore, PCSK1 deficiency leads to a broad phenotype characterized by endocrine deficiencies and gastro-intestinal symptoms, such as severe neonatal diarrhea. In the hypothalamus, PCSK1 deficiency leads to impaired cleavage of pro-TRH (thyrotropin-releasing hormone) into TRH, leading to central hypothyroidism [1, 12]. In the SON, PCSK1 deficiency leads to aberrant processing of provasopressin, resulting in AVP deficiency (formerly known as central diabetes insipidus) [1]. In the pituitary gland, reduced production of pro-ACTH and ACTH from POMC lead to a phenotype of central adrenal insufficiency [1, 9]. Moreover, impaired activation of pro-GnRH (gonadotropin-releasing hormone) and kisspeptin can ultimately cause hypogonadotropic hypogonadism [1, 10]. Moreover, PCSK1 is needed

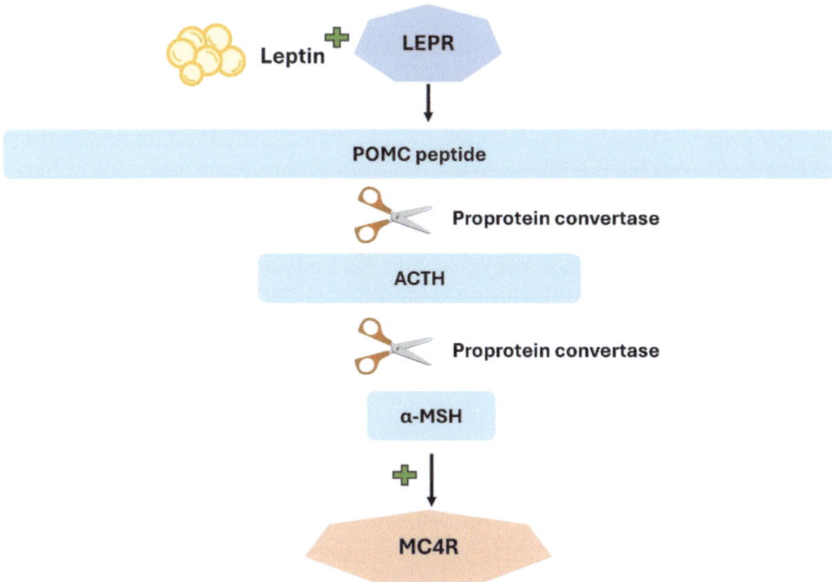

Fig. 1 Simplified overview of prohormone processing by proprotein convertase 1, the enzyme for which the PCSK1 gene encodes. As an example, the processing of POMC to alpha-MSH is shown via the cleavage of POMC into (among others) ACTH. Similar processing is performed by PCSK1 to produce other hormones, e.g. insulin from pro-insulin (see full text for details). Abbreviations: *LEPR* leptin receptor, *POMC* proopiomelanocortin, *PCSK1* proprotein convertase subtilisin/kexin type 1, *ACTH* adrenocorticotropic hormone, *α-MSH* alpha-melanocyte stimulating hormone, *MC4R* melanocortin-4-receptor

for the processing of pro-growth hormone releasing hormone (GHRH) to GHRH, and PCSK1 deficiency can lead to growth hormone deficiency [1, 11]. In the endocrine pancreas, reduced cleavage of proinsulin into insulin causes abnormal glucose metabolism characterized by hyperglycemia followed by reactive hypoglycemia hours after meals and ultimately diabetes mellitus [1, 13, 14]. In the small intestine, defective processing of several gut hormones and gut peptides involved in digestion, especially in the enteroendocrine cells, results in intestinal malabsorption and severe congenital diarrhea [1, 4].

2.2 *Molecular Genetics*

Complete PCSK1 deficiency is caused by biallelic (homozygous or compound heterozygous) loss-of-function *PCSK1* variants. Several pathogenic variants in *PCSK1* have been described, including missense variants. There appears to be no clear genotype-phenotype correlation [15]. Heterozygous carriers of a complete loss-of-function *PCSK1* variants have an increased risk of developing obesity [5]. Rare heterozygous variants in *PCSK1* that lead to complete loss-of-function (e.g. nonsense or missense variants that show complete loss of function *in vitro)* are associated with obesity (odds ratio of having obesity 9.3 compared to non-carriers) and higher BMI (on average + 4.7 kg/m^2), whereas missense variants with residual activity *in vitro* did not show a clear association with obesity [5]. Common variants in *PCSK1* are associated with increased BMI and slightly increased odds of having obesity, and with increased circulating proinsulin levels and alterations in glucose homeostasis [1, 16].

There is one case report of a child with PCSK1 deficiency caused by a maternal uniparental isodisomy (UPD) with a homozygous pathogenic variant in the *PCSK1* gene [17].

3 Clinical Presentation

The clinical manifestations of PCSK1 deficiency can vary greatly between patients. The patients generally are born at full term with a normal birth weight, but typically present in the neonatal period or shortly thereafter with early-onset severe malabsorptive diarrhea and/or severe hypoglycemia [1]. The gastrointestinal symptoms can last for several months, and prolonged hospital admission is often needed [1]. Over 90% of the patients need parenteral nutrition in early childhood [2]. Early-onset obesity and hyperphagia are reported in 79% of the published cases [2].

To our knowledge, 30 patients, with complete PCSK1 deficiency have been described in literature. The most recent overview of the clinical phenotypes was published in 2021 by Duclaux-Loras et al., which included data on 28 patients [2]. The clinical features are shown in Table 1 sorted by frequency.

Table 1 Clinical features of PCSK1 deficiency and their frequency in cases reported in literature

Feature	Frequency in reported cases [2]
Diarrhea	96%
Receiving parenteral nutrition	92%
Polyuria-polydipsia	86%
Early-onset obesity	79%
AVP deficiency (central diabetes insipidus)	61%
Hypocortisolism	57%
Hypothyroidism	56%
Growth hormone deficiency	44%
Hypogonadism	44%

4 Differential Diagnosis

Other non-syndromic genetic obesity disorders, for example LEP and LEPR deficiency, should be considered when there is early-onset severe obesity. Furthermore, consider multifactorial obesity including use of obesogenic medication, polygenic obesity, syndromic obesity, overgrowth, hypothalamic obesity, and endocrine obesity. For more details regarding the differential diagnosis, see the differential diagnosis paragraph in Chapter "Non-syndromic Leptin Melanocortin Pathway Disorders".

The most important key symptoms for the differential diagnosis of PCSK1 deficiency are neonatal diarrhea and the various hormonal deficiencies. A comprehensive overview of the differential diagnoses associated with these symptoms falls beyond the scope of this book. Non-exhaustive examples of important diagnoses to consider are given below.

4.1 Neonatal or Congenital Diarrhea

For the neonatal phase with malabsorptive diarrhea, other genes that are involved in the enteroendocrine development should be considered. For example, *NEUROG3* and *PERCC1* [18].

4.2 Endocrinopathies

The diverse endocrinopathies that can be seen in PCSK1 deficiency all have their own differential diagnoses. However, the combination with congenital diarrhea and early-onset obesity makes many of these diagnoses less likely. Some diagnosis to consider are:

- LEP and LEPR deficiency: Patients with leptin or leptin receptor deficiency can also have hypogonadism, growth hormone deficiency, and hypothyroidism. Adrenal insufficiency, however, is not seen in LEP and LEPR deficiency. See Chapter "Leptin and Leptin Receptor Deficiency" for more information.
- POMC deficiency: overlapping phenotype of obesity and adrenal failure. See Chapter "POMC Deficiency" for further clinical features of this disorder (such as pale skin and red hair)

5 Molecular Diagnosis

PCSK1 deficiency is caused by biallelic loss-of-function (likely) pathogenic variants in the *PCSK1* gene. The molecular diagnosis of PCSK1 deficiency can be made by sequencing of the *PCSK1* gene. In the neonatal phase, NGS gene panels for congenital diarrhea can lead to this diagnosis. *PCSK1* is also included in many gene panels for early-onset obesity, but the disease is rarely diagnosed in children with only early-onset obesity as their main or only complaint. Heterozygous carriers of a complete loss-of-function variant in *PCSK1* have an increased risk of developing obesity [5].

6 Therapy

An individualized tailored treatment plan should be made for every patient with genetic obesity including PCSK1 deficiency. It should be appropriate for age, culturally sensitive, and family-centered. Adhering to a healthy diet can be especially challenging for children with complete PCSK1 deficiency because of their intestinal symptoms. For example, there is a case report on a 2-year-old child with PCSK1 deficiency who had a diet without fruit and vegetables to prevent diarrhea. At that time, he had a BMI of 19 kg/m^2 (+3SD) [5].

Little is known about the effectiveness of anti-obesity medication for PCSK1 deficiency, probably because of the rarity of the disorder. MC4R agonist setmelanotide is approved for patients with PCSK1 deficiency and obesity. The approval application for PCSK1 deficiency was combined with data from POMC deficiency because of their overlapping mechanisms and the very low prevalence of PCSK1 deficiency. The phase 3 trial included only 1 patient with PCSK1 deficiency [19, 20]. He initially lost 7.1% body weight on setmelanotide. During the placebo-controlled withdrawal phase, he regained weight and developed depression, for which the obesogenic drug risperidone was prescribed. After restarting the setmelanotide at the end of the withdrawal phase, the researchers noted that he did not lose any additional weight, even when his risperidone was eventually stopped. After study completion, the patient had a 2.4% weight reduction from baseline owing to the initial rapid weight loss at the start of the study. It is unknown whether the loss of effect of setmelanotide treatment was caused by the depression and risperidone treatment, or by the placebo-controlled withdrawal phase. As far as we are aware, there are no publications on the effects of other anti-obesity drugs, such as GLP-1 agonist treatment, naltrexone/bupropione, phentermine, or central stimulants (methylphenidate and dexamphetamine) in patients with PCSK1 deficiency. Furthermore, no gene therapy possibilities restoring *PCSK1* function *in vivo* have been published to date.

There is one case report on a patient with biallelic PCSK1 deficiency that underwent bariatric surgery. He underwent a Roux-en-Y gastric bypass with good effect, resulting in >25% body weight loss and reversal of his type 2 diabetes [1]. Five patients with heterozygous complete or partial loss-of-function variants in *PCSK1* who underwent bariatric surgery have also been described in literature. They appear to have similar weight loss results two years after bariatric surgery as patients who do not have genetic obesity [21]. No long-term data are available as of yet.

In addition to the obesity treatment, it is important to treat the associated endocrinopathies by supplementing the hormonal deficiencies. As an example, desmopressin is used to treat the AVP deficiency, while the adrenal insufficiency is treated with oral glucocorticoids. Recombinant growth hormone may be given in patients with growth hormone deficiency, as well as levothyroxine and insulin to treat the hypothyroidism and diabetes mellitus, respectively. In patients with stagnating pubertal development, sex hormone replacement therapy is given.

7 Follow-up Advices

Management of PCSK1 deficiency requires multidisciplinary long-term care. There is no uniform follow-up or screening recommendation.

Follow-up monitoring that could be considered:

- Height, weight, and puberty
- Gastrointestinal symptoms and dietary status
- Associated endocrine deficiencies and evaluation of hormonal treatment
- Endocrine evaluation for hormonal disturbances and screening for comorbidities (signs of hepatic steatosis, lipid profile, hyperglycemia, and/or postprandial hypoglycemia)
- Body composition and of resting energy expenditure to guide tailored dietary advice
- Cardiovascular screening according to severity of the obesity and presence of comorbidities

8 Family Screening

Since PCSK1 deficiency is an autosomal recessive genetic disorder, siblings of an affected child have a 25% chance of having the same condition. Because heterozygous carriers of loss-of-function variants are likely more at risk to develop obesity, one could consider family screening for heterozygotes as well, especially if available treatment options depend on the genetic diagnosis.

Take Home Messages

- PCSK1 deficiency is a rare genetic obesity disorder with an autosomal recessive inheritance pattern.
- Key clinical characteristics are severe diarrhea and failure to thrive in infancy, followed by hyperphagia and obesity in childhood. Several hormonal disturbances (complete or partial), such as AVP deficiency, growth hormone deficiency, and adrenal insufficiency are also associated with PCSK1 deficiency.

- Heterozygous carriers of pathogenic loss-of-function variants in *PSCK1* are at risk to develop obesity, but they do not have the complete (severe) phenotype of hormonal deficiencies seen in PCSK1 deficiency.
- PCSK1 deficiency can be treated with MC4R agonist setmelanotide. If indicated, hormonal deficiencies should be treated with hormone replacement therapy.

References

1. Stijnen P, Ramos-Molina B, O'Rahilly S, Creemers JW. PCSK1 mutations and human endocrinopathies: from obesity to gastrointestinal disorders. Endocr Rev. 2016;37(4):347–71.
2. Duclaux-Loras R, Bourgeois P, Lavrut PM, Charbit-Henrion F, Bonniaud-Blot P, Maudinas R, et al. A novel mutation of PCSK1 responsible for PC1/3 deficiency in two siblings. Clin Res Hepatol Gastroenterol. 2021;45(6):101640.
3. Jackson RS, Creemers JW, Ohagi S, Raffin-Sanson ML, Sanders L, Montague CT, et al. Obesity and impaired prohormone processing associated with mutations in the human prohormone convertase 1 gene. Nat Genet. 1997;16(3):303–6.
4. Martín MG, Lindberg I, Solorzano-Vargas RS, Wang J, Avitzur Y, Bandsma R, et al. Congenital proprotein convertase 1/3 deficiency causes malabsorptive diarrhea and other endocrinopathies in a pediatric cohort. Gastroenterology. 2013;145(1):138–48.
5. Folon L, Baron M, Toussaint B, Vaillant E, Boissel M, Scherrer V, et al. Contribution of heterozygous PCSK1 variants to obesity and implications for precision medicine: a case-control study. Lancet Diabetes Endocrinol. 2023;11(3):182–90.
6. Karczewski KJ, Francioli LC, Tiao G, Cummings BB, Alföldi J, Wang Q, et al. The mutational constraint spectrum quantified from variation in 141,456 humans. Nature. 2020;581(7809):434–43.
7. Baxter S, Grant R, Lee J, Watts N, Chan Zuckerberg initiative rare as one network, O'Donnell-Luria A, Rehm H. GeniE, the Genetic Prevalence Estimator: Broad Institute; 2024. [updated 06/04/2024]. Available from: https://genie.broadinstitute.org/.
8. Harno E, Gali Ramamoorthy T, Coll AP, White A. POMC: the physiological power of hormone processing. Physiol Rev. 2018;98(4):2381–430.
9. Jackson RS, Creemers JW, Farooqi IS, Raffin-Sanson ML, Varro A, Dockray GJ, et al. Small-intestinal dysfunction accompanies the complex endocrinopathy of human proprotein convertase 1 deficiency. J Clin Invest. 2003;112(10):1550–60.
10. Wetsel WC, Liposits Z, Seidah NG, Collins S. Expression of candidate pro-GnRH processing enzymes in rat hypothalamus and an immortalized hypothalamic neuronal cell line. Neuroendocrinology. 1995;62(2):166–77.
11. Posner SF, Vaslet CA, Jurofcik M, Lee A, Seidah NG, Nillni EA. Stepwise posttranslational processing of progrowth hormone-releasing hormone (proGHRH) polypeptide by furin and PC1. Endocrine 2004;23(2–3):199–213.
12. Wardman JH, Zhang X, Gagnon S, Castro LM, Zhu X, Steiner DF, et al. Analysis of peptides in prohormone convertase 1/3 null mouse brain using quantitative peptidomics. J Neurochem. 2010;114(1):215–25.
13. O'Rahilly S, Gray H, Humphreys PJ, Krook A, Polonsky KS, White A, et al. Brief report: impaired processing of prohormones associated with abnormalities of glucose homeostasis and adrenal function. N Engl J Med. 1995;333(21):1386–90.

14. Bandsma RH, Sokollik C, Chami R, Cutz E, Brubaker PL, Hamilton JK, et al. From diarrhea to obesity in prohormone convertase 1/3 deficiency: age-dependent clinical, pathologic, and enteroendocrine characteristics. J Clin Gastroenterol. 2013;47(10):834–43.
15. Pépin L, Colin E, Tessarech M, Rouleau S, Bouhours-Nouet N, Bonneau D, Coutant R. A new case of PCSK1 pathogenic variant with congenital proprotein convertase 1/3 deficiency and literature review. J Clin Endocrinol Metab. 2019;104(4):985–93.
16. Nead KT, Li A, Wehner MR, Neupane B, Gustafsson S, Butterworth A, et al. Contribution of common non-synonymous variants in PCSK1 to body mass index variation and risk of obesity: a systematic review and meta-analysis with evidence from up to 331 175 individuals. Hum Mol Genet. 2015;24(12):3582–94.
17. Qian Y, Wu B, Liu R, Lu Y, Zhang P, Shao C, et al. Case report: complete maternal uniparental isodisomy of chromosome 5 (iUPD(5)mat) with PCSK1 nonsense variant in an infant with recurrent diarrhea. Front Genet. 2021;12:668326.
18. Esposito MV, Comegna M, Cernera G, Gelzo M, Paparo L, Berni Canani R, Castaldo G. NGS gene panel analysis revealed novel mutations in patients with rare congenital diarrheal disorders. Diagnostics (Basel). 2021;11(2)
19. Wabitsch M, Farooqi S, Flück CE, Bratina N, Mallya UG, Stewart M, et al. Natural history of obesity due to POMC, PCSK1, and LEPR deficiency and the impact of setmelanotide. J Endocr Soc 2022;6(6):bvac057.
20. Clément K, van den Akker E, Argente J, Bahm A, Chung WK, Connors H, et al. Efficacy and safety of setmelanotide, an MC4R agonist, in individuals with severe obesity due to LEPR or POMC deficiency: single-arm, open-label, multicentre, phase 3 trials. Lancet Diabetes Endocrinol. 2020;8(12):960–70.
21. Cooiman MI, Kleinendorst L, Aarts EO, Janssen IMC, van Amstel HKP, Blakemore AI, et al. Genetic obesity and bariatric surgery outcome in 1014 patients with morbid obesity. Obes Surg. 2020;30(2):470–7.

Methylation Analysis in Diagnostics; the Episignature

Liselot van der Laan, Peter Henneman, and Mariëlle Alders

1 Principles of Epigenetics

Epigenetic changes are reversible alterations that modify the activity of a gene without changing the genetic code. They are chemical modifications to the DNA and the protein structures around which the DNA is wound, called histones. DNA and histones together form nucleosomes, the basic unit that makes up chromatin. The epigenetic modifications regulate whether the chromatin becomes more or less condensed or 'folded', thus regulate accessibility of genes and thereby expression of genes. An open DNA structure is associated with increased gene activity, while a closed DNA structure is associated with reduced gene activity. The most commonly studied epigenetic change is the attachment of a methyl group to the cytosine base in the DNA. Other epigenetic features involve chemical changes possible at the histone tails, such as acetylation, phosphorylation, and methylation, which can occur at many different positions on the histone tail. The collective epigenetic changes to the genome are referred to as the epigenome. Epigenetic changes are reversible, modifications are actively added or erased, and therefore the epigenome is more flexible than the genome. The epigenome is also responsive to environmental factors, such as diet and stress or exposure to chemicals [1–3].

L. van der Laan (✉) · P. Henneman · M. Alders
Department of Human Genetics, Amsterdam University Medical Center, Amsterdam, The Netherlands

Amsterdam Reproduction & Development Research Institute, Amsterdam, The Netherlands
e-mail: l.vanderlaan@amsterdamumc.nl; p.henneman@amsterdamumc.nl; m.alders@amsterdamumc.nl

M. van Haelst, E. van den Akker (eds.), *Clinical Obesity Genetics*,
https://doi.org/10.1007/978-3-032-04095-4_14

2 Epigenetic Signatures

Numerous genes are intricately connected to epigenetic regulation, specifically those associated with the epigenetic machinery. These genes encode proteins categorized as writers, erasers, readers, and remodelers, with writers modifying specific regions of the genome, erasers removing epigenetic marks, readers recognizing these marks and recruiting other enzymes, and remodelers facilitating access to chromatin regions and aiding in protein-DNA interactions [1]. Variants in such genes that affect normal function affect the epigenome and results in specific consistent and reproducible DNA methylation patterns, also detectable in peripheral blood, called episignatures [4]. In recent years, numerous epigenetic signatures based on DNA methylation have been discovered by various research groups. Among the first known episignatures published were those associated with Floating-Harbor syndrome (*SRCAP),* Claes Jensen syndrome (*KDM5C),* Kabuki syndrome 1 & 2 (*KMT2D, KDM6A),* Helsmoortel-Van der Aa syndrome (*ADNP)* and Charge syndrome (*CHD7*) [5–10]. The number of disorder linked episignatures continues to grow annually, with today over 100 episignatures identified, spanning more than 120 genes or genomic regions [11]. The more episignature are established, the more is learned about epigenetic processes. It was shown that multiple genes (mostly connected in the same pathway) display (partly) identical or overlapping episignatures. An example is the overlapping signatures of BAFopathies (*ARID1A, ARID1B, SMARCB1, SMARCA4, SMARCA2*) and Börjeson-Forssman-Lehmann, Chung-Jansen and White-Kernohan syndromes (*resp. PHF6, PHIP, DDB1*) [12, 13]. It has also been shown that some genes have multiple episignatures, or that only certain regions of the gene exhibit episignatures. For instance, Rubinstein-Taybi syndrome has two episignatures RTS1 and RTS2, caused by loss of function variants in *CREBBP* or *EP300.* However, patients with Menke-Hennekam syndrome, caused by variants in the ID4 regions of these two genes have a different phenotype, each associated with a different but specific episignature. Similarly, for Helsmoortel-van der AA syndrome, caused by in *ADNP* variants, two distinct and partially opposing episignatures have been identified [14, 15]. In addition to variants in genes affecting the epigenetic machinery, environmental factors can also result in specific episignatures [16].

Episignatures can serve as highly sensitive and specific biomarkers that can be used in diagnostics. They have been shown to be a valuable tool in resolving Variants of Uncertain Significance (VUS) that are being identified in diagnostic genetic testing [2]. Standard diagnostic testing, typically, sequencing methods such as Whole Exome Sequencing (WES), often yield these inconclusive results that do match the phenotype of the patient. The presence of a specific epigenetic signature in a patient can subsequently supports the associated diagnosis and provides evidence for pathogenicity of the variant. However, it is important to note that a negative episignature, can not be considered as conclusive evidence for lack of pathogenicity. As highlighted before, multiple episignature profiles may exist for a single gene, related to different protein domains or variant types. In case of a negative result, it can not be completely ruled out that the variant results in another, yet undiscovered episignature [16, 17]. In addition, episignatures can be used in cases where standard genetics testing for example WES, did not reveal a causal variant. They can even be used as first tier test for patients with a striking phenotype suggestive of a syndrome diagnosis of whom parental samples are unavailable or when parents do not have queries regarding recurrence risks for future children. In such cases, an episignature can help provide personalized care. Even without a positive episignature, it offers clues about which genes to analyze in more detail, potentially leading to the identification of the causal variant without needing parental samples when a VUS is identified through regular Sanger sequencing.

3 Case Example Episignature

Exome sequencing in a 17-year-old boy presenting with intellectual deficit (ID), obesity, and behavior problems revealed a VUS in *PHIP* (c.2200A > G, p.Ser734Gly). Pathogenic variants in this gene cause Chung-Jansen syndrome (OMIM #617991).

PHIP encodes the Pleckstrin homology domain-interacting protein. This protein is integral to an epigenetic modifier protein complex. *PHIP* is also associated with for ID-overweight syndromes [18]. A combined episignature for Börjeson-Forssman-Lehmann (BFLS), Chung-Jansen (CHUJANS) and White Kernohan (WHIKERS) syndromes (*PHF6*, *PHIP*, *DDB1*) has recently been identified. These syndromes also show overlapping clinical features and manifests as neurodevelopmental disorders marked by intellectual disability, behavioural issues, obesity, and distinctive dysmorphic features.

The DNA methylation profile in peripheral blood of our overlapped with the BFLS/CHUJANS/WHIKERS combined episignature and with this CHUJANS (*PHIP*) sub-signature we could subsequently, reclassify the VUS to a likely pathogenic *PHIP* variant (Fig. 1).

4 Imprinting Disorders

Another group of disorders where epigenetics plays an important role are imprinting disorders. Imprinting disorders are a group of rare genetic conditions characterized by abnormal gene expression of genes that are subject to genomic imprinting. Genomic imprinting describes the that the difference in expression of some genes depending on parental origin. Some genes are expressed only from the paternal or the maternal allele. At present there are around 100 imprinted genes known and they tend to be clustered in the genome. An epigenetic methylation mark can identify an allele as being maternally or paternally inherited. This mark is set during gametogenesis and remains throughout the development of the individual. Imprinting disorders typically arise from deletions or uniparental disomy (UPD) (see Chap. 5). At

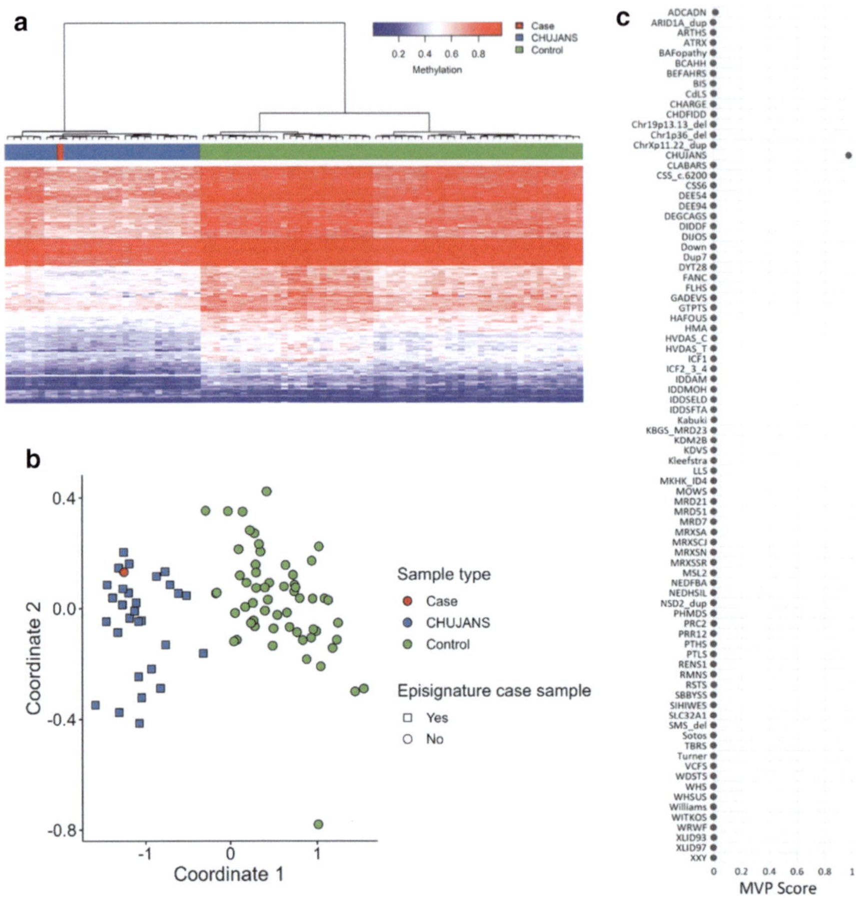

Fig. 1 Confirmed episignature for our case with three different methods. (**a**) Euclidean hierarchical clustering (heatmap): each column represents a single case (blue) or control (green), and the red row represents our case, clustering between the CHUJANS patients. (**b**) multidimensional scaling plots indicate that the case (red) clusters with the CHUJANS cases (blue), away from controls (green) (**c**) methylation variant pathogenicity (MVP) score range between 0 and 1, with scores close to 1 indicating a high probability of a methylation pattern for the target syndrome (CHUJANS), and scores close to 0 indicating a methylation profile similar to controls. Our case is showing a high MVP score, indicating the presence of the CHUJANS episignature

times, defects in imprint establishment or maintenance can disrupt parent-of-origin-specific gene expression patterns. Phenotypes of most imprinting disorders include abnormal growth, either reduced or enhanced. Imprinting disorders in which obesity is one of the key features include Prader- Willi syndrome and Pseudohypoparathyroidism (PHP) syndrome. They each exhibit apart from the obesity distinct clinical features and are associated with specific genetic loci. Prader-Willi syndrome is caused by the loss of function of certain genes on chromosome 15q11-q13, see chap. 5. PHP is often caused by pathogenic variants or affecting the imprinting *GNAS* located on chromosome 20q13.32. This gene encodes the alpha subunit of the stimulatory G protein, which plays a crucial role in transmitting signals from certain G-coupled hormone receptors including the MC4R [19, 20]. The diagnosis of an imprinting disorders is made by identifying abnormal methylation at the imprinting control regions of the chromosomal locus involved. A targeted, commonly used test for Imprinting disorders is Methylation specific Multiplex Ligation-dependent Probe Amplification (MLPA). However, a genome wide methylation analysis approach can also be used to determine abnormal methylation at imprinted loci.

5 EpiSign™ Method

The incorporation of episignatures into diagnostics has been pioneered by EpiSign™, a diagnostic test utilizing the Illumina microarray (Illumina, CA, USA) as its primary platform for profiling DNA methylation episignatures [21, 22]. Leveraging bioinformatic and machine learning applications enables the assessment of DNA methylation profiles simultaneously. In its latest version (version 5 (February 2024), it can detect 96 different episignatures, 10 imprinting disorders and the trinucleotide repeat expansion in males with Fragile X syndrome. Disorders associated with episignatures, categorized by their function in the epigenetic machinery (writers, readers, erasers and remodelers) screened with the EpiSign™ test, are shown in Fig. 2.

6 Environmental Factors

As described above, the epigenome is a highly dynamic molecular mechanism that regulates gene expression. It is controlled by genetic factors and can also be affected by environmental influences, such as lifestyle and traumatic events. It has therefore been suggested that epigenetics may represent the missing genetic variance (heritability) for common disease such as complex obesity and other non-communicable disease. In addition, accumulating evidence also suggests a role of epigenetic mechanisms in post-traumatic stress syndrome and its related traits. Studying these multifactorial epigenetic mechanisms are however rather complex. Although, strong associations between DNA methylation and disease have been reported is such studies [23–25], conclusions regarding whether such association is causal or a consequence of the disease remains a challenge in most studies for the following reasons. Firstly, the most commonly applied study design follows a cross-sectional approach, wherein cases and controls express differential DNA methylation at only one time point. Secondly, epigenetics, by definition, is highly tissue-specific, and most studies typically rely on DNA extracted from whole blood rather than the diseased tissue of interest. A striking example of such causality or consequence

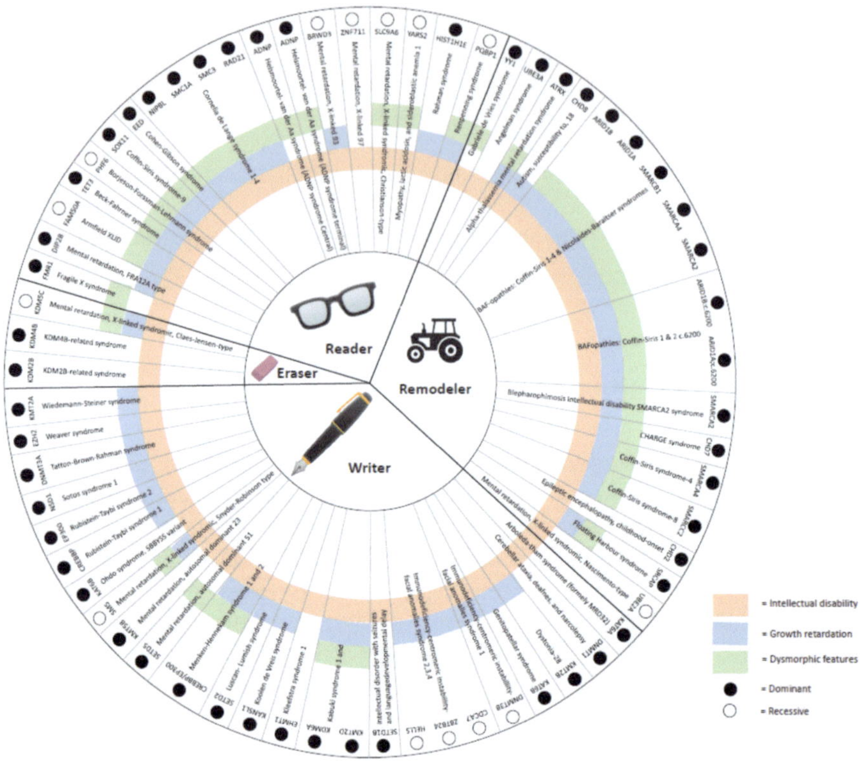

Fig. 2 Episignatures detectable by EpiSign™ V3. Four distinct categories are delineated: reader, eraser, writer, and remodeler proteins. The outer circles represent inheritance patterns, with open circles indicating recessive inheritance and closed circles signifying dominant inheritance. Disorder phenotypes are depicted in various colors: dysmorphic features (green), growth retardation (blue), and intellectual disability (orange). (This figure is added with permission from van der Laan et al. [1])

question is illustrated by the epigenome-wide association analysis of obesity traits that detected (among many others) aberrant DNA methylation of the *ABCG1* gene. Follow-up translational studies reported that this gene is indeed functionally active in fat storage and fat mass growth. However, whether the aberrant methylation is a consequence of unfavourable lifestyle factors, or that it represents a causal link to be susceptible to become obese, remains so far unclear [26, 27].

The role of the environment affecting the human epigenome includes more than just external factors such as lifestyle and traumatic events. The microbiome, defined as a collection of bacteria, viruses, and fungi that inhabit a specific part of the body, has also been shown to interact with the human epigenome. The most commonly studied microbiome in relation to the epigenome is that of the gut. For example, several studies in obese subjects *per se*, or those who were following a weight loss intervention program, have demonstrated an association between the epigenome and the gut microbiome [28, 29].

In addition, *in utero* exposure to environmental stressors such as famine has been associated with an increased susceptibility to high blood pressure, Diabetes Mellitus and obesity in later life [30]. Epigenetic surveys in this context, based on genome-wide DNA methylation profiles, have suggested that aberrant DNA methylation serves as a mediator for metabolic diseases, including obesity [31]. Interestingly, all aforementioned studies suggest that the fetus is particularly at risk during exposures in early gestation.

Exposure to substances during pregnancy is a particular environmental exposure that may represent a phenotype comparable with previously described rare disorders. Important examples of such *in utero* exposures include Valproic acid and Alcohol. Alcohol, in this sense, is a known factor that impairs the folate pathway, which is involved in the general production of methyl groups, which also are required as an epigenetic mark, i.e., to methylate DNA [32–35]. Similarly, Valproic acid is a known inhibitor of histone deacetylase and therefore also directly affects epigenetic programming. *In utero* Valproic acid is linked to adverse effects in the foetus, but it also has been reported to be associated with weight gain and insulin resistance in patients with neurological or psychiatric disorders [36]. The exact molecular mechanism(s), linking valpoic acid administration to epigenetic aberrations and weight gain are poorly understood. However, recently it was shown that this compound was epigenetically and functionally associated with the *FTO* gene, an, from the early days, obesity-linked GWAS locus [37, 38].

Altogether, there is substantial evidence that environmental factors play a significant role in affecting the human epigenome and may, in turn, cause adverse affects like obesity.

The future of episignatures in medicine holds great promise, particularly with the ongoing discovery of epigenetically active compounds and their role in disease pathology. With more and more rapidly discovered episignatures becoming available in diagnostic testing, the power of episignature testing will increase accordingly. As we delve deeper into understanding how episignatures function within the body, we anticipate not only improved diagnosis but also the development of tailored therapies that address the affected mechanism causing the diseases. Moreover, advancements in epigenetic editing techniques provide unprecedented opportunities to target and modify specific epigenetic marks, potentially leading to the development of novel and more precise treatments [39]. Furthermore, we foresee a shift towards the integration of episignatures into routine medical practice, with clinicians utilizing them as diagnostic tools to predict treatment responses and personalize patient care effectively. In summary, the future of episignatures offers a wealth of opportunities for advancing medical understanding, refining diagnostics, and revolutionizing personalized treatment strategies for epigenetic diseases to meet the unique needs of each patient [4, 16].

7 Conclusion

In conclusion, DNA methylation analyses stands as a powerful and versatile tool in the realm of genomic diagnostics. Its capability to identify a wide range of episignatures, including those associated with specific disorders such as imprinting defects and obesity-related conditions, underscores its strength in establishing precise diagnoses.

References

1. Bjornsson HT. The Mendelian disorders of the epigenetic machinery. Genome Res. 2015;25(10):1473–81.
2. Mannens M, Lombardi MP, Alders M, Henneman P, Bliek J. Further introduction of DNA methylation (DNAm) arrays in regular diagnostics. Front Genet. 2022;13:831452.
3. van der Laan L, Rooney K, Trooster TM, Mannens MM, Sadikovic B, Henneman P. DNA methylation episignatures: insight into copy number variation. Epigenomics. 2022;14(21):1373–88.
4. Sadikovic B, Aref-Eshghi E, Levy MA, Rodenhiser D. DNA methylation signatures in mendelian developmental disorders as a diagnostic bridge between genotype and phenotype. Epigenomics. 2019;11(5):563–75.
5. Breen MS, Garg P, Tang L, Mendonca D, Levy T, Barbosa M, et al. Episignatures stratifying Helsmoortel-Van Der Aa syndrome show modest correlation with phenotype. Am J Hum Genet. 2020;107(3):555–63.
6. Hood RL, Schenkel LC, Nikkel SM, Ainsworth PJ, Pare G, Boycott KM, et al. The defining DNA methylation signature of Floating-Harbor Syndrome. Sci Rep. 2016;6:38803.
7. Schenkel LC, Aref-Eshghi E, Skinner C, Ainsworth P, Lin H, Paré G, et al. Peripheral blood epi-signature of Claes-Jensen syndrome enables sensitive and specific identification of patients and healthy carriers with pathogenic mutations in KDM5C. Clin Epigenetics. 2018;10:21.
8. Lee S, Ochoa E, Badura-Stronka M, Donnelly D, Lederer D, Lynch SA, et al. Germline pathogenic variants in HNRNPU are associated with alterations in blood methylome. Eur J Hum Genet. 2023;31(9):1040–7.
9. Awamleh Z, Choufani S, Wu W, Rots D, Dingemans AJM, Nadif Kasri N, et al. A new blood DNA methylation signature for Koolen-de Vries syndrome: classification of missense KANSL1 variants and comparison to fibroblast cells. Eur J Hum Genet. 2024;
10. Choufani S, McNiven V, Cytrynbaum C, Jangjoo M, Adam MP, Bjornsson HT, et al. An HNRNPK-specific DNA methylation signature makes sense of missense variants and expands the phenotypic spectrum of Au-Kline syndrome. Am J Hum Genet. 2022;109(10):1867–84.
11. Kerkhof J, Rastin C, Levy MA, Relator R, McConkey H, Demain L, et al. Diagnostic utility and reporting recommendations for clinical DNA methylation episignature testing in genetically undiagnosed rare diseases. Genet Med. 2024;26(5):101075.
12. Aref-Eshghi E, Bend EG, Hood RL, Schenkel LC, Carere DA, Chakrabarti R, et al. BAFopathies' DNA methylation epi-signatures demonstrate diagnostic utility and functional continuum of Coffin-Siris and Nicolaides-Baraitser syndromes. Nat Commun. 2018;9(1):4885.
13. Vos N, Haghshenas S, van der Laan L, Russel PKM, Rooney K, Levy MA, et al. The detection of a strong episignature for Chung-Jansen syndrome, partially overlapping with Börjeson-Forssman-Lehmann and White-Kernohan syndromes. Hum Genet. 2024;143:761–73.
14. Bend EG, Aref-Eshghi E, Everman DB, Rogers RC, Cathey SS, Prijoles EJ, et al. Gene domain-specific DNA methylation episignatures highlight distinct molecular entities of ADNP syndrome. Clin Epigenetics. 2019;11(1):64.

15. Sarli C, van der Laan L, Reilly J, Trajkova S, Carli D, Brusco A, et al. Blepharophimosis with intellectual disability and Helsmoortel-Van Der Aa Syndrome share episignature and phenotype. Am J Med Genet C Semin Med Genet. 2024;196:e32089.
16. Sadikovic B, Levy MA, Kerkhof J, Aref-Eshghi E, Schenkel L, Stuart A, et al. Clinical epigenomics: genome-wide DNA methylation analysis for the diagnosis of Mendelian disorders. Genet Med. 2021;23(6):1065–74.
17. Aref-Eshghi E, Kerkhof J, Pedro VP, France GD, Barat-Houari M, Ruiz-Pallares N, et al. Evaluation of DNA methylation episignatures for diagnosis and phenotype correlations in 42 mendelian neurodevelopmental disorders. Am J Hum Genet. 2021;108(6):1161–3.
18. Jansen S, Hoischen A, Coe BP, Carvill GL, Van Esch H, Bosch DGM, et al. A genotype-first approach identifies an intellectual disability-overweight syndrome caused by PHIP haploinsufficiency. Eur J Hum Genet. 2018;26(1):54–63.
19. Li T, Vu TH, Zeng ZL, Nguyen BT, Hayward BE, Bonthron DT, et al. Tissue-specific expression of antisense and sense transcripts at the imprinted Gnas locus. Genomics. 2000;69(3):295–304.
20. Vos N, Menke LA, Mooij CF, van den Akker ELT, Alders M, van Haelst MM. Severe early-onset overgrowth in a case of pseudohypoparathyroidism type 1b, caused by STX16 deletion. Am J Med Genet A. 2023;191(5):1476–8.
21. Levy MA, McConkey H, Kerkhof J, Barat-Houari M, Bargiacchi S, Biamino E, et al. Novel diagnostic DNA methylation episignatures expand and refine the epigenetic landscapes of Mendelian disorders. HGG Adv. 2022;3(1):100075.
22. Aref-Eshghi E, Bend EG, Colaiacovo S, Caudle M, Chakrabarti R, Napier M, et al. Diagnostic utility of genome-wide DNA methylation testing in genetically unsolved individuals with suspected hereditary conditions. Am J Hum Genet. 2019;104(4):685–700.
23. Manolio TA, Collins FS, Cox NJ, Goldstein DB, Hindorff LA, Hunter DJ, et al. Finding the missing heritability of complex diseases. Nature. 2009;461(7265):747–53.
24. Oliva M, Demanelis K, Lu Y, Chernoff M, Jasmine F, Ahsan H, et al. DNA methylation QTL mapping across diverse human tissues provides molecular links between genetic variation and complex traits. Nat Genet. 2023;55(1):112–22.
25. Tammen SA, Friso S, Choi SW. Epigenetics: the link between nature and nurture. Mol Asp Med. 2013;34(4):753–64.
26. Frisdal E, Le Lay S, Hooton H, Poupel L, Olivier M, Alili R, et al. Adipocyte ATP-binding cassette G1 promotes triglyceride storage, fat mass growth, and human obesity. Diabetes. 2015;64(3):840–55.
27. Geurts YM, Dugué PA, Joo JE, Makalic E, Jung CH, Guan W, et al. Novel associations between blood DNA methylation and body mass index in middle-aged and older adults. Int J Obes. 2018;42(4):887–96.
28. Qin Y, Roberts JD, Grimm SA, Lih FB, Deterding LJ, Li R, et al. An obesity-associated gut microbiome reprograms the intestinal epigenome and leads to altered colonic gene expression. Genome Biol. 2018;19(1):7.
29. Hill EB, Konigsberg IR, Ir D, Frank DN, Jambal P, Litkowski EM, et al. The microbiome, epigenome, and diet in adults with obesity during behavioral weight loss. Nutrients. 2023;15(16)
30. Bleker LS, de Rooij SR, Painter RC, Ravelli AC, Roseboom TJ. Cohort profile: the Dutch famine birth cohort (DFBC)- a prospective birth cohort study in The Netherlands. BMJ Open. 2021;11(3):e042078.
31. Tobi EW, Slieker RC, Luijk R, Dekkers KF, Stein AD, Xu KM, et al. DNA methylation as a mediator of the association between prenatal adversity and risk factors for metabolic disease in adulthood. Sci Adv. 2018;4(1):eaao4364.
32. Cobben JM, Krzyzewska IM, Venema A, Mul AN, Polstra A, Postma AV, et al. DNA methylation abundantly associates with fetal alcohol spectrum disorder and its subphenotypes. Epigenomics. 2019;11(7):767–85.
33. Lussier AA, Morin AM, JL MI, Salmon J, Weinberg J, Reynolds JN, et al. DNA methylation as a predictor of fetal alcohol spectrum disorder. Clin Epigenetics. 2018;10:5.

34. Portales-Casamar E, Lussier AA, Jones MJ, MacIsaac JL, Edgar RD, Mah SM, et al. DNA methylation signature of human fetal alcohol spectrum disorder. Epigenetics Chromatin. 2016;9:25.
35. Collins NJ, Zimmerman CW, Phillips NLH, Fern S, Doherty TS, Roth TL. Developmental administration of valproic acid alters DNA methylation and maternal behavior. Dev Psychobiol. 2022;64(3):e22231.
36. Masuccio F, Verrotti A, Chiavaroli V, de Giorgis T, Giannini C, Chiarelli F, Mohn A. Weight gain and insulin resistance in children treated with valproate: the influence of time. J Child Neurol. 2010;25(8):941–7.
37. Zhang H, Lu P, Tang HL, Yan HJ, Jiang W, Shi H, et al. Valproate-induced epigenetic upregulation of hypothalamic Fto expression potentially linked with weight gain. Cell Mol Neurobiol. 2021;41(6):1257–69.
38. Loos RJ, Yeo GS. The bigger picture of FTO: the first GWAS-identified obesity gene. Nat Rev Endocrinol. 2014;10(1):51–61.
39. Fahrner JA, Bjornsson HT. Mendelian disorders of the epigenetic machinery: postnatal malleability and therapeutic prospects. Hum Mol Genet. 2019;28(R2):R254–r64.

Clinical Obesity Treatment

Anti-obesity Pharmacotherapy for Patients with Genetic Obesity Disorders

Mila Welling, Elisabeth van Rossum, and Erica van den Akker

1 Introduction

Reducing weight is essential in obesity treatment as it is associated with numerous co-morbidities, such as cardiovascular and metabolic diseases, depression, and various types of cancer. Several studies have shown an association between higher BMI categories and the number of years of life lost [1–3]. For example, in women and men with obesity between 20 to 29 years of age, life expectancy is predicted to be decreased with 8.1–10.3 and 5.6–7.6 years, respectively [2]. This shows that there

M. Welling
Obesity Center CGG, Erasmus MC, University Medical Center Rotterdam, Rotterdam, The Netherlands

Division of Endocrinology, Department of Pediatrics, Erasmus MC-Sophia Children's Hospital, University Medical Center Rotterdam, Rotterdam, The Netherlands

Division of Endocrinology, Department of Internal Medicine, Erasmus MC, University Medical Center Rotterdam, Rotterdam, The Netherlands
e-mail: m.welling@erasmusmc.nl

E. van Rossum
Obesity Center CGG, Erasmus MC, University Medical Center Rotterdam, Rotterdam, The Netherlands

Division of Endocrinology, Department of Pediatrics, Erasmus MC-Sophia Children's Hospital, University Medical Center Rotterdam, Rotterdam, The Netherlands
e-mail: e.vanrossum@erasmusmc.nl

E. van den Akker (✉)
Obesity Center CGG, Erasmus MC, University Medical Center Rotterdam, Rotterdam, The Netherlands

Division of Endocrinology, Department of Internal Medicine, Erasmus MC, University Medical Center Rotterdam, Rotterdam, The Netherlands
e-mail: e.l.t.vandenakker@erasmusmc.nl

M. van Haelst, E. van den Akker (eds.), *Clinical Obesity Genetics*,
https://doi.org/10.1007/978-3-032-04095-4_15

is an urgent need for preventing the development of obesity as well as efficient treatments in patients who suffer from obesity already.

The cornerstone of obesity treatment, including genetic obesity, is combined lifestyle interventions, focusing on nutrition and physical activity. In some treatment strategies, cognitive behavioural therapy can be included as well. In addition, children with genetic obesity and severe hyperphagia, along with their families, frequently require a multidisciplinary team approach to tackle all associated problems. This team typically comprises a paediatrician, dietician, physiotherapist, psychologist, or family therapist, who collaboratively guide and offer advice on managing the extreme food-seeking behaviour. These conventional lifestyle treatments often have insufficient long-term effects in patients with genetic obesity, as their hyperphagia remains untreated [4].

Additional pharmacotherapy, specifically targeting the hyperphagia, is often needed. Reducing hyperphagia not only leads to weight loss and enhanced mobility, but also significantly improves patients' quality of life [5–7]. Continuing with lifestyle guidance is essential, as multiple studies have shown the additive value of lifestyle interventions in addition to anti-obesity pharmacotherapy [8–10]. Importantly, treatment goals for patients with genetic obesity may differ from those with common (multifactorial) obesity. Firstly, achieving weight stabilization by halting the progressive weight gain can also be considered a treatment goal. Secondly, ameliorating the hyperphagia and consequently improving their quality of life is already an important treatment goal on its own. Another treatment option would be bariatric surgery, however, the long-term effects of bariatric surgery remain questionable in patients with genetic obesity as it does not treat the hyperphagia [11, 12]. This demonstrates that non-invasive appetite-suppressing agents are needed in this groups of patients to induce weight loss, ameliorate hyperphagia, and improve their quality of life.

Several anti-obesity medications (AOMs) are available nowadays. The targeted pharmacotherapies, i.e., leptin replacement therapy and MC4R agonists, are only FDA and EMA approved and available for patients with certain types of genetic obesity. Both leptin analogues and MC4R-agonists activate important receptors (the leptin receptor and melanocortin-4 receptor) of the hypothalamic leptin-melanocortin pathway respectively. In case of a more upstream gene defect impairing this pathway, these two receptors can be activated which on its turn restore the function of the leptin-melanocortin pathway as it bypasses the defect gene [13]. Additionally, it is suggested that it also affects other neuronal populations of the dopaminergic reward system [14].

Several non-targeted AOMs are approved for obesity, regardless of the underlying cause. Therefore, they can also be used for genetic obesity. Lipase inhibitors were first on the market. These agents induce weight loss by reducing the dietary fat absorption within the intestinal tract [15]. Subsequently, nervous system stimulants, such as phentermine and phentermine-topiramate, became available for obesity treatment. Phentermine is thought to mainly act on the reward system, specifically the nucleus accumbens, by enhancing the release of norepinephrine, and to a lesser extent serotonin and dopamine [16, 17]. By increasing these neurotransmitter concentrations they mediate the reward value of food and, consequently, affect appetite [18]. By adding topiramate, a carbonic anhydrase inhibitor and glutamate receptor antagonist, to phentermine, the effects on appetite suppression and increasing satiety seem to be enhanced [19]. Naltrexone-bupropion is another anti-obesity agents which targets both the homeostatic leptin-melanocortin pathway and the hedonic reward-related pathway [20]. Bupropion is thought to act on the arcuate hypothalamic nucleus by stimulating the melanocortin-4 receptor via the induced secretion of alpha-melanocyte stimulating hormone (α-MSH) by proopiomelanocortin (POMC) neurons, while naltrexone blocks the POMC auto-inhibitory loop and hereby enhances the bupropion induced POMC activation [20]. Both naltrexone and bupropion also affect the reward system via increasing the catecholamines dopamine and norepinephrine in the nucleus accumbens [20].

Glucagon-like peptide-1 (GLP-1) analogues mimic the effects of endogenous glucagon-like peptide-1, resulting in an increased glucose-dependent release of insulin. It inhibits the glucose-dependent release of glucagon, delays gastric emptying, and reduces appetite via hypothalamic neuronal pathways [11, 21]. Additionally, it has anti-inflammatory, anti-addictive and protective cardiovascular effects [22–28]. Currently, two types of GLP-1 analogues, short-acting 3.0 mg liraglutide and long-acting 2.4 mg semaglutide, are available. Recently, tirzepatide has been approved by the FDA and EMA for obesity treatment as the first long-acting dual glucose-dependent insulinotropic polypeptide (GIP) and GLP-1 receptor agonist. Next to the anorexigenic actions of GLP-1, activation of GIP improves glycaemic control and insulin sensitivity, regulates glucagon release, enhances clearing of dietary triglycerides by adipocytes, and enhances lipid-buffering capacity of the white adipose tissue [29]. Additionally, GIP appears to act centrally in the hypothalamus affecting appetite [29].

In this chapter, we will discuss the effects of the currently EMA and FDA approved AOMs in patients with multifactorial obesity and in patients with genetic obesity. Additionally, we provide a summary of off-label drugs which have been used in the past to treat the hyperphagia and obesity in patients with genetic obesity. Lastly, some of the new expected anti-obesity agents and their future role will be described.

2 Currently Approved Targeted Anti-obesity Agents

Two targeted AOMs, i.e. MC4R-agonist and metreleptin, that specifically target the leptin-melanocortin pathway are currently available. Only setmelanotide has been approved by the FDA and EMA and is currently available for patients with a selection of specific genetic obesity disorders (Table 1).

Table 1 Overview of available targeted anti-obesity agents

Anti-obesity medication	Mechanism of action	For genetic obesity disorders	Approved age categories by EMA	Approved age categories by FDA
Metreleptin	Leptin analogue	Congenital leptin deficiency	Adults Children ≥6 years	Adults Children ≥6 years
Setmelanotide	MC4R agonist	Biallelic POMC, LEPR, PCSK1 deficiency Bardet Biedl syndrome	Adults Children ≥6 years	Adults Children ≥6 years

Abbreviations: *MC4R* melanocortin-4 receptor, *POMC* pro-opiomelanocortin, *LEPR* leptin receptor, *PiCSK1* proprotein convertase subtilisin and kexin type 1, *EMA* European Medicines Agency, *FDA* U.S. Food and Drug Administration

2.1 Leptin

Leptin replacement therapy was first reported in children with congenital leptin deficiency (CLD). These showed beneficial effects on weight (ranges −3.4% to −24.8%), BMI (ranges −12.4% to −44.2%), fat mass (ranges −4.1% to −20.8%), metabolic parameters and appetite after six to 48 months of treatment [30–33]. Similar effects of leptin treatment were observed in a three-year-old patient with biologically inactive leptin [34]. Increased physical activity and improvement of psychological wellbeing were observed during four months of leptin treatment in seven children with CLD [35]. Also, adults with CLD respond to leptin replacement therapy on the short-term (weight loss ranges −11.9% to −13.9% after nineteen weeks of treatment) and long-term (weight loss ranges −41.7% to −55.3% after eightteen to 72 months of treatment) [36–38]. So far, studies involving patients with CLD have not reported any side effects from leptin replacement therapy. Reported side effects in patients with lipodystrophy were nausea and hypoglycaemia, specifically in patients with type 2 diabetes as comorbidity [39]. Importantly, neutralizing leptin antibodies have been reported, leading to loss of efficacy [40]. Since fat cells secrete leptin, patients with multifactorial obesity have high leptin levels and leptin resistance. Consequently, leptin replacement therapy had minimal impact on weight in patients with multifactorial obesity and, therefore, has no role in treatment of multifactorial obesity [41–43].

2.2 MC4R Agonist

The MC4R agonist setmelanotide is approved by the European Medical association for treatment of obesity and hunger in patients with POMC, PCSK1 and LEPR deficiency, and Bardet Biedl syndrome. Although studies in rodents with diet-induced obesity treated with MC4R agonists have shown promising results, these were not observed in humans with multifactorial obesity [44]. Additional studies followed in which specifically patients with certain types of genetic obesity were treated. A phase three non-randomized controlled trial (NRCT), including twelve adults and nine children ≥6 years with POMC, PCSK1, and LEPR deficiency, showed a mean weight decrease of −25.6% ± 9.9 in all patients with POMC or PCSK1 deficiency and −12.5% ± 8.9 in all patients with LEPR deficiency [45]. In children with POMC and LEPR deficiency a decrease in BMI z-score was observed after twelve months of treatment, −1.6 ± 0.9 and −0.5 ± 0.4 ($n = 3$), respectively [45]. Moreover, improved appetite regulation and quality of life were reported during setmelanotide treatment in these patients [46, 47]. Setmelanotide might also be safe and effective to treat children with genetic obesity younger than six years [48]. Two longer-term studies showed sustained weight-reducing effects of setmelanotide in both POMC deficiency and LEPR deficiency after at least four years of treatment [49, 50]. Patients with Bardet-Biedl syndrome (BBS) and Alström syndrome (AS) that were treated with setmelanotide also showed weight reductions. The phase three NRCT, including adults and children aged ≥6 years with BBS, showed a mean weight decrease of −7.6% ± 7.1 in the adults and a −17.3% ± 7.7 decrease in BMI percent of the 95th percentile (BMI%P95) in children, decreases in maximal hunger score, and improvements in health-related quality of life measures [51, 52]. In patients with AS, the results of setmelanotide treatment were inconclusive. Importantly, this weight-reducing potential of setmelanotide was not observed in a study including nine patients with heterozygous MC4R deficiency (mean weight loss of −3.1% (95% CI of −4.11 to −2.04) after 29 days of treatment) [53]. The most frequently reported side-effect is hyperpigmentation of skin, lips, and naevi, which is related to cross stimulation of the melanocortin-1 receptor [54]. This has, until now, not evolved into increased risk of malignant lesions, however studies with longer follow-up are needed [49]. Other reported side-effects are injection site reactions, such as pain, erythema and pruritus, nausea, and vomiting [45, 51, 53, 55, 56].

Currently, multiple phase two and three trials are being performed to investigate the impact of setmelanotide treatment in patients with obesity due to defects in other genes that are part of the leptin-melanocortin pathway. These studies include patients with pathogenic *SH2B1* or *SRC1* variants who have shown varying effects on weight during setmelanotide treatment [57, 58]. The patients who continued treatment due to experienced clinical benefit demonstrated a sustained weight loss after twelve months of treatment (mean percent BMI change of −10.1% ± 9.4 in *SRC1* and −9.7% ± 8.0 in *SH2B1*) [59, 60].

3 Currently Approved Non-targeted Anti-obesity Agents

An overview of the approved non-targeted anti-obesity agents by the EMA and FDA is shown in Table 2. The effects of these AOMs have mostly been described in observational studies, including case reports, case series and small cohort studies, which are prone to publication bias. Consequently, long-term placebo-controlled randomized controlled trials (RCT) are needed in future.

Table 2 Overview of available regular non-targeted anti-obesity agents

Anti-obesity medication	Mechanism of action	Approved age categories by EMA	Approved age categories by FDA
Lipase inhibitors	Lipase inhibition	Adults	Adults Children ≥12 years
Phentermine	Noradrenergic sympathomimetic amine	n.a.	Adults Children ≥16 years
Phentermine-topiramate	Noradrenergic sympathomimetic amine (phentermine) and carbonic anhydrase inhibitor and glutamate receptor antagonist (topiramate)	n.a.	Adults Children ≥12 years
Naltrexone-bupropion	μ-opioid antagonist (naltrexone) and selective inhibitor of neuronal dopamine and norepinephrine reuptake (bupropion)	Adults	Adults
Liraglutide	GLP-1 receptor agonist, short-acting	Adults Children ≥12 years	Adults Children ≥12 years
Semaglutide	GLP-1 receptor agonist, long-acting	Adults Children ≥12 years	Adults Children ≥12 years
Tirzepatide	Dual GIP and GLP-1 receptor agonist, long-acting	Adults	Adults

Abbreviations: *GLP-1* glucagon-like peptide-1, *GIP* glucose-dependent insulinotropic polypeptide, *EMA* European Medicines Agency, *n.a.* not approved, *FDA* U.S. Food and Drug Administration

3.1 Lipase Inhibitor

Orlistat is the most well-known lipase inhibitor. Several meta-analyses reported modest effects of orlistat on weight in patients with multifactorial obesity [61, 62]. The most recent meta-analysis, including 49,810 adults, showed a decrease in body weight of −3.16% (95% CI −3.53 to −2.78) at follow-up after twelve to 104 weeks of treatment [61]. Similar results were observed in a long-term study of four years [63]. A meta-analysis of the effects of orlistat in children with obesity showed no significant effect of orlistat on body weight, BMI or metabolic parameters [64]. In these studies, a large proportion (ranges 6.4% to 48.5%), discontinued treatment due to lack of therapeutic response and/or side-effects [61–63, 65]. One reported seventeen-year-old adolescent with heterozygous MC4R deficiency did not show any weight loss during lifestyle changes, metformin, and orlistat treatment [66]. No other studies investigating the effect of orlistat in patients with genetic obesity disorders are available. The side effects include mainly gastrointestinal symptoms, such as flatulence, diarrhoea, mild steatorrhea, and faecal incontinence [67]. Furthermore, it is recommended to monitor fat-soluble vitamins levels, as these can decrease due to the reduced fat absorption [67]. The combination of minimal therapeutic response together with significant side-effects, has resulted in orlistat not being frequently prescribed in clinical practice.

3.2 *Short-Term Phentermine*

Adults with obesity were treated with phentermine for twelve weeks, which showed placebo-subtracted weight losses of −3.0 to −6.4 kg [19]. Patients reported significantly larger reduction of cravings for fats and sweets [68]. One study has investigated phentermine in six patients with heterozygous MC4R deficiency, showing a significant mean weight loss of −15.5% ± 2.9 after six months of treatment [69]. Additionally, non-significant improvements of percentage fat mass and muscle mass, several glucose indices, and leptin levels were observed [69]. Similar side-effects as in patients with multifactorial obesity were observed. Commonly reported side-effects are dry mouth, insomnia, dizziness, palpitations, constipation, and psychiatric adverse effects such as agitation, irritability and anxiety [19, 70].

3.3 *Phentermine-Topiramate*

There are two large RCTs with phentermine-topiramate treatment reported. Adults with obesity or overweight in combination with more than two obesity-related co-morbidities who were treated with phentermine-topiramate for 56 weeks, showed placebo-subtracted weight losses at maximum dose of −9.3% and −8.6% [71, 72]. A sustained effect was observed in a long-term study of 106 weeks of treatment [73, 74]. Children aged ≥12 years with obesity have also been treated with phentermine-topiramate, demonstrating a −10.4% (95% CI of −13.9 to −6.9) decrease in BMI after 56 week of treatment at maximum dose [75]. Interestingly, weight-related quality of life did not improve. No literature is available about the effects of phentermine-topiramate treatment in patients with genetic obesity. Phentermine-topiramate might be effective as well for patients with genetic obesity disorders, as the study of Salazar et al. showed beneficial effects of phentermine treatment as monotherapy in patients with heterozygous MC4R deficiency [69]. Frequently reported side effects are constipation, paraesthesia, dry mouth, dysgeusia, and psychiatric adverse events such as insomnia and anxiety [71–74].

3.4 *Naltrexone-Bupropion*

A large study, including 1496 adults with overweight or obesity, revealed a −6.4% weight loss after 56 weeks of treatment with naltrexone-bupropion [76]. Additionally, improvements in cardiometabolic risk factors, such as waist circumference, lipids, and fasting insulin, weight-related quality of life and control of eating were observed [76]. The effects of naltrexone-bupropion in patients with genetic obesity disorders have been investigated in two separate studies. In the largest study, eleven patients with molecularly-confirmed genetic obesity (specific gene defects not reported) were treated with naltrexone-bupropion. This study demonstrated a weight loss of −5.2% ± 5.8, a fat mass decrease of −3.9% ± 2.8, improved self-reported appetite in 90.9%, and improved obesity-related comorbidities in significant proportions of patients. There was no placebo or control group [77]. Similar results were seen in 22 patients suspected for a genetic obesity disorder, but without definite diagnosis [77]. This study includes the patient described in a separate case report [7]. Evidently, more research is needed to evaluate the effectiveness of naltrexone-bupropion on weight and hyperphagia in patients with genetic obesity. Commonly reported side-effects were nausea, constipation, headache, insomnia, dry mouth, and dizziness [76]. Importantly, possible psychiatric adverse effects, such as anxiety, depression and sleep disorders, can occur [78]. Naltrexone-bupropion is not approved by the FDA and EMA for obesity treatment in children (<18 years).

3.5 Liraglutide and Semaglutide

The first RCT with once daily 3.0 mg liraglutide showed a mean reduction of −8.0% ± 6.7 of body weight after 56 weeks of treatment in adults with obesity [79]. Similar results were observed in a long-term study of 160 weeks in adults with pre-diabetes with obesity or overweight combined with one or more obesity-related co-morbidity, including a 66% risk reduction for progression to type 2 diabetes [80]. Also in children with obesity, these beneficial effects have been reported: after liraglutide treatment, the BMI SD-score decreased with −0.22 (95% CI, −0.37 to −0.08) with a relative BMI change of −4.64% (95% CI, −7.14 to −2.14), compared to placebo [81]. Studies with once weekly 2.4 mg semaglutide followed, showing stronger effect on weight reduction. Mean body weight in adults with obesity decreased with −14.9% and −15.2% after resp. 68 and 104 weeks of treatment [82, 83]. Additionally, semaglutide led to a sustained suppressed appetite resulting in an improved control of eating and reduced food cravings in the two years of treatment [84, 85]. In adolescents (aged twelve to <18 years) with obesity, similar weight reductions (−16.1%) were observed. In both adults and adolescents, improvements in cardiometabolic risk factors, such as waist circumference, glycaemic indices and lipids, were reported during semaglutide treatment [23, 86]. The cardioprotective potency of semaglutide was also shown in two studies reporting a reduced incidence of death from cardiovascular causes in patients with obesity who had pre-existing cardiovascular disease and improved exercise function in patients with obesity-related heart failure with preserved ejection fraction [22, 24]. GLP-1 analogues are the most studied non-targeted anti-obesity agents in patients with genetic obesity. The largest real-world study was performed in 30 adults with Alström syndrome, reporting a mean body weight decrease of −5.4 kg (−6%) ± 1.7 and improved satiety using a VAS-score after six months of treatment [87]. Another observational study in eighteen adults with molecularly confirmed genetic obesity treated with 3.0 mg liraglutide for four months, demonstrated a −4.7% (IQR −6.0 to −1.5%) decrease in body weight, −0.9% ± 2.7 decrease in fat mass, improved self-reported appetite in 83.3%, and improved obesity-related comorbidities in significant proportions of patients [77]. Similar results were seen in 59 patients suspected for a genetic obesity disorder, but without molecularly confirmed diagnosis [77]. Another study in patients with obesity, including fourteen adults with heterozygous MC4R deficiency, treated with 3.0 mg liraglutide for sixteen weeks reported a weight loss of −5.7% ± 1.4 and improved cardiometabolic factors, such as fat mass, waist circumference and fasting glucose [88]. Similar weight-reducing effects and appetite suppressing potential were reported in smaller case series, including a case series of four adults with 16p11.2 deletion syndrome ($n = 2$) and heterozygous MC4R deficiency ($n = 2$) and several case reports in children with heterozygous or homozygous MC4R deficiency, an adult with biallelic MC4R deficiency, and a patient with molecularly confirmed BBS type 10 [5, 66, 89–91]. Frequently reported side effects of GLP-1 analogues are gastro-intestinal, such as nausea, vomiting, constipation, and diarrhoea [79, 81, 82, 86]. A severe but rare adverse effect of GLP-1 analogues is pancreatitis [92], which has not been observed in children so far.

3.6 Tirzepatide

Jastreboff et al. evaluated the effect of 15 mg tirzepatide for 72 weeks in 2539 adults with obesity [93]. They showed a weight decrease of −20.9% (95% CI, −21.8 to −19.9), next to improvements in cardiometabolic risk parameters, such as waist circumference, blood pressure, insulin and lipids. In 95.3% of patients with prediabetes, tirzepatide was able to convert glucose levels to normoglycemia, compared to 61.9% patients in the placebo-treated group [93]. No literature is available yet about the effects of tirzepatide on weight in genetic obesity, besides one conference paper reporting a −28.0 kg (−20%) decrease of excess body weight during three months of treatment in an adult with a heterozygous VUS in *MC4R* [94]. Commonly reported side-effects of tirzepatide were nausea, diarrhoea, constipation, dyspepsia, vomiting, and headache [93]. Episodes of hypoglycaemia may arise when sulphonylurea, insulin, or metformin are used concurrently [95].

4 Off-Label Use of Other Pharmacological Agents

Several non-targeted pharmacological agents have been used off-label for obesity treatment in patients with genetic obesity. This is particularly the case in paediatric obesity treatment, as for a long time no anti-obesity agents were approved for children. The most described off-label pharmacotherapeutical agents are central nervous stimulants, such as dextroamphetamine, methylphenidate, sibutramine, and fluvoxamine. These are thought to affect the hedonic dopaminergic system and the homeostatic leptin-melanocortin pathway [96, 97]. Multiple case series have described beneficial effects of these agents on weight, BMI, and appetite in both children and adults [98–103]. Clinicians should be aware of possible increase in blood pressure, necessitating appropriate treatment. Future research is needed to evaluate the long-term efficacy and side effects of these agents. Metformin is also being used as off-label pharmacotherapeutical agent for obesity treatment. On group level, metformin has modest effects on weight in both adults and children with obesity [104, 105]. There are three case reports on the effect of metformin on weight and appetite in patients with genetic obesity: one reports weight stabilization in a child with POMC deficiency and otherwise progressive weight gain, while the two other case reports, including two children with heterozygous or homozygous MC4R deficiency, report no effect [66, 90, 106]. Lastly, growth hormone has been used to effectively improve body composition and reduce weight in patients with Prader Willi Syndrome, Temple syndrome and Schaaf- Yang syndrome [107–111].

5 Summary

Patients with genetic obesity and/ or hyperphagia require pharmacotherapy in addition to multidisciplinary lifestyle interventions. In these patients, treatment aims may be different compared to patients with multifactorial obesity. Treatment may also be considered successful when the progressive weight gain halts or when hyperphagia is reduced leading to an improved quality of life. Since they suffer from chronic and relapsing obesity, a trial-and-error treatment approach appears to be most appropriate. If a particular anti-obesity agent fails to yield the desired effects, the decision can be made to switch to an alternative anti-obesity agent or to start an additional anti-obesity agent. Great advances have been made in pharmacotherapeutical options for obesity in the last couple of years, with the availability of several anti-obesity agents as result. Currently, patients with certain genetic obesity disorders can be treated with targeted pharmacotherapy, such as leptin replacement therapy and setmelanotide. Now that these targeted pharmacotherapies are available, it is of utmost importance to test patients who are highly suspected of these genetic obesity disorders. Additionally, non-targeted anti-obesity pharmacotherapies, such as GLP-1 analogues and naltrexone-bupropion, are available for patients with obesity, with or without a molecularly confirmed genetic obesity gene defects. In the future, novel and innovative pharmacotherapeutical options, including gene therapy, will emerge, offering promising and possibly long-term effects on body weight, hyperphagia, and, most importantly, health and quality of life.

References

1. Kitahara CM, Flint AJ, Berrington de Gonzalez A, Bernstein L, Brotzman M, MacInnis RJ, et al. Association between class III obesity (BMI of 40–59 kg/m^2) and mortality: a pooled analysis of 20 prospective studies. PLoS Med. 2014;11(7):e1001673.
2. Lung T, Jan S, Tan EJ, Killedar A, Hayes A. Impact of overweight, obesity and severe obesity on life expectancy of Australian adults. Int J Obes. 2019;43(4):782–9.

3. Nagai M, Kuriyama S, Kakizaki M, Ohmori-Matsuda K, Sone T, Hozawa A, et al. Impact of obesity, overweight and underweight on life expectancy and lifetime medical expenditures: the Ohsaki Cohort Study. BMJ Open. 2012;2(3):e000940.
4. Trier C, Hollensted M, Schnurr TM, Lund MAV, Nielsen TRH, Rui G, et al. Obesity treatment effect in Danish children and adolescents carrying Melanocortin-4 receptor mutations. Int J Obes. 2021;45(1):66–76.
5. Welling MS, de Groot CJ, Kleinendorst L, van der Voorn B, Burgerhart JS, van der Valk ES, et al. Effects of glucagon-like peptide-1 analogue treatment in genetic obesity: a case series. Clin Obes. 2021;11(6):e12481.
6. Welling MS, Kleinendorst L, van Haelst MM, van den Akker ELT. The narrative of a patient with leptin receptor deficiency: personalized medicine for a rare genetic obesity disorder. Obes Facts. 2023;16(5):514–8.
7. Welling MS, Mohseni M, van der Valk ES, van Hagen JM, Burgerhart JS, van Haelst MM, van Rossum EFC. Successful naltrexone-bupropion treatment after several treatment failures in a patient with severe monogenic obesity. iScience. 2023;26(3):106199.
8. Wadden TA, Bailey TS, Billings LK, Davies M, Frias JP, Koroleva A, et al. Effect of subcutaneous Semaglutide vs placebo as an adjunct to intensive behavioral therapy on body weight in adults with overweight or obesity: the STEP 3 randomized clinical trial. JAMA. 2021;325(14):1403–13.
9. Wadden TA, Hollander P, Klein S, Niswender K, Woo V, Hale PM, et al. Weight maintenance and additional weight loss with liraglutide after low-calorie-diet-induced weight loss: the SCALE maintenance randomized study. Int J Obes. 2013;37(11):1443–51.
10. Wadden TA, Foreyt JP, Foster GD, Hill JO, Klein S, O'Neil PM, et al. Weight loss with naltrexone SR/bupropion SR combination therapy as an adjunct to behavior modification: the COR-BMOD trial. Obesity (Silver Spring). 2011;19(1):110–20.
11. Cooiman MI, Alsters SIM, Duquesnoy M, Hazebroek EJ, Meijers-Heijboer HJ, Chahal H, et al. Long-term weight outcome after bariatric surgery in patients with melanocortin-4 receptor gene variants: a case-control study of 105 patients. Obes Surg. 2022;32(3):837–44.
12. Vos N, Oussaada SM, Cooiman MI, Kleinendorst L, Ter Horst KW, Hazebroek EJ, et al. Bariatric surgery for monogenic non-syndromic and syndromic obesity disorders. Curr Diab Rep. 2020;20(9):44.
13. Kuhnen P, Krude H, Biebermann H. Melanocortin-4 receptor signalling: importance for weight regulation and obesity treatment. Trends Mol Med. 2019;25(2):136–48.
14. Farr OM, Tsoukas MA, Mantzoros CS. Leptin and the brain: influences on brain development, cognitive functioning and psychiatric disorders. Metabolism. 2015;64(1):114–30.
15. Guerciolini R. Mode of action of orlistat. Int J Obes Relat Metab Disord. 1997;21(Suppl 3):S12–23.
16. Rothman RB, Baumann MH. Appetite suppressants, cardiac valve disease and combination pharmacotherapy. Am J Ther. 2009;16(4):354–64.
17. Kalyanasundar B, Perez CI, Luna A, Solorio J, Moreno MG, Elias D, et al. D1 and D2 antagonists reverse the effects of appetite suppressants on weight loss, food intake, locomotion, and rebalance spiking inhibition in the rat NAc shell. J Neurophysiol. 2015;114(1):585–607.
18. Lewis RG, Florio E, Punzo D, Borrelli E. The brain's reward system in health and disease. Adv Exp Med Biol. 2021;1344:57–69.
19. Pilitsi E, Farr OM, Polyzos SA, Perakakis N, Nolen-Doerr E, Papathanasiou AE, Mantzoros CS. Pharmacotherapy of obesity: available medications and drugs under investigation. Metabolism. 2019;92:170–92.
20. Billes SK, Sinnayah P, Cowley MA. Naltrexone/bupropion for obesity: an investigational combination pharmacotherapy for weight loss. Pharmacol Res. 2014;84:1–11.
21. He Z, Gao Y, Lieu L, Afrin S, Cao J, Michael NJ, et al. Direct and indirect effects of liraglutide on hypothalamic POMC and NPY/AgRP neurons—implications for energy balance and glucose control. Mol Metab. 2019;28:120–34.
22. Kosiborod MN, Abildstrom SZ, Borlaug BA, Butler J, Rasmussen S, Davies M, et al. Semaglutide in patients with heart failure with preserved ejection fraction and obesity. N Engl J Med. 2023;389(12):1069–84.

23. Kosiborod MN, Bhatta M, Davies M, Deanfield JE, Garvey WT, Khalid U, et al. Semaglutide improves cardiometabolic risk factors in adults with overweight or obesity: STEP 1 and 4 exploratory analyses. Diabetes Obes Metab 2023;25(2):468–478.
24. Lincoff AM, Brown-Frandsen K, Colhoun HM, Deanfield J, Emerson SS, Esbjerg S, et al. Semaglutide and cardiovascular outcomes in obesity without diabetes. N Engl J Med. 2023;389(24):2221–32.
25. Bendotti G, Montefusco L, Lunati ME, Usuelli V, Pastore I, Lazzaroni E, et al. The anti-inflammatory and immunological properties of GLP-1 receptor agonists. Pharmacol Res. 2022;182:106320.
26. Aranas C, Edvardsson CE, Shevchouk OT, Zhang Q, Witley S, Blid Skoldheden S, et al. Semaglutide reduces alcohol intake and relapse-like drinking in male and female rats. EBioMedicine. 2023;93:104642.
27. Chuong V, Farokhnia M, Khom S, Pince CL, Elvig SK, Vlkolinsky R, et al. The glucagon-like peptide-1 (GLP-1) analogue semaglutide reduces alcohol drinking and modulates central GABA neurotransmission. JCI. Insight. 2023;8(12)
28. Drucker DJ. The cardiovascular biology of glucagon-like Peptide-1. Cell Metab. 2016;24(1):15–30.
29. Samms RJ, Coghlan MP, Sloop KW. How may GIP enhance the therapeutic efficacy of GLP-1? Trends Endocrinol Metab. 2020;31(6):410–21.
30. Farooqi IS, Jebb SA, Langmack G, Lawrence E, Cheetham CH, Prentice AM, et al. Effects of recombinant leptin therapy in a child with congenital leptin deficiency. N Engl J Med. 1999;341(12):879–84.
31. Farooqi IS, Matarese G, Lord GM, Keogh JM, Lawrence E, Agwu C, et al. Beneficial effects of leptin on obesity, T cell hyporesponsiveness, and neuroendocrine/metabolic dysfunction of human congenital leptin deficiency. J Clin Invest. 2002;110(8):1093–103.
32. Gibson WT, Farooqi IS, Moreau M, DePaoli AM, Lawrence E, O'Rahilly S, Trussell RA. Congenital leptin deficiency due to homozygosity for the Δ133G mutation: report of another case and evaluation of response to four years of leptin therapy. J Clin Endocrinol Metab. 2004;89(10):4821–6.
33. von Schnurbein J, Heni M, Moss A, Nagel SA, Machann J, Muehleder H, et al. Rapid improvement of hepatic steatosis after initiation of leptin substitution in a leptin-deficient girl. Horm Res Paediatr. 2013;79(5):310–7.
34. Wabitsch M, Funcke JB, Lennerz B, Kuhnle-Krahl U, Lahr G, Debatin KM, et al. Biologically inactive leptin and early-onset extreme obesity. N Engl J Med. 2015;372(1):48–54.
35. Von Schnurbein J, Remy M, Brandt S, Manzoor J, Kohlsdorf K, Mahmood S, et al. Preliminary evidence for a strong effect of leptin on mood and behaviour in patients with congenital leptin deficiency. Horm Res Paediatr. 2022;95:223.
36. Licinio J, Caglayan S, Ozata M, Yildiz BO, de Miranda PB, O'Kirwan F, et al. Phenotypic effects of leptin replacement on morbid obesity, diabetes mellitus, hypogonadism, and behavior in leptin-deficient adults. Proc Natl Acad Sci USA. 2004;101(13):4531–6.
37. Paz-Filho G, Esposito K, Hurwitz B, Sharma A, Dong C, Andreev V, et al. Changes in insulin sensitivity during leptin replacement therapy in leptin-deficient patients. Am J Physiol Endocrinol Metab. 2008;295(6):E1401–8.
38. Galgani JE, Greenway FL, Caglayan S, Wong ML, Licinio J, Ravussin E. Leptin replacement prevents weight loss-induced metabolic adaptation in congenital leptin-deficient patients. J Clin Endocrinol Metab. 2010;95(2):851–5.
39. Ajluni N, Dar M, Xu J, Neidert AH, Oral EA. Efficacy and safety of metreleptin in patients with partial lipodystrophy: lessons from an expanded access program. J Diabetes Metab. 2016;7(3)
40. Chan JL, Koda J, Heilig JS, Cochran EK, Gorden P, Oral EA, Brown RJ. Immunogenicity associated with metreleptin treatment in patients with obesity or lipodystrophy. Clin Endocrinol. 2016;85(1):137–49.
41. Zelissen PM, Stenlof K, Lean ME, Fogteloo J, Keulen ET, Wilding J, et al. Effect of three treatment schedules of recombinant methionyl human leptin on body weight in obese adults: a randomized, placebo-controlled trial. Diabetes Obes Metab. 2005;7(6):755–61.

42. Moon HS, Matarese G, Brennan AM, Chamberland JP, Liu X, Fiorenza CG, et al. Efficacy of metreleptin in obese patients with type 2 diabetes: cellular and molecular pathways underlying leptin tolerance. Diabetes. 2011;60(6):1647–56.
43. Shetty GK, Matarese G, Magkos F, Moon HS, Liu X, Brennan AM, et al. Leptin administration to overweight and obese subjects for 6 months increases free leptin concentrations but does not alter circulating hormones of the thyroid and IGF axes during weight loss induced by a mild hypocaloric diet. Eur J Endocrinol. 2011;165(2):249–54.
44. Fani L, Bak S, Delhanty P, van Rossum EF, van den Akker EL. The melanocortin-4 receptor as target for obesity treatment: a systematic review of emerging pharmacological therapeutic options. Int J Obes. 2014;38(2):163–9.
45. Clement K, van den Akker E, Argente J, Bahm A, Chung WK, Connors H, et al. Efficacy and safety of setmelanotide, an MC4R agonist, in individuals with severe obesity due to LEPR or POMC deficiency: single-arm, open-label, multicentre, phase 3 trials. Lancet Diabetes Endocrinol. 2020;8(12):960–70.
46. Kuhnen P, Wabitsch M, von Schnurbein J, Chirila C, Mallya UG, Callahan P, et al. Quality of life outcomes in two phase 3 trials of setmelanotide in patients with obesity due to LEPR or POMC deficiency. Orphanet J Rare Dis. 2022;17(1):38.
47. Wabitsch M, Fehnel S, Mallya UG, Sluga-O'Callaghan M, Richardson D, Price M, Kuhnen P. Understanding the patient experience of hunger and improved quality of life with setmelanotide treatment in POMC and LEPR deficiencies. Adv Ther. 2022;39(4):1772–83.
48. Dubern B, Lourdelle A, Clement K. Beneficial effects of setmelanotide in a 5-year-old boy with POMC deficiency and on his caregivers. JCEM Case Rep. 2023;1(3):luad041.
49. Kühnen P, Clément K. Long-term MC4R agonist treatment in POMC-deficient patients. N Engl J Med. 2022;387(9):852–4.
50. Wendy Chung JS, Peter Kühnen, Martin Wabitsch, Erica van den Akker, Jill Garrison, Guojun Yuan, Jesús Argente, Karine Clément, Sadaf Farooqi. 4-year setmelanotide weight outcomes of patients with POMC and LEPR deficiency obesity. ECE 20242024.
51. Haqq AM, Chung WK, Dollfus H, Haws RM, Martos-Moreno GA, Poitou C, et al. Efficacy and safety of setmelanotide, a melanocortin-4 receptor agonist, in patients with Bardet-Biedl syndrome and Alstrom syndrome: a multicentre, randomised, double-blind, placebo-controlled, phase 3 trial with an open-label period. Lancet Diabetes Endocrinol. 2022;10(12):859–68.
52. Forsythe E, Haws RM, Argente J, Beales P, Martos-Moreno GA, Dollfus H, et al. Quality of life improvements following one year of setmelanotide in children and adult patients with Bardet-Biedl syndrome: phase 3 trial results. Orphanet J Rare Dis. 2023;18(1):12.
53. Collet TH, Dubern B, Mokrosinski J, Connors H, Keogh JM, Mendes de Oliveira E, et al. Evaluation of a melanocortin-4 receptor (MC4R) agonist (Setmelanotide) in MC4R deficiency. Mol Metab. 2017;6(10):1321–9.
54. Kanti V, Puder L, Jahnke I, Krabusch PM, Kottner J, Vogt A, et al. A Melanocortin-4 receptor agonist induces skin and hair pigmentation in patients with monogenic mutations in the leptin-melanocortin pathway. Skin Pharmacol Physiol. 2021;34(6):307–16.
55. Haws R, Brady S, Davis E, Fletty K, Yuan G, Gordon G, et al. Effect of setmelanotide, a melanocortin-4 receptor agonist, on obesity in Bardet-Biedl syndrome. Diabetes Obes Metab. 2020;22(11):2133–40.
56. Argente J, Clément K, Van Den Akker E, Wabitsch M, Kühnen P, Farooqi S, et al. Clinical safety summary of setmelanotide in healthy volunteers with obesity and patients with rare genetic diseases of obesity. Horm Res Paediatr. 2022;95:180–2.
57. Argente J, Farooqi S, Oral E, Goldstone A, Ohayon O, Scimia C, et al. Efficacy and safety results of a phase 2 trial of setmelanotide in obesity due to SH2B1 variants and 16p11.2 deletion syndrome. Horm Res Paediatr. 2021;94(SUPPL 1):30.
58. Farooqi S, Argente J, Martos-Moreno G, Oral E, Spiliotis B, Kostopoulou E, et al. A phase 2 trial of the melanocortin-4 receptor agonist setmelanotide in obesity due to src1 insufficiency: body weight, body mass index z score, and safety results. Horm Res Paediatr. 2021;94(SUPPL 1):31–2.

59. Martos-Moreno GÁ, Argente J, Scimia C, Ohayan O, Yuan G, Farooqi S. Body mass index and weight reductions in patients with SRC1 genetic variant obesity after 1 year of Setmelanotide. J Endocr Soc. 2022;6:A13–A4.
60. Argente J, Farooqi S, Chung W, Wabitsch M, Scimia C, Srinivasan M, Hu S. Body mass index and weight reduction in patients with SH2B1 genetic variant obesity after one year of Setmelanotide. J Endocr Soc. 2022;6:A35.
61. Shi Q, Wang Y, Hao Q, Vandvik PO, Guyatt G, Li J, et al. Pharmacotherapy for adults with overweight and obesity: a systematic review and network meta-analysis of randomised controlled trials. Lancet. 2022;399(10321):259–69.
62. Singh AK, Singh R. Pharmacotherapy in obesity: a systematic review and meta-analysis of randomized controlled trials of anti-obesity drugs. Expert Rev Clin Pharmacol. 2020;13(1):53–64.
63. Torgerson JS, Hauptman J, Boldrin MN, Sjostrom L. XENical in the prevention of diabetes in obese subjects (XENDOS) study: a randomized study of orlistat as an adjunct to lifestyle changes for the prevention of type 2 diabetes in obese patients. Diabetes Care. 2004;27(1):155–61.
64. Nikniaz Z, Nikniaz L, Farhangi MA, Mehralizadeh H, Salekzamani S. Effect of Orlistat on anthropometrics and metabolic indices in children and adolescents: a systematic review and meta-analysis. BMC Endocr Disord. 2023;23(1):142.
65. Dong Z, Xu L, Liu H, Lv Y, Zheng Q, Li L. Comparative efficacy of five long-term weight loss drugs: quantitative information for medication guidelines. Obes Rev. 2017;18(12):1377–85.
66. Çamtosun E, Akıncı A, Kayaş L, Çiftçi N, Tekedereli İ. Liraglutide treatment experience in morbid obese adolescent with a MC4R gene variant: side effects reduce success. J Clin Res Pediatr Endocrinol. 2021;
67. Filippatos TD, Derdemezis CS, Gazi IF, Nakou ES, Mikhailidis DP, Elisaf MS. Orlistat-associated adverse effects and drug interactions: a critical review. Drug Saf. 2008;31(1):53–65.
68. Moldovan CP, Weldon AJ, Daher NS, Schneider LE, Bellinger DL, Berk LS, et al. Effects of a meal replacement system alone or in combination with phentermine on weight loss and food cravings. Obesity (Silver Spring). 2016;24(11):2344–50.
69. Salazar-Valencia IG, Villamil-Ramirez H, Barajas-Olmos F, Guevara-Cruz M, Macias-Kauffer LR, Garcia-Ortiz H, et al. Effect of the Melanocortin 4-receptor Ile269Asn mutation on weight loss reşponse to dietary, phentermine and bariatric surgery interventions. Genes (Basel). 2022;13(12)
70. Munro JF, MacCuish AC, Wilson EM, Duncan LJ. Comparison of continuous and intermittent anorectic therapy in obesity. Br Med J. 1968;1(5588):352–4.
71. Allison DB, Gadde KM, Garvey WT, Peterson CA, Schwiers ML, Najarian T, et al. Controlled-release phentermine/topiramate in severely obese adults: a randomized controlled trial (EQUIP). Obesity (Silver Spring). 2012;20(2):330–42.
72. Gadde KM, Allison DB, Ryan DH, Peterson CA, Troupin B, Schwiers ML, Day WW. Effects of low-dose, controlled-release, phentermine plus topiramate combination on weight and associated comorbidities in overweight and obese adults (CONQUER): a randomised, placebo-controlled, phase 3 trial. Lancet. 2011;377(9774):1341–52.
73. Smith SM, Meyer M, Trinkley KE. Phentermine/topiramate for the treatment of obesity. Ann Pharmacother. 2013;47(3):340–9.
74. Garvey WT, Ryan DH, Look M, Gadde KM, Allison DB, Peterson CA, et al. Two-year sustained weight loss and metabolic benefits with controlled-release phentermine/topiramate in obese and overweight adults (SEQUEL): a randomized, placebo-controlled, phase 3 extension study. Am J Clin Nutr. 2012;95(2):297–308.
75. Kelly AS, Bensignor MO, Hsia DS, Shoemaker AH, Shih W, Peterson C, Varghese ST. Phentermine/topiramate for the treatment of adolescent obesity. NEJM Evid. 2022;1(6)
76. Apovian CM, Aronne L, Rubino D, Still C, Wyatt H, Burns C, et al. A randomized, phase 3 trial of naltrexone SR/bupropion SR on weight and obesity-related risk factors (COR-II). Obesity (Silver Spring). 2013;21(5):935–43.

77. Welling MS, dGCJ, Mohseni M, Meeusen REH, Boon MR, van Haelst MM, van den Akker ELT, van Rossum EFC. Treatment with liraglutide or naltrexone-bupropion in patients with genetic obesity: a real-world study. eClin Med. 2024;74:102709.
78. Pi-Sunyer X, Apovian CM, McElroy SL, Dunayevich E, Acevedo LM, Greenway FL. Psychiatric adverse events and effects on mood with prolonged-release naltrexone/bupropion combination therapy: a pooled analysis. Int J Obes. 2019;43(10):2085–94.
79. Pi-Sunyer X, Astrup A, Fujioka K, Greenway F, Halpern A, Krempf M, et al. A randomized, controlled trial of 3.0 mg of Liraglutide in weight management. N Engl J Med. 2015;373(1):11–22.
80. le Roux CW, Astrup A, Fujioka K, Greenway F, Lau DCW, Van Gaal L, et al. 3 years of liraglutide versus placebo for type 2 diabetes risk reduction and weight management in individuals with prediabetes: a randomised, double-blind trial. Lancet. 2017;389(10077):1399–409.
81. Kelly AS, Auerbach P, Barrientos-Perez M, Gies I, Hale PM, Marcus C, et al. A randomized, controlled trial of Liraglutide for adolescents with obesity. N Engl J Med. 2020;382(22):2117–28.
82. Wilding JPH, Batterham RL, Calanna S, Davies M, Van Gaal LF, Lingvay I, et al. Once-weekly Semaglutide in adults with overweight or obesity. N Engl J Med. 2021;384(11):989–1002.
83. Garvey WT, Batterham RL, Bhatta M, Buscemi S, Christensen LN, Frias JP, et al. Two-year effects of semaglutide in adults with overweight or obesity: the STEP 5 trial. Nat Med. 2022;28(10):2083–91.
84. Friedrichsen M, Breitschaft A, Tadayon S, Wizert A, Skovgaard D. The effect of semaglutide 2.4 mg once weekly on energy intake, appetite, control of eating, and gastric emptying in adults with obesity. Diabetes Obes Metab. 2021;23(3):754–62.
85. Wharton S, Batterham RL, Bhatta M, Buscemi S, Christensen LN, Frias JP, et al. Two-year effect of semaglutide 2.4 mg on control of eating in adults with overweight/obesity: STEP 5. Obesity (Silver Spring). 2023;31(3):703–15.
86. Weghuber D, Barrett T, Barrientos-Perez M, Gies I, Hesse D, Jeppesen OK, et al. Once-weekly Semaglutide in adolescents with obesity. N Engl J Med. 2022;387(24):2245–57.
87. Ali S, Baig S, Wanninayake S, da Silva Xavier G, Dawson C, Paisey R, Geberhiwot T. Glucagon-like peptide-1 analogues in monogenic syndromic obesity: real-world data from a large cohort of Alstrom syndrome patients. Diabetes Obes Metab. 2023;
88. Iepsen EW, Zhang J, Thomsen HS, Hansen EL, Hollensted M, Madsbad S, et al. Patients with obesity caused by melanocortin-4 receptor mutations can be treated with a glucagon-like peptide-1 receptor agonist. Cell Metab 2018;28(1):23–32.e23.
89. Iepsen EW, Have CT, Veedfald S, Madsbad S, Holst JJ, Grarup N, et al. GLP-1 receptor agonist treatment in morbid obesity and type 2 diabetes due to pathogenic homozygous melanocortin-4 receptor mutation: a case report. Cell Rep Med. 2020;1(1):100006.
90. Zaitoon H, Lubetzky R, Amir AZ, Moran-Lev H, Sagi L, Yacobi-Bach M, et al. Glucagon-like peptide-1 analog therapy in rare genetic diseases: monogenic obesity, monogenic diabetes, and spinal muscular atrophy. Acta Diabetol. 2023;60:1099–108.
91. Ganawa S, Santhosh SH, Parry L, Syed AA. Weight loss with glucagon-like peptide-1 receptor agonists in Bardet-Biedl syndrome. Clin Obes. 2022;12(5)
92. Sodhi M, Rezaeianzadeh R, Kezouh A, Etminan M. Risk of gastrointestinal adverse events associated with glucagon-like Peptide-1 receptor agonists for weight loss. JAMA. 2023;330(18):1795–7.
93. Jastreboff AM, Aronne LJ, Ahmad NN, Wharton S, Connery L, Alves B, et al. Tirzepatide once weekly for the treatment of obesity. N Engl J Med. 2022;387(3):205–16.
94. Mubeen F, Andre KS, Shakil J. Abstract #1411741: genetic obesity case with 2 heterozygote variants: MKS1 and MC4R in which weight loss managed with Tirzepatide. Endocr Pract. 2023;29(5):S39.

95. Tang Y, Zhang L, Zeng Y, Wang X, Zhang M. Efficacy and safety of tirzepatide in patients with type 2 diabetes: a systematic review and meta-analysis. Front Pharmacol. 2022;13:1016639.
96. Lau J, Farzi A, Qi Y, Heilbronn R, Mietzsch M, Shi YC, Herzog H. CART neurons in the arcuate nucleus and lateral hypothalamic area exert differential controls on energy homeostasis. Mol Metab. 2018;7:102–18.
97. Seiden LS, Sabol KE, Ricaurte GA. Amphetamine: effects on catecholamine systems and behavior. Annu Rev Pharmacol Toxicol. 1993;33:639–77.
98. Albayrak O, Albrecht B, Scherag S, Barth N, Hinney A, Hebebrand J. Successful methylphenidate treatment of early onset extreme obesity in a child with a melanocortin-4 receptor gene mutation and attention deficit/hyperactivity disorder. Eur J Pharmacol. 2011;660(1):165–70.
99. Brandt S, von Schnurbein J, Lennerz B, Kohlsdorf K, Vollbach H, Denzer C, et al. Methylphenidate in children with monogenic obesity due to LEPR or MC4R deficiency improves feeling of satiety and reduces BMI-SDS—A case series. Pediatr Obes. 2020;15(1)
100. Menendez A, Williams J, Trapp C. BMI Z-score reduction following combination therapy with topiramate and lisdexamfetamine in a pediatric patient with hyperphagia and early onset obesity due to a novel variant of uncertain significance in the BDNF gene. Horm Res Paediatr. 2023;96:264–6.
101. van Schaik J, Welling MS, de Groot CJ, van Eck JP, Juriaans A, Burghard M, et al. Dextroamphetamine treatment in children with hypothalamic obesity. Front Endocrinol. 2022:13.
102. Kor Y, Kor D. Can obesity associated with LEPR gene mutations be treated with fluvoxamine? A case report. Horm Res Paediatr. 2017;88:533–4.
103. Hainerová IA, Zamrazilová H, Sedláčková D, Hainer V. Hypogonadotropic hypogonadism in a homozygous MC4R mutation carrier and the effect of sibutramine treatment on body weight and obesity-related health risks. Obes Facts. 2011;4(4):324–8.
104. Lentferink YE, Knibbe CAJ, van der Vorst MMJ. Efficacy of metformin treatment with respect to weight reduction in children and adults with obesity: a systematic review. Drugs. 2018;78(18):1887–901.
105. Pu R, Shi D, Gan T, Ren X, Ba Y, Huo Y, et al. Effects of metformin in obesity treatment in different populations: a meta-analysis. Ther Adv Endocrinol Metab. 2020;11:2042018820926000.
106. Hilado MA, Randhawa RS. A novel mutation in the proopiomelanocortin (POMC) gene of a Hispanic child: metformin treatment shows a beneficial impact on the body mass index. J Pediatr Endocrinol Metab. 2018;31(7):815–9.
107. Hebach NR, Caro P, Martin-Giacalone BA, Lupo PJ, Marbach F, Choukair D, Schaaf CP. A retrospective analysis of growth hormone therapy in children with Schaaf–Yang syndrome. Clin Genet 2021;100(3):298–307.
108. Juriaans AF, Trueba-Timmermans DJ, Kerkhof GF, Grootjen LN, Walet S, Sas TCJ, et al. The effects of 5 years of growth hormone treatment on growth and body composition in patients with Temple syndrome. Horm Res Paediatr. 2023;96(5):483–94.
109. Stalman SE, Kamp GA, Hendriks YMC, Hennekam RCM, Rotteveel J. Positive effect of growth hormone treatment in maternal uniparental disomy chromosome 14. Clin Endocrinol. 2015;83(5):671–6.
110. Passone CGB, Franco RR, Ito SS, Trindade E, Polak M, Damiani D, Bernardo WM. Growth hormone treatment in Prader-Willi syndrome patients: systematic review and meta-analysis. BMJ Paediatr Open. 2020;4(1):e000630.
111. Rosenberg AGW, Passone CGB, Pellikaan K, Damiani D, van der Lely AJ, Polak M, et al. Growth hormone treatment for adults with Prader-Willi syndrome: a meta-analysis. J Clin Endocrinol Metab. 2021;106(10):3068–91.

Metabolic Bariatric Surgery

Mellody Cooiman, Edo Aarts, Frits Berends, and Mieke van Haelst

1 Introduction

Since obesity is a potential life threatening condition, it is of the utmost importance to offer a sustainable treatment. Previous chapters shed light on non-invasive obesity treatment options, such as improvement of physical activity, lower energy consumption, lifestyle changes and pharmacotherapy to induce weight loss and improve obesity associated disorders. However, in some patients with severe (genetic) obesity these adjustments lack the ability of achieving durable weight loss with relapsing cardiovascular or metabolic complications as a result. Metabolic surgery (previously named bariatric surgery) is currently the most effective option for common (severe) obesity in adults. The results in genetic obesity disorders are less studied. This chapter will highlight the working mechanisms of Metabolic Bariatric Surgery (MBS) and gives an overview of weight outcomes in patients with genetic obesity, as described in the other chapters.

2 Changing Normal Anatomy

MBS involves procedures to the gastro-intestinal tract inducing metabolic changes and thereby weight loss. The National Institutes of Health (NIH) and the International Federation for the Surgery of Obesity and Metabolic Disorders (IFSO) composed

M. Cooiman (✉) · M. van Haelst
Department of Human Genetics, Section Clinical Genetics, Amsterdam University Medical Center, Amsterdam, The Netherlands
e-mail: m.vanhaelst@amsterdamumc.nl

E. Aarts · F. Berends
WeightWorks Amersfoort, Amersfoort, The Netherlands

M. van Haelst, E. van den Akker (eds.), *Clinical Obesity Genetics*,
https://doi.org/10.1007/978-3-032-04095-4_16

international guidelines for surgical obesity interventions. In 1991 the first NIH consensus statement, confined MBS surgery to patients with a BMI of at least 40 kg/m^2 or a BMI of ≥35 kg/m^2 and at least one obesity associated condition such as type 2 diabetes mellitus or hypertension [1, 2]. Recently, the American Society for Metabolic and Bariatric Surgery (ASMBS) and IFSO published new recommendations according the eligibility for MBS (October 2022) [3]. These guidelines now recommend MBS for patients with a BMI ≥35 kg/m^2 regardless of presence/absence or severity of obesity associated conditions. Also, patients with type 2 diabetes mellitus (T2DM) and a BMI ≥30 kg/m^2 are now regarded suitable to undergo MBS. Besides these numerical prerequisites, patients have to change their eating behavior and lifestyle for the rest of their lives. Combined lifestyle intervention before and after surgery, is recommended to improve lifestyle and decrease body weight through professional guidance, is recommended [4].

The choice of intervention depends on the evaluation of several (individual) patient characteristics and often on the patients' and surgeons' preference and varies greatly regionally. Worldwide, approximately 90%, undergo either a Sleeve Gastrectomy (SG) or a Roux-en-Y Gastric Bypass (RYGB).

2.1 *Surgical Techniques*

The SG is currently the most performed procedure worldwide [5]. By removing 2/3 part (or 70–80%) of the greater curvature section of the stomach through a longitudinal resection, it restricts dietary intake (Fig. 1). The diameter of the 'tube'

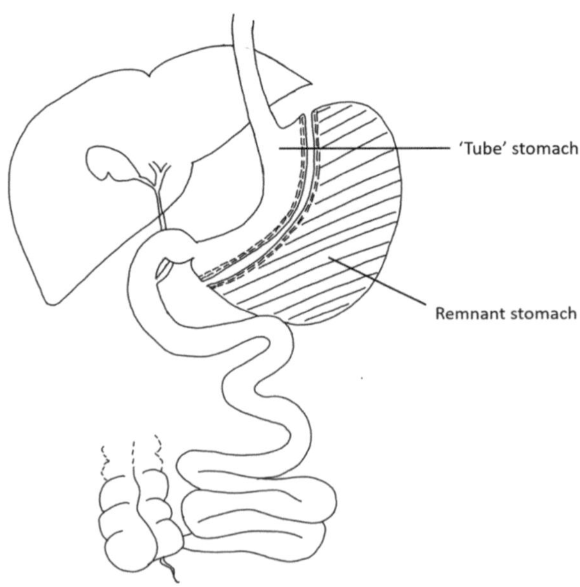

Fig. 1 Sleeve Gastrectomy

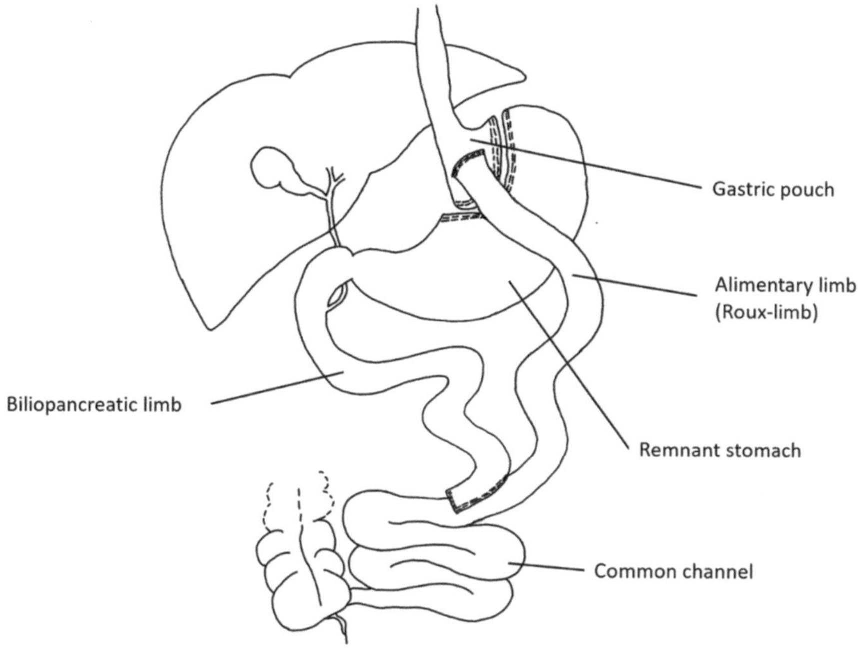

Fig. 2 Roux-en-Y Gastric Bypass

stomach that is left is calibrated along a bougie, ensuring the possibility of food passage [6].

The RYGB includes a restriction in dietary intake by the creation of a gastric 'pouch' of approximately 30 cc (Fig. 2) [7]. The remnant stomach is left in situ but is disconnected from the normal route of ingested nutrients. This is combined with a change in the normal anatomy of the small bowel, by bypassing approximately 150 cm (varying between 50 and 250 cm worldwide) of the distal part of the stomach, duodenum and proximal part of the small bowel. The actual digestion of ingested nutrients is theoretically delayed to the part of the small bowel where these nutrients are joined by the digestive peptides and cholic acids, i.e. in the (middle) jejunum [5, 7].

3 Metabolic Effects

Previously it was thought that the primary aim of a RYGB was to induce weight loss through mechanical restriction of dietary intake, combined with micronutrient malabsorptive aspects, which alter eating behaviours, such as volume and food choice [5, 8]. However, recent research has highlighted the significant role of MBS in changing incretine levels, modifying complex gut-brain-endocrine and adipose-brain-endocrine signalling pathways that regulate hunger, satiety, body weight, as well as glucose- and immunometabolism [8].

The postoperative changes in various components within these pathways, including incretins, gut hormones, bile acids, and gut microbiota, have been extensively studied. Below is a brief overview, though not exhaustive, of these changes.

1. Incretines and gut hormones

Removing 2/3 part of the greater curvature section of the stomach during SG surgery results in short-term lower levels of the hunger hormone ghrelin. An increased postprandial secretion of glucagon-like-peptide 1 (GLP-1), glucagon-like-peptide 2 (GLP-2), peptide YY (PYY) and cholecystokinin (CCK) is reported after both SG and RYGB [9, 10]. GLP-1 and GLP-2 are produced by L-cells in the (distal) ileum, resulting in delayed gastric emptying, increased insulin secretion (by GLP-1), increased mucosal crypt depth and absorptive surface area of the gut (by GLP-2) [11–13].

L-cells are an important part of the enteroendocrine cell population of the lower gastrointestinal tract. CCK is produced by L-cells in the duodenum and proximal part of the intestines, regulating increased food satiety, energy expenditure and insulin secretion after SG. CCK also stimulates gallbladder contraction and thereby bile acid production [14, 15]. PYY is produced by L-cells of the ileum and colon, regulating increased food satiety and decreased food intake [12, 16, 17]. All above mentioned effects induce a decrease in body weight and food intake, diabetes resolution and an increase in metabolic control.

2. Bile acids

In the normal situation, bile acids will be mixed with ingested nutrients in the duodenum, i.e. after the papilla of Vater (major duodenal papilla). However, after RYGB surgery bile acids will be mixed with ingested nutrients in the common channel, after flowing down the biliopancreatic limb (BPL) (Fig. 3). Results from mice studies suggested that the bile acids in the BPL might have a signaling role. With a direct effect in insulin resistance by increasing energy expenditure in brown adipose tissue [18, 19]. Bile acid synthesis in the liver is regulated via Farnesoid X receptor (FXR), G protein-coupled bile acid receptor−1 (Gpbar-1, also known as TGR5), and Fibroblast Growth Factor 19 and 21 (FGF-19 and FGF-21) [20, 21]. Besides the role in the negative feedback loop, FGF-19 is thought to contribute to the increased metabolic rate and decreased adiposity seen after RYGB [22]. Furthermore, animal studies suggested that bile acids might have a direct and indirect effect on the gut microbiota [19, 22].

The role of bile acids in the improved metabolic state following MBS is not yet fully understood. However, it is likely that the combined effects of changes in bile acids and gut hormone levels/functions contribute to the long-term metabolic benefits seen after these surgical procedures.

3. Gut microbiota

The human gut is the host of more than trillions of microbes with a collective genome, also named the gut microbiome [23]. The gut microbiome is thought to be

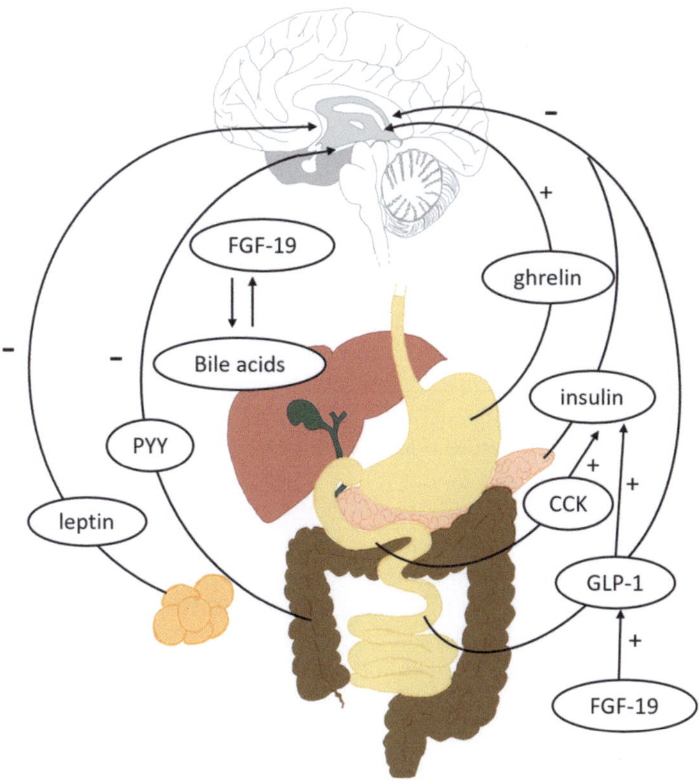

Fig. 3 Gut hormones, incretines. + anorexigenic by stimulating alpha-melanocyt-stimulating hormone.—orexigenic by stimulating neuropeptide-Y. Peptide-YY anorexigenic by blocking neuropeptide-Y

a linking factor between food intake resulting in obesity, metabolic alterations such as insulin resistance and intestinal inflammation [24]. For example, some microbes produce lipopolysaccharides which are pro-inflammatory molecules, affecting metabolism by mediating the immune response [24, 25].

Analysis of the gut microbiome of patients with (severe) obesity revealed an alteration in composition with reduced microbial diversity and reduced gene richness compared to lean patients [26–31]. Both dietary and surgically induced weight loss, have been reported to result in an increase in microbial gene richness and a shift in the microbial composition towards a lean composition [26, 28, 32]. The gut microbiome also play an important role in bile acid regulation, via FXR (farnesoid X- receptor), and the glucose and lipid metabolism [23, 33].

Further research is needed to explore the specific interactions between the gut microbiome and bile acids and their significant role in metabolism, particularly in cases following metabolic bariatric surgery.

4 (Weight) Outcome

Both SG and RYGB result in durable weight loss and remission of obesity complications in the majority of patients. Weight loss after MBS is often reported as percentage Excess Body Weight Loss (%EWL), and preferably as percentage Total Weight Loss (%TWL). The mean %TWL that has been reported in the long term varies between 25–30% for SG and 30–35% for RYGB [4, 34–37]. As stated earlier in this chapter, obesity is associated with varying obesity complications, in particular T2DM. A large number of patients experience improvement or even remission of their T2DM, i.e. discontinuation of anti-diabetic medication, shortly after MBS, in particular after RYGB [4, 37]. The remission rate depends on several factors, such as the duration and severity of the T2DM and dependence on insulin treatment and is correlated with the amount of weight loss in the long term [38].

Weight outcome after MBS varies widely and is thought to be a dynamic process. The initial maximum weight loss response is generally achieved within the first 2 years after the procedure [39, 40]. However, the majority of patients tend to regain 5–10% of their total weight loss within the first decade [39, 41]. This is illustrated by large long-term studies, such as the Swedish Obese Subjects (SOS) study, which reported a decrease in %TWL from 32 to 25% within 10 years after RYGB [39]. Overall, it seems that some recurrent weight gain after MBS is common. Previous mentioned weight loss percentages are the result of studies among large metabolic bariatric cohorts worldwide. However, the percentage of patients with genetic obesity in these cohorts is unknown. In 2020 a study was published reporting the first MBS cohort in which the prevalence of genetic obesity was established. It showed a proven molecular genetic obesity diagnosis of 3% [42]. Since then, the field of genetic obesity research expanded enormously, with many 'new' genetic obesity diagnoses as a result. Given these developments, it is anticipated that the prevalence of genetic obesity diagnoses in metabolic bariatric cohorts will be higher than previously thought.

4.1 Syndromic Obesity

4.1.1 Prader-Willi Syndrome (PWS)

Six studies investigated RYGB surgery outcomes in 11 patients with Prader-Willi syndrome (PWS) [43–47]. Their mean age was 25.1 years, and their initial BMI was 50.3 kg/m^2 (ranging from 42.3 to 68.7 kg/m^2). Among them, three pediatric patients, averaging 15 years of age, had a mean baseline BMI of 55.9 kg/m^2 (47.0 to 69.0 kg/m^2). Within 48 months after surgery, PWS patients showed significantly less weight loss compared to controls (−7.0% (95% CI: −13·6 to −0·5%; $p = 0.034$). Adjustments for age, sex, and baseline T2DM did not alter these outcomes. Short-term complications, such as aspiration pneumonia and intestinal perforation, were reported in two patients, with no long-term complications noted. However, the resolution of obesity-associated complications was not described.

Seven studies examined the effects of SG in 34 patients with PWS [48–54]. The majority of the patients were male (59%), with an average age of 12.9 years (range 4.9–23 years) and baseline BMI of 49.3 kg/m^2 (range 30.1–80.9 kg/m^2). In comparison to the control group, patients with PWS showed lower %TBWL) (−12.9; 95% CI:-19.6 to −6.2; $p \leq 0.001$) within 36 months of follow-up.

The rate of complications and (resolution of) obesity-related complications were not reported.

4.1.2 16p11.2 Microdeletion Syndrome

RYGB surgery outcomes were documented in two individuals with 16p11.2 microdeletion syndrome [55]. One of the patients died 2 days after surgery; the cause of death was not specified. The other patient achieved a 37.5% weight loss after 1 year, maintaining a substantial 27.2% decrease from baseline weight during a 10-year follow-up period.

4.1.3 Bardet-Biedl Syndrome (BBS)

Two case reports detailed uncomplicated RYGB surgery in two individuals with Bardet Biedl syndrome (BBS-gene variants not reported). In the first case, a 16-year-old boy had a BMI reduction from 52.3 to 34.8 kg/m^2 over 42 months, along with improved hypertension control and mobility [56]. Similarly, a 17-year-old BBS patient undergoing RYGB surgery achieved an excess weight loss (EWL) of 28.1% after 12 months. The impact on comorbidity resolution was not discussed [57]. Additionally, the effects of SG were documented in three patients with BBS [50, 58, 59]. These patients exhibited similar responses to SG on weight-related parameters compared to controls, with one patient followed for 36 months after surgery. However, there is limited data available following both types of MBS in genetic obesity regarding complication rates and the resolution of obesity-related complications.

4.2 Monogenic Non-syndromic Obesity

4.2.1 Leptin Receptor (LEPR)

A single case report outlined the weight loss trajectory of a 24-year-old woman with bi-allelic pathogenic *LEPR* variants and a baseline BMI of 81 kg/m^2 [60]. Following uneventful RYGB surgery, she achieved a 15% weight loss within 6 months but experienced a 5% weight regain over the subsequent 12 months.

Additionally, a case report details an eight-year-old girl with a homozygous pathogenic variant in *LEPR* who underwent surgery twice, first at 11 months and subsequently at the age of eight [61]. By the age of eight, she had developed hypertension, dyslipidemia, and T2DM, with a BMI of 35.2 kg/m^2. Following surgery, her BMI decreased significantly to 25.1 kg/m^2 within 3 months and continued to decline over the 3-year follow-up, reaching 22.7 kg/m^2. Notably, while she still exhibited hypertension, she no longer had dyslipidemia or T2DM.

4.2.2 Pro-opiomelanocortin (POMC)—Obesity Risk Factor

Fifteen patients with (likely) pathogenic monoallelic *POMC* variants undergoing RYGB surgery were studied across two case series [42, 62]. Predominantly female (75%), this cohort held an average age of 44.7 years and a BMI of 47.6 kg/m^2 (ranging from 38.0 to 70.6 kg/m^2). Over a follow-up period of up to 60 months, they achieved weight loss similar to that of the control group. Comparative data on short- and long-term complications and resolution of obesity complications post-surgery are lacking.

Two patients (a 28-year-old female and a 57-year-old male) were previously reported with (likely) pathogenic monoallelic *POMC* variants who underwent uncomplicated SG surgery [42]. After 24 months post-surgery, their BMI decreased from 43.2 to 28.5 kg/m^2 and from 56.5 to 28.3 kg/m^2, respectively. No information on the resolution of obesity-related complications was available.

4.2.3 Melanocortin-4 Receptor (MC4R)

One report described weight loss outcomes following RYGB surgery in a family with pathogenic bi-allelic *MC4R* variants [63]. Two family members, aged 16 and 17, exhibited contrasting results with baseline BMIs of 40.8 kg/m^2 and 81.1 kg/m^2, respectively. While the first patient regained all the lost weight and reverted to baseline weight, the other achieved a significant weight loss of 30.9%. Post-surgery, hypertension resolved in the first patient, and both remained free of complications.

In seven publications 31 patients with (likely) pathogenic monoallelic *MC4R* variants were reported [42, 62, 64–68]. Within this cohort the majority was female (73%) with a mean age of 42.6 years and a baseline BMI of 48.8 kg/m^2 (range 38.5–76.7 kg/m^2). Weight loss outcomes were comparable to those of the control group post-RYGB surgery during the total follow-up period. Documentation of post-surgical complications was limited; however, three case reports indicated no complications.

Two case series report the effect of SG in five children (2 boys, 3 girls) with bi-allelic pathogenic *MC4R* variants, with an average age of 11.7 years (range 8–11 years) and BMI of 65.1 kg/m^2 (range 52.0–73.0 kg/m^2) [63, 69]. Within 1 year, they experienced a mean TWL of 21.5%. However, this percentage decreased to a

TWL of −1.9% after 24 months. No information regarding the resolution of obesity complications post-surgery was provided.

Three studies examined the weight outcomes of 12 patients who underwent SG with a (likely) pathogenic monoallelic *MC4R* variant [42, 65, 70]. Of these patients, 55% was female, with an average age of 37 years at baseline. Their baseline BMI ranged from 37.3 to 72.2 kg/m^2, with a mean of 53 kg/m^2. They reported a significantly lower %TBWL compared to the control group (−35.5; 95% CI: −49.7 to −21.4; $p \leq 0.001$). This effect was observed up to a 60-month follow-up period and remained consistent across other weight metrics. Adjustments for age, sex, and baseline T2DM did not alter these results. However, no information regarding complications or the post-surgical resolution of obesity complications was provided.

5 Discussion

5.1 MBS in Syndromic Obesity (Prader Willi Syndrome and Bardet Biedl Syndrome)

Metabolic bariatric surgery in syndromic obesity, particularly in patients with Prader-Willi syndrome (PWS), presents distinct challenges. These patients are characterized by a profound hyperphagic drive, which leads to early-onset obesity [71]. Cases have shown that while procedures like RYGB and SG can help with weight loss, they tend to result in less weight loss for patients with PWS compared to common obesity. In addition, the effects on hyperphagia and complications is not described. This suggests that a more personalized treatment approach is needed.

A review examining weight outcomes from various MBS procedures in 104 cases of PWS showed that the most significant weight loss occurred at one-year after the procedure, regardless of the type of surgery [71]. However, the positive effects were not sustained over time. After 5 years, there were no significant changes compared to baseline, indicating that while MBS may prevent further weight gain in some patients, it is not a long-term solution. The challenge of managing hyperphagia, especially when combined with the altered anatomy post-surgery, raises concerns about the risk of life-threatening complications associated with surgical intervention. Despite this, advancements in pharmacological treatments for hyperphagia, as well as interventions like dietary modifications and growth hormone supplementation, have helped reduce the prevalence of class III obesity in this patient group [72].

Similarly, Bardet Biedl Syndrome (BBS), is also associated with obesity in the majority of cases (72–86%) [73, 74]. MBS procedures, including RYGB and SG, have shown promise in addressing class III obesity and improving related complications in the short term for cases with BBS. However, the long-term effectiveness of these surgeries remains to be validated through further studies.

5.2 MBS in Monogenic Non-syndromic Obesity

The impact of MBS in patients with monogenic non-syndromic obesity is mostly studied in those with (likely) pathogenic *MC4R* variants. MC4R is pivotal in regulating food intake and energy balance, with dysfunctions leading to hyperphagia and varying degrees of obesity severity [75]. Bi-allelic pathogenic *MC4R* variants are rare and associated with severe obesity phenotypes [75], resulting in less weight loss following both RYGB [63] and SG [63, 69] procedures compared to control groups. The suitability of MBS for these patients remains debatable, although it may be considered in individual cases when other interventions fail. Future research, particularly exploring new pharmacotherapeutic options, could help to bridge this therapeutic gap.

In patients with (likely) pathogenic monoallelic *MC4R* variants, RYGB [42, 62, 64–68, 70] can induce weight loss comparable to the control group in the short term, but long-term maintenance poses challenges. Conversely, SG procedures show significantly less weight loss compared to controls over the total follow-up period up to 60 months [42, 65, 70]. Despite recurrent weight gain, RYGB surgery still results in weight loss up to 6 years of follow-up, suggesting it may be a preferable option for these patients. However, managing expectations regarding long-term weight maintenance is crucial.

Bi-allelic (likely) pathogenic *LEPR* variants are extremely rare and give rise to an extreme obesity phenotype [60]. MBS, such as RYGB, can lead to initial weight loss in some individuals with this condition. However, maintaining this progress can be challenging, as seen in one case report where the patient experienced a 5% recurrent weight gain after losing 15% within a year following surgery [76]. Currently, investigational pharmacotherapeutic options, such as setmelanotide, are being explored in individuals with bi-allelic pathogenic *LEPR* variants, showing promising weight reduction of up to 10% after 1 year [77]. These drugs, either as an addition to existing therapies or as standalone options, have the potential to significantly improve outcomes for (these) patients [77]. Further research into novel therapeutic strategies, including drugs targeting multiple receptors, remains crucial in the ongoing fight against obesity.

Initially, only bi-allelic (likely) pathogenic variants in genes like *POMC* and *PCSK1* were known to cause obesity, but (likely) pathogenic monoallelic variants are now recognised as risk factors [78–81]. In two studies, the weight outcomes following RYGB and SG surgeries were examined in 17 patients with monoallelic (likely) pathogenic *POMC* variants [42, 62]. However, the findings revealed no significant difference in weight loss compared to the control group, after a follow-up period of up to 60 months. Additional research is essential to better understand and demonstrate the outcomes of MBS in this particular patient group.

6 Summary

Metabolic bariatric surgery has been shown to induce long-term, durable weight loss in the majority of the general population who suffer from obesity. However, for patients with molecularly confirmed genetic obesity, the results are more variable, depending on the underlying obesity gene defect—i.e. monogenic syndromic or non-syndromic obesity.

In patients with syndromic obesity, MBS may play a modest role in weight reduction, especially in the long term. In the light of potential life threatening side effects, other interventions, such as lifestyle coaching and medication, should be considered as first line of treatment in weight management for these individuals.

For those with monogenic non-syndromic obesity, MBS may offer additional benefits, especially in certain cases where RYGB procedures are performed in patients with mono-allelic (likely) pathogenic *MC4R* variants. However, it's important to be mindful of a potential trend toward weight gain over time, which could be mitigated by incorporating pharmacological interventions.

In the case of patients with genetic obesity caused by rarer genetic variants, such as bi-allelic *MC4R* or *LEPR* variants, it is anticipated that future pharmacological treatments will play a crucial role in weight reduction. MBS, in this specific group of patients, appears to have a limited effect on weight loss.

Take Home Message

- MBS in patients with rare genetic variants, such as bi-allelic *MC4R* or *LEPR* variants, appears to have a limited effect on weight loss. It is anticipated that future pharmacological treatments will play a crucial role in weight reduction.
- In patients with (likely) pathogenic monoallelic *MC4R* variants, RYGB surgery is suggested to be a preferable option, compared to SG surgery. However, managing expectations regarding long-term weight maintenance is crucial.
- Promising pharmacotherapeutic agents like GLP1-agonists and setmelanotide offer hope for expanded treatment options in managing genetic obesity, as standalone therapy or in addition to existing therapies, such as MBS.

References

1. Consensus statement, NIH consensus development conference, gastrointestinal surgery for severe obesity, March 25–27, 1991.
2. Fried M, Yumuk V, Opperts JM, et al. Interdisciplinary European guidelines on metabolic and bariatric surgery. Obes Facts. 2013:449–68.
3. Eisenberg D, Shikora SA, Aarts E, et al. 2022 American society for metabolic and bariatric surgery (ASMBS) and International federation for the surgery of obesity and metabolic

disorders (IFSO): indications for metabolic and bariatric surgery. Surg Obes Relat Dis. 2022;18:1345–56. https://doi.org/10.1016/j.soard.2022.08.013.
4. Mechanick JI, Apovian C, Brethauer S, et al. Clinical practice guidelines for the perioperative nutrion, metabolic, and nonsurgical support of patients undergoing bariatric procedures—2019 update. Obesity. 2020;28(4):1–58.
5. Xu G, Song M. Recent advances in the mechanisms underlying the beneficial effects of bariatric and metabolic surgery. Surg Obes Relat Dis. 2020;17(1):231–8.
6. Angrisani L, Santonicola A, Ionovo P, et al. Bariatric surgery worldwide 2013. Obes Surg. 2015;25:1822–32.
7. Buchwald H. The evolution of metabolic/bariatric surgery. Obes Surg. 2014;24:1026–35.
8. Sinclair P, Brennan DJ, Roux le CW. Gut adaption after metabolic surgery and its influences on the brain, liver and cancer. Nat Rev Gastroenterol Hepatol. 2018;15:606–24.
9. Le Roux CW, et al. Gut hormone profiles following bariatric surgery favor an anorectic state, facilitate weight loss, and improve metabolic parameters. Ann Surg. 2006;243:108–14.
10. Albaugh VL, Flynn RC, Tamboli RA, et al. Recent advances in metabolic and bariatric surgery. F1000Res. 2016:5.
11. Russell-Jones D, Gough S. Recent advances in incretin-based therapies. Clin Endocrinol. 2012;77:489–99.
12. le Roux CW, et al. Gut hypertrophy after gastric bypass is associated with increased glucagon-like peptide 2 and intestinal crypt cell proliferation. Ann Surg. 2010;252:50–6.
13. Romero F, et al. Comparable early changes in gastrointestinal hormones after sleeve gastrectomy and Roux-En-Y gastric bypass surgery for morbidly obese type 2 diabetic subjects. Surg Endosc. 2012;26:2231–9.
14. Kellum JM, et al. Gastrointestinal hormone responses to meals before and after gastric bypass and vertical banded gastroplasty. Ann Surg. 1990;211:763–70.
15. Cote CD, Zadeh-Tahmasebi M, Rasmussen BA, et al. Hormonal signaling in the gut. J Biol Chem. 2014;289:11642–9.
16. Sumithran P, et al. Long-term persistence of hormonal adaptations to weight loss. N Engl J Med. 2011;365:1597–604.
17. Batterham RL, et al. Inhibition of food intake in obese subjects by peptide YY3–36. N Engl J Med. 2003;349:941–8.
18. Brighton CA, et al. Bile acids trigger GLP-1 release predominantly by accessing basolaterally located G protein-coupled bile acid receptors. Endocrinology. 2015;156:3961–70.
19. Watanabe M, et al. Bile acids induce energy expenditure by promoting intracellular thyroid hormone activation. Nature. 2006;439:484–9.
20. Ding L, Sousa KM, Jin L, et al. Vertical sleeve gastrectomy activates GPBAR-1/TGR5 to sustain weight loss, improve fatty liver, and remit insulin resistance in mice. Hepatology. 2016;64:760–73.
21. Li K, Zou J, Song L, et al. Farnesoid X receptor contributes to body weight independent improvement in glycemic control after Roux-en-Y Gastric bypass surgery in diet-induced obese mice. Mol Metab. 2020;37:100980.
22. Begley M, Gahan CGM, Hill C. The interaction between bacteria and bile. FEMS Microbiol Rev. 2005;29:625–51.
23. Brahe LK, Chatelier le E, Prifti E, Pons N, Kennedy S, Hansen T, Pedersen O, Astrup A, Ehrlich SD, Larsen LH. Specific gut microbiotica features and metabolic markers in postmenopausal women with obesity. Nutr Diabetes. 2015;5:e159.
24. Tremaroli V, Backhed F. Functional interactions between the gut microbiota and host metabolism. Nature. 2012;489:242–9.
25. Cani PD, Amar J, Iglesias MA, et al. Metabolic endotoxemia initiates obesity and insulin resistance. Diabetes. 2007;56:1761–72.
26. Palleja A, Kashani A, Allin KH, et al. Roux-en-Y gastric bypass surgery of morbidly obese patients induces swift and persistant changes of the individual gut microbiota. Genome Med. 2016;6:67.

27. Ley RE, Backhed F, Turnbaugh P, et al. Obesity alters gut microbial ecology. Proc Natl Acad Sci USA. 2005;102:11070–5.
28. Ley RE, Turnbaugh PJ, Klein S, et al. Microbial ecology: human gut microbes associated with obesity. Nature. 2006;444:1022–3.
29. Turnbaugh PJ, Ley RE, Mahowald MA, et al. An obesity-associated gut microbiome with increased capacity for energy harvest. Nature. 2006;444:1027–31.
30. Turnbaugh PJ, Hamady M, Yatsunenko T, et al. A core gut microbiome in obese and lean twins. Nature. 2009;457:480–4.
31. Le Chatelier E, Nielsen T, Qin J, et al. Richness of human gut microbiome correlates with metabolic markers. Nature. 2013;500:541–6.
32. Cotillard A, Kennedy SP, Kong LC, et al. Dietary intervention impact on gut microbial gene richness. Nature. 2013;500:585–8.
33. Ocana-Wilhelmi L, Martin-Nunez GM, Ruiz-Limon P, et al. Gut microbiota metabolism of bile acids could contribute to the bariatric surgery improvements in extreme obesity. Meta. 2021;11(11):733.
34. le Roux CW, Heneghan HM. Bariatric surgery for obesity. Med Clin North Am. 2018;108:165–82.
35. Dogan K, Betzel B, Homan J, et al. Long-term effect of laparoscopic Roux-en-Y gastric bypass on diabetes mellitus, hypertension and dyslipidaemia in morbidly obese patients. Obes Surg. 2014;24:1835–42.
36. Homan J, Boerboom A, Aarts E, et al. A longer biliopancreatic limb in Roux-enY gastric bypass improves weight loss in the first years after surgery: results of a randomized controlled trial. Obes Surg. 2018;28(12):3744–55.
37. Peterli R, Wolnerhanssen BK, Vetter D. Laparoscopic sleeve gastrectomy versus Roux-en-Y gastric bypass for morbid obesity-3- year outcomes of the prospective randomized Swiss multicenter bypass or sleeve study (SMBOSS). Ann Surg. 2017;265:466–73.
38. Thereaux J, Lesuffleur T, Czernichow S, et al. Association between bariatric surgery and rates of continuation, discontinuation or initiation of antidiabetic treatment 6 years later. JAMA. 2018;153(6):526–33.
39. Sjöström L. Review of the key results from the Swedish obese subjects (SOS) trial—a prospective controlled intervention study of bariatric surgery. J Intern Med. 2013;273(3):219–34.
40. Adams TD, Davidson LE, Litwin SE, et al. Weight and metabolic outcomes 12 years after gastric bypass. N Engl J Med. 2017;377(12):1143–55.
41. Courcoulas AP, King WC, Belle SH, et al. Seven-year weight trajectories and health outcomes in the longitudinal assessment of bariatric surgery (labs) study. JAMA Surg. 2017;153(5):427–34.
42. Cooiman MI, et al. Genetic obesity and bariatric surgery outcome in 1014 patients with morbid obesity. Obes Surg. 2020;30(2):470–7.
43. Braghetto I, et al. Prader-Willi syndrome (PWS) associated to morbid obesity: surgical treatment. Rev Med Chile. 2003;131(4):427–31.
44. Lujan HG, et al. Gastric bypass in a patient presenting prader willi syndrome. Case report with a 12 year follow-up. Obes Surg. 2015;25(11):1990.
45. Rivas A, et al. Long-term results of laparoscopic Roux-en-Y gastric bypass in two patients with prader-willi syndrome. Obes Surg. 2009;19(8):1053.
46. Hu S, Yang W, Jiang S, Wang C. 6 cases follow up of Prader-Willi syndrome patients after bariatric surgery. Surg Obes Relat Dis. 2019;15(10 Supplement):S232.
47. Wittert GA, Game P, Thompson C. Roux-en-Y gastric bypass for the management of Prader-Willi syndrome. Obes Res Clin Pract. 2013;2:e108–9.
48. Alqahtani AR, et al. Laparoscopic sleeve gastrectomy in children and adolescents with Prader-Willi syndrome: a matched-control study. Surg Obes Relat Dis. 2016;12(1):100–10.
49. Fong AK, Wong SK, Lam CC, Ng EK. Ghrelin level and weight loss after laparoscopic sleeve gastrectomy and gastric mini-bypass for Prader-Willi syndrome in Chinese. Obes Surg. 2012;22(11):1742–5.

50. Iossa A, et al. Laparoscopic sleeve gastrectomy in adolescents with or without syndromic obesity: two years follow-up. Eat Weight Disord. 2017;09:09.
51. Martinelli V, et al. Laparoscopic sleeve gastrectomy in an adolescent with Prader-Willi syndrome: psychosocial implications. Nutrition. 2019;61:67–9.
52. Yu H, Di J, Jia W. Laparoscopic sleeve gastrectomy in Chinese female patient with Prader-Willi syndrome and diabetes. Surg Obes Relat Dis. 2013;9(2):e25–7.
53. Soomro FH, Razzaq A, Siddiq G. Effects of restrictive bariatric surgery on congenital Prader-Willi syndrome: a case report. Cureus. 2022;14(8):e27955.
54. Hu S, et al. Patients with Prader-Willi syndrome (PWS) underwent bariatric surgery benefit more from high-intensity home care. Obes Surg. 2022;32(5):1631–40.
55. Kristensson FM, et al. Long-term effects of bariatric surgery in patients with obesity and chromosome 16 p11.2 microdeletion. Surg Obes Relat Dis. 2017;13(8):1321–5.
56. Daskalakis M, et al. Roux-en-Y gastric bypass in an adolescent patient with Bardet-Biedl syndrome, a monogenic obesity disorder. Obes Surg. 2010;20(1):121–5.
57. Raj PKS, Perumal S, Palanivelu C. Roux en y gastric bypass as a treatment option for obesity in underlying bardet biedl syndrome-first case report. Obes Surg. 2014:1303.
58. Ates U, et al. Pediatric laparoscopic sleeve gastrectomy in Turkey: short-term results. Pediatr Int. 2018;60(5):461–6.
59. Boscolo M, Fery F, Cnop M. Beneficial outcomes of sleeve gastrectomy in a morbidly obese patient with Bardet-Biedl syndrome. J Endocr Soc. 2017;1(4):317–22.
60. Le Beyec J, et al. Homozygous leptin receptor mutation due to uniparental disomy of chromosome 1: response to bariatric surgery. J Clin Endocrinol Metab. 2013;98(2):E397–402.
61. Patil PP, Rajagara S, Dhamankar S, Yalamgonde M, Thakare P. Congenital leptin receptor deficiency: a novel leptin receptor gene mutation in an Indian family producing severe early-onset monogenic obesity. J Pediatr Endocrinol Diabet. 2023;3:29–33.
62. Campos A, et al. Effects of heterozygous variants in the leptin-Melanocortin pathway on Roux-en-Y gastric bypass outcomes: a 15-year case-control study. Obes Surg. 2022;32(8):2632–40.
63. Grinbaum R, et al. The obesogenic and glycemic effect of bariatric surgery in a family with a Melanocortin 4 receptor loss-of-function mutation. Meta. 2022;12(5)
64. Aslan IR, et al. Weight loss after Roux-en-Y gastric bypass in obese patients heterozygous for MC4R mutations. Obes Surg. 2011;21(7):930–4.
65. Cooiman MI, et al. Long-term weight outcome after bariatric surgery in patients with Melanocortin-4 receptor gene variants: a case-control study of 105 patients. Obes Surg. 2022;32(3):837–44.
66. Elkhenini HF, New JP, Syed AA. Five-year outcome of bariatric surgery in a patient with melanocortin-4 receptor mutation. Clin Obes. 2014;4(2):121–4.
67. Bonnefond A, et al. Eating behavior, low-frequency functional mutations in the Melanocortin-4 receptor (MC4R) gene, and outcomes of bariatric operations: a 6-year prospective study. Diabetes Care. 2016;39(8):1384–92.
68. Moore BS, et al. Long-term weight-loss in gastric bypass patients carrying melanocortin 4 receptor variants. PLoS ONE [Electronic Resource]. 2014;9(4):e93629.
69. Jelin EB, et al. Melanocortin-4 receptor signaling is not required for short-term weight loss after sleeve gastrectomy in pediatric patients. Int J Obes. 2016;40(3):550–3.
70. Censani M, et al. Weight loss after bariatric surgery in morbidly obese adolescents with MC4R mutations. Obesity. 2014;22(1):225–31.
71. Gantz MG, et al. Critical review of bariatric surgical outcomes in patients with Prader-Willi syndrome and other hyperphagic disorders. Obesity (Silver Spring). 2022;30(5):973–81.
72. Passone CGB, et al. Growth hormone treatment in Prader-Willi syndrome patients: systematic review and meta-analysis. BMJ Paediatr Open. 2020;4(1):e000630.
73. Forsythe E, Beales PL. Bardet-Biedl syndrome. Eur J Hum Genet. 2013;21(1):8–13.
74. Dollfus H, Lilien MR, Maffei P, et al. Bardet-Biedl syndrome improved diagnosis criteria and management: inter European Reference Networks consensus statement and recommendations. Eur J Hum Genet. 2024;32(11):1347–60.

75. Tao YX. The melanocortin-4 receptor: physiology, pharmacology, and pathophysiology. Endocr Rev. 2010;31(4):506–43.
76. Clement K, Vaisse C, Lahlou N, Cabrol S, Pelloux V, Cassuto D, et al. A mutation in the human leptin receptor gene causes obesity and pituitary dysfunction. Nature. 1998;392(6674):398–401.
77. Clement K, Akker van den E, Argente J, et al. Efficacy and safety of setmelanotide, an MC4R agonist, in individuals with severe obesity due to LEPR or POMC deficiency: single-arm, open-label, multicenter, phase 3 trials. Lancet Diabetes Endocrinol. 2020;8(12):960–70.
78. Creemers JW, Choquet H, Stijnen P, Vatin V, Pigeyre M, Beckers S, et al. Heterozygous mutations causing partial prohormone convertase 1 deficiency contribute to human obesity. Diabetes. 2012;61(2):383–90.
79. Folon L, Baron M, Toussaint B, Vaillant E, Boissel M, Scherrer V, et al. Contribution of heterozygous PCSK1 variants to obesity and implications for precision medicine: a case-control study. Lancet Diabetes Endocrinol. 2023;11(3):182–90.
80. Faccioli N, et al. Current treatments for patients with genetic obesity. J Clin Res Pediatr Endocrinol. 2023;15(2):108–19.
81. Courbage S, et al. Implication of heterozygous variants in genes of the leptin-Melanocortin pathway in severe obesity. J Clin Endocrinol Metab. 2021;106(10):2991–3006.

Future Directions

Circadian Clock Genes

Susanne la Fleur and Lotte Kleinendorst

1 Introduction

Obesity is a multifactorial disease and to understand mechanisms underlying the development of obesity, focus has been on energy intake and energy expenditure as too much food and too little activity contribute to weight gain. Evidence is emerging that not only total intake or expenditure is an important factor for obesity development but also the timing of energy intake and expenditure (thus when you eat or are active) can affect weight gain, and also affect weight loss effectiveness [1]. For example, eating late at night has been associated with weight gain whereas when in a weight loss program eating your lunch late impairs the success of the weight loss therapy [2]. Also people that regularly eat at night, like during shift work, are at increased risk of developing obesity [3]. It has been proposed that the link between shift work and obesity is due to circadian disruption, when your internal biological clock is out of sync with the environment.

S. la Fleur (✉)
Department of Laboratory Medicine, Endocrine Laboratory, Amsterdam Medical Center, University of Amsterdam, Amsterdam, The Netherlands
e-mail: s.e.lafleur@amsterdamumc.nl

L. Kleinendorst
Department of Human Genetics, Section Clinical Genetics, Amsterdam University Medical Center, Amsterdam, The Netherlands

Emma Center for Personalized Medicine, Amsterdam University Medical Center, Amsterdam, The Netherlands
e-mail: L.Kleinendorst@amsterdamumc.nl

M. van Haelst, E. van den Akker (eds.), *Clinical Obesity Genetics*,
https://doi.org/10.1007/978-3-032-04095-4_17

2 Circadian Rhythms

The rotation of the earth around its own axis generates the day-night cycle with a period length of exactly 24 h. To adjust to this environment most living organisms developed a temporal organization of their behavior, as well as their internal physiology. This internal temporality allows an optimal adaptation to the environmental light-dark cycle, for instance, by keeping the organisms awake and aroused at times of food availability and reduced risks from predators and other dangers, thereby increasing the chances of survival [4]. The internal cyclic changes that happen in a cycle of about 24 h are known as 'circadian', a word which comes from Latin meaning around (circa) and day (dies).

Within the body, nearly all processes exhibit circadian fluctuations. This includes metabolic processes, peptide and hormonal production, or gene expression [5, 6]. It's important to note that these cellular rhythms are not operating independently; there is a cell synchronization within tissues and among organs to regulate both physiology and behavior [7]. At the core of the circadian system's hierarchy is the suprachiasmatic nucleus (SCN), situated in the hypothalamus and often referred to as the central brain clock, whereas other brain areas and peripheral organs and tissues that display rhythmic functions are known as peripheral oscillators. The SCN plays a crucial role in coordinating all the oscillators in other parts of the brain and body. This coordination among peripheral clocks results in an internal synchronization, where various cycles are interconnected with each other and synchronized with the SCN.

When the internal rhythmicity is coupled to the external cyclic environment, it is called external synchronization [7]. This circadian rhythmicity of the SCN is synchronized to the exact 24 h rhythm of the external environment through different cues with light being the most potent stimulus [5]. These stimuli that are able to entrain circadian rhythms are referred to as Zeitgeber, which in German means: time-giver. Beyond light, other Zeitgebers such as temperature fluctuations, fasting/feeding cycles, arousal and social cues also play a role in synchronizing circadian rhythms [8–11]. Maintaining proper synchronization between internal and external rhythms is crucial for maintaining a healthy state, while disruptions in this synchronization—whether internally among different organs or externally due to factors like shift work or frequent jet lag—have been associated with an increased susceptibility for various diseases including obesity, type 2 diabetes and cardiovascular disease [12–14].

The SCN generates its rhythm though a group of genes forming a transcriptional-translational feedback loop, known as clock-genes [15]. It is not only the clock genes themselves that are expressed in a circadian fashion, but they also control the rhythmicity of many so-called clock-controlled genes, thereby modifying rhythmic gene expression patterns throughout the whole organism including in metabolic tissues such as muscle, liver, and adipose tissue. However, at the same time, many non-photic environmental factors are also able to regulate the intrinsic expression patterns of the (non-SCN) peripheral clocks.

In a simplified model of the molecular clock, the core components of this system are represented by a positive and a negative limb that signal each other. The positive limb of the loop includes the genes *Clock* and *Bmal1,* whose protein products form a dimer in the cytoplasm (Fig. 1). This dimer moves to the nucleus and binds to the promoter region of the *Per* and *Cry* genes, which are part of the negative limb. Subsequently, these genes are translated into proteins in the cytoplasm that form a dimer and enter back into the nucleus where they act as a repression signal to the different components of the positive limb. When PER/CRY dimers degrade, the transcription of *Clock* and *Bmal1* restarts [15]. Interestingly, the function of the canonical genes in the feedback loop, i.e. *Clock, Bmal1, Per* and *Cry*, can be taken over by homologue genes. For example, the *Npas2* gene can substitute *Clock* in the SCN when it is genetically knocked down [16], and there is evidence of a hierarchy in clock-gene function dependent on the brain area. In the SCN, the proteins encoded from clock genes form a BMAL1/CLOCK dimer, although NPAS2 can substitute.

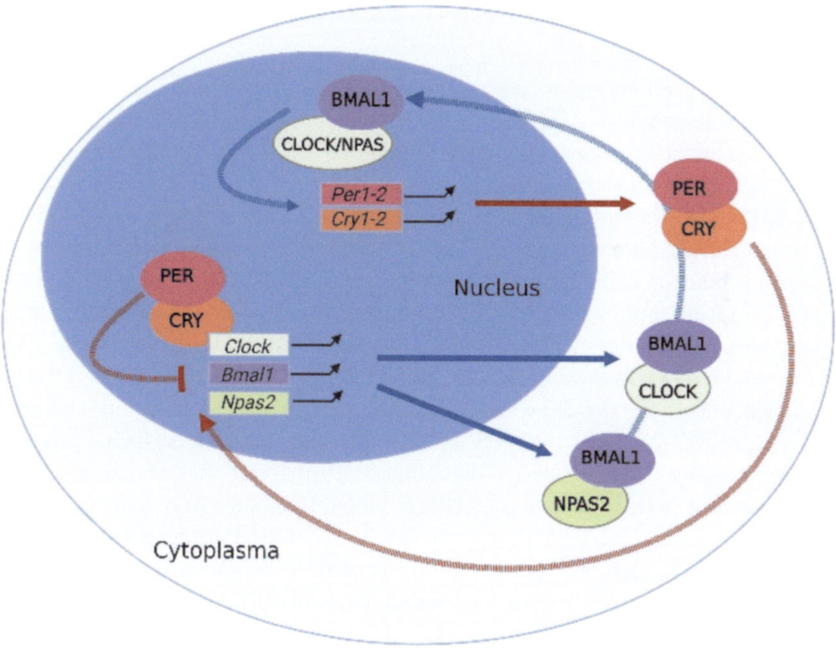

Fig. 1 Simplified model of clock-gene expression. *CLOCK*, *BMAL1* and *NPAS2* genes (rectangles) form the positive limb of the feedback loop, its proteins (ovals) form dimers in the cytoplasm and are translocated into the nucleus (the long blue dashed arrow). In the nucleus, the BMAL1/CLOCK or BMAL/NPAS2 dimer bind to the negative limb (the short blue arrow) elements of the clock-gene loop, *PER* and *CRY* genes (rectangles). The proteins PER and CRY will dimerize in the cytoplasm and translocate to the nucleus (the long red dashed arrow) and inhibit the expression of the clock-gene positive limb elements (the short red blind-ended dashed arrow). (Figure made with Biorender)

In the forebrain, however, NPAS2 has a more important role than BMAL1 in dimer formation [17].

3 Genetic Defects in Clock Genes

Evidence for functional connections between circadian clock genes and the development of obesity and metabolic disorders is emerging. One of the first models to show this connection was that of mice with a disruption of the *Clock* gene which are prone to develop obesity with characteristics of the metabolic syndrome. Moreover, mutations in *Clock* and *Bmal* genes are associated with impaired glucose tolerance and mutant mice show altered daily variation in feeding behavior with higher intake during the inactive (light) period, glucose and triglyceride levels [18–20].

4 Human Polymorphisms in Clock Genes

In line with several animal models, genetic polymorphisms in human clock genes have been associated with increased obesity incidence in epidemiological studies. *PER2* variants were associated with abdominal obesity and different psycho-behavioral factors related to the success of weight loss [21]. In a group of Brazilian individuals, a *PER3* variant showed a significant association with extreme obesity and some *PER3* SNPs were more prevalent in a group of individuals with obesity [22]. And, humans carrying the genetic variant C at the circadian gene *CLOCK* (3111 T/C) were more likely to be obese, had more difficulties in controlling body weight than non-carriers (TT) and had a worse prognosis in dietary weight loss treatments [23–27]. Interestingly, one particular *CLOCK* 3111C SNP (rs1801260) was independently associated with total weight loss in a dietary program with the C carriers loosing ~23% less with the same weight loss intervention than T carriers) [24]. Importantly, the effect of this particular SNP on obesity has also been demonstrated and replicated in several populations with different environment and genetic background [23, 26, 28]. Given that the *CLOCK* 3111C SNP is present in half of the U.S. population [25], it is of great interest for public health to understand underlying mechanisms how this genetic variation impacts obesity.

5 Conclusion

Several studies have shown evidence that circadian disruption can contribute to the development of obesity and related metabolic disorders. Genetic deletion experiments in animals have shown the functional role of different clock genes in obesity development. In humans, several clock gene polymorphisms have been shown to correlate with obesity and the effectiveness of weight loss therapy.

References

1. Mihaylova MM, Chaix A, Delibegovic M, Ramsey JJ, Bass J, Melkani G, et al. When a calorie is not just a calorie: diet quality and timing as mediators of metabolism and healthy aging. Cell Metab. 2023;35(7):1114–31.
2. Garaulet M, Gomez-Abellan P, Alburquerque-Bejar JJ, Lee YC, Ordovas JM, Scheer FA. Timing of food intake predicts weight loss effectiveness. Int J Obes. 2013;37(4):604–11.
3. Sooriyaarachchi P, Jayawardena R, Pavey T, King NA. Shift work and the risk for metabolic syndrome among healthcare workers: a systematic review and meta-analysis. Obes Rev. 2022;23(10):e13489.
4. DeCoursey PJ, Walker JK, Smith SA. A circadian pacemaker in free-living chipmunks: essential for survival? J Comp Physiol A. 2000;186(2):169–80.
5. Dibner C, Schibler U, Albrecht U. The mammalian circadian timing system: organization and coordination of central and peripheral clocks. Annu Rev Physiol. 2010;72:517–49.
6. Kalsbeek A, Perreau-Lenz S, Buijs RM. A network of (autonomic) clock outputs. Chronobiol Int. 2006;23(1–2):201–15.
7. Welsh DK, Logothetis DE, Meister M, Reppert SM. Individual neurons dissociated from rat suprachiasmatic nucleus express independently phased circadian firing rhythms. Neuron. 1995;14(4):697–706.
8. Tahara Y, Shiraishi T, Kikuchi Y, Haraguchi A, Kuriki D, Sasaki H, et al. Entrainment of the mouse circadian clock by sub-acute physical and psychological stress. Sci Rep. 2015;5:11417.
9. Rensing L, Ruoff P. Temperature effect on entrainment, phase shifting, and amplitude of circadian clocks and its molecular bases. Chronobiol Int. 2002;19(5):807–64.
10. Landry GJ, Mistlberger RE. Food entrainment: methodological issues. J Biol Rhythm. 2007;22(6):484–7.
11. Hirao A, Nagahama H, Tsuboi T, Hirao M, Tahara Y, Shibata S. Combination of starvation interval and food volume determines the phase of liver circadian rhythm in Per2::Luc knock-in mice under two meals per day feeding. Am J Physiol Gastrointest Liver Physiol. 2010;299(5):G1045–53.
12. Wyse CA, Selman C, Page MM, Coogan AN, Hazlerigg DG. Circadian desynchrony and metabolic dysfunction; did light pollution make us fat? Med Hypotheses. 2011;77(6):1139–44.
13. Voigt RM, Forsyth CB, Green SJ, Mutlu E, Engen P, Vitaterna MH, et al. Circadian disorganization alters intestinal microbiota. PLoS One. 2014;9(5):e97500.
14. Scheer FA, Hilton MF, Mantzoros CS, Shea SA. Adverse metabolic and cardiovascular consequences of circadian misalignment. Proc Natl Acad Sci USA. 2009;106(11):4453–8.
15. Takahashi JS. Molecular components of the circadian clock in mammals. Diabetes Obes Metab. 2015;17 Suppl 1(0 1):6–11.
16. DeBruyne JP, Weaver DR, Reppert SM. CLOCK and NPAS2 have overlapping roles in the suprachiasmatic circadian clock. Nat Neurosci. 2007;10(5):543–5.
17. Reick M, Garcia JA, Dudley C, McKnight SL. NPAS2: an analog of clock operative in the mammalian forebrain. Science. 2001;293(5529):506–9.
18. Turek FW, Joshu C, Kohsaka A, Lin E, Ivanova G, McDearmon E, et al. Obesity and metabolic syndrome in circadian Clock mutant mice. Science. 2005;308(5724):1043–5.
19. Rudic RD, McNamara P, Curtis AM, Boston RC, Panda S, Hogenesch JB, Fitzgerald GA. BMAL1 and CLOCK, two essential components of the circadian clock, are involved in glucose homeostasis. PLoS Biol. 2004;2(11):e377.

20. Kennaway DJ, Owens JA, Voultsios A, Boden MJ, Varcoe TJ. Metabolic homeostasis in mice with disrupted Clock gene expression in peripheral tissues. Am J Physiol Regul Integr Comp Physiol. 2007;293(4):R1528–37.
21. Garaulet M, Corbalan-Tutau MD, Madrid JA, Baraza JC, Parnell LD, Lee YC, Ordovas JM. PERIOD2 variants are associated with abdominal obesity, psycho-behavioral factors, and attrition in the dietary treatment of obesity. J Am Diet Assoc. 2010;110(6):917–21.
22. Azevedo PG, Miranda LR, Nicolau ES, Alves RB, Bicalho MAC, Couto PP, et al. Genetic association of the PERIOD3 (PER3) Clock gene with extreme obesity. Obes Res Clin Pract. 2021;15(4):334–8.
23. Bandin C, Martinez-Nicolas A, Ordovas JM, Ros Lucas JA, Castell P, Silvente T, et al. Differences in circadian rhythmicity in CLOCK 3111T/C genetic variants in moderate obese women as assessed by thermometry, actimetry and body position. Int J Obes. 2013;37(8):1044–50.
24. Garaulet M, Corbalan MD, Madrid JA, Morales E, Baraza JC, Lee YC, Ordovas JM. CLOCK gene is implicated in weight reduction in obese patients participating in a dietary programme based on the Mediterranean diet. Int J Obes. 2010;34(3):516–23.
25. Garaulet M, Lee YC, Shen J, Parnell LD, Arnett DK, Tsai MY, et al. CLOCK genetic variation and metabolic syndrome risk: modulation by monounsaturated fatty acids. Am J Clin Nutr. 2009;90(6):1466–75.
26. Monteleone P, Tortorella A, Docimo L, Maldonato MN, Canestrelli B, De Luca L, Maj M. Investigation of 3111T/C polymorphism of the CLOCK gene in obese individuals with or without binge eating disorder: association with higher body mass index. Neurosci Lett. 2008;435(1):30–3.
27. Sookoian S, Gemma C, Gianotti TF, Burgueno A, Castano G, Pirola CJ. Genetic variants of Clock transcription factor are associated with individual susceptibility to obesity. Am J Clin Nutr. 2008;87(6):1606–15.
28. Tsuzaki K, Kotani K, Sano Y, Fujiwara S, Takahashi K, Sakane N. The association of the Clock 3111 T/C SNP with lipids and lipoproteins including small dense low-density lipoprotein: results from the Mima study. BMC Med Genet. 2010;11:150.

Functional Assessment of G-Protein Coupled Receptor Variants Associated with Genetic Obesity

Alejandra Rodriguez Rondon, Karina Prins, Patric Delhanty, and Jenny Visser

1 Cellular Signalling

The mammalian cell is a well-organized, stream-lined unit able to respond in a coordinated way to external influences. Signalling molecules are present in the fluids outside this unit and may either be derived from neighbouring cells, in the case of α-melanocyte stimulating hormone (α-MSH), or the circulation, for example leptin. Once these molecules or ligands bind to their dedicated receptor on the cell surface, an intracellular signalling cascade is set in motion. The activated receptor will start to recruit and activate second messengers. These messenger molecules will carry the signal further down into the cell, amplifying the signal and affecting the activity of other proteins and/or changing the ion balance in the cytoplasm. Eventually, this cascade may affect a broad range of cellular outputs, from secretion of neurotransmitters to alterations in gene expression.

Three main classes of receptors reside at the cell membrane: ligand-gated ion channels, G-protein coupled receptors (GPCRs), and receptor kinases (RKs) [1]. As the name implies, ligand-gated ion channels are proteins that allow ions, such as Ca^{2+}, Na^{2+}, and K^{+}, to pass the cell membrane upon ligand binding. These proteins have been associated with obesity [2, 3], but their role in monogenetic obesity is minor. More important in relation to monogenic obesity are the receptor kinases, exemplified by the leptin receptor, but particularly the GPCRs, which are the focus of this book chapter.

A. Rodriguez Rondon · K. Prins · P. Delhanty · J. Visser (✉)
Department of Internal Medicine, Division of Endocrinology, Erasmus MC, University Medical Center Rotterdam, Rotterdam, The Netherlands
e-mail: a.rodriguezrondon@erasmusmc.nl; k.prins@erasmusmc.nl; p.delhanty@erasmusmc.nl; j.visser@erasmusmc.nl

M. van Haelst, E. van den Akker (eds.), *Clinical Obesity Genetics*,
https://doi.org/10.1007/978-3-032-04095-4_18

1.1 G-Protein Coupled Receptors

The G-protein coupled receptor (GPCR) superfamily is one of the most abundant protein classes, comprising approximately 800 membrane bound cell-surface receptors in the human genome [4]. Dysfunction in GPCR signalling can cause diverse pathological conditions, and their vital physiological functions make them important targets for drug development. In addition, variants in several GPCRs are reported to be causative or associated with monogenic obesity [4]. The most common cause of monogenic obesity is due to variants in the *MC4R* gene that encodes the melanocortin 4 G-protein coupled receptor [5, 6]. Gene variants affecting other GPCRs that regulate energy expenditure and metabolism have also been found to be associated with obesity, such as *MC3R* (melanocortin 3 receptor), *ADRB3* (adrenoceptor β3), glucagon receptors (eg. *GCGR*, *GLP1R* and *GIPR*) and *HTR2C* (5-hydroxytryptamine receptor 2c) (Table 1) [4, 7].

GPCRs are structurally characterised as having seven transmembrane domains comprised of hydrophobic α-helices of 25–35 amino acids with an extracellular amino-terminus and intracellular carboxyl-terminus. The site at which ligands bind for many GPCRs occurs within the transmembrane domain. GPCRs are also characterized by their second messenger system. They are coupled via a cytoplasmic crevice to a heterotrimeric G protein complex in an inactive state that is activated upon ligand binding [8]. The G-protein complex consists of Gα and a Gβγ dimer, of which there are 15 Gα, 5 Gβ, and 11 Gγ subunits in humans. Based on the nature of the downstream signalling cascade, Gα subunits are divided into four families:

Table 1 Main GPCRs involved in energy homeostasis and associated in genetic obesity

GPCR	Chromosome	Ligand	Canonical signaling
Body weight regulatory GPCRs with variants associated with obesity[1]			
5-HT2CR [7]	X	Serotonin	$G\alpha_{q/11}$
MC3R [4, 81]	20q13.2	MSH	$G\alpha_s$
MC4R [4, 81]	18q21.3	MSH	$G\alpha_s$
Additional GPCRs involved in body weight regulation[2]			
FFAR1 (GPR40) [4]	19q13.1	Medium–/long-chain FFA	$G\alpha_s/G\alpha_{q/11}$
FFAR4 (GPR120) [4]	10q23.33	Medium–/long-chain FFA	$G\alpha_{q/11}$
GCGR [4, 81]	17q25	Glucagon	$G\alpha_s/G\alpha_{q/11}$
GHSR1a [4, 81]	3q26.2	Ghrelin	$G\alpha_{q/11}$
GIPR [4, 81]	19q13	GIP	$G\alpha_s$
GLP1R [4, 81]	6p21	GLP-1	$G\alpha_s$
MCHR1 [82]	22q13	MCH	$G\alpha_{i/o}/G\alpha_{q/11}$

[1]Variants found in these GPCRs have been associated with obesity in humans
[2]GPCRs involved in metabolic homeostasis and/or potential targets for anti-obesity treatment
Abbreviations: *5-HTR2C* 5-hydroxytryptamine receptor 2 C, *MC3R* melanocortin 3 receptor, *MC4R* melanocortin 4 receptor, *FFA* free fatty acids, *GHSR* growth hormone secretagogue receptor, *GCGR* glucagon receptor, *GLP-1R* glucagon-like peptide-1 receptor, *GIPR* glucose-dependent insulinotropic polypeptide, *MCH1R* melanin concentrating hormone receptor 1, *MCH* melanin concentrating hormone

$G\alpha_{i/o}$, $G\alpha_s$, $G\alpha_{q/11}$, and $G\alpha_{12/13}$ [9]. Each receptor-ligand combination has a preference for one or more of these Gα families, thereby showing a signalling bias. For example, the melanocortin 4 receptor (MC4R) mainly signals through $G\alpha_s$ when stimulated by α-MSH, but can also signal through $G\alpha_q$ upon α-MSH or pharmacological stimulation [10].

Below, we describe GPCR signalling from membrane localization to the Gα subunit-mediated signalling cascades that are initiated by GPCR activation upon ligand binding, also illustrated in Fig. 1. The Gβγ dimer can also activate signalling pathways independently of Gα [11]. However, in this chapter we will mainly focus on the Gα subunit-induced signalling cascade and β-arrestin signalling, because these are currently considered the main signalling pathways of GPCRs.

1.1.1 Cell Membrane Trafficking

After synthesis, GPCRs undergo a process of quality control before being trafficked to the cell membrane. This quality control takes place in the endoplasmic reticulum (ER), where GPCRs interact with chaperones, proteins that assist in folding the GPCR. These chaperones are able to retain the GPCR in the ER when it is misfolded. There, it is either refolded correctly or degraded. This means that variants that result in a misfolded protein can reduce cell membrane availability of the receptor, thereby reducing responsivity of the cell to a ligand [12].

1.1.2 Ligand Binding

On the cell membrane, the receptor can bind its ligand, present in the extracellular space. Ligands bind in a dedicated ligand binding pocket in the receptor. This pocket contains several amino acids that are critical for ligand interaction and bind the ligand primarily through ionic and hydrogen bonds. Binding of the ligand results in a conformational shift of the receptor allowing the activation of the G-protein complex. Ligand binding to the receptor can be inhibited or prevented by the binding of high affinity receptor antagonists, which block access to the ligand binding pocket [13]. Altogether, the binding of ligands and other molecules from the extracellular space are pivotal for GPCR function.

1.1.3 G-Protein Signalling

The Gα subunit plays an important role in mediating downstream signalling of the receptor through binding of either guanosine triphosphate (GTP) or guanosine diphosphate (GDP). When inactive, the Gα-GDP and Gβγ complex are bound to the receptor. The GPCR can be activated by ligand binding, but some receptors also show constitutive activity, i.e. activity without a ligand present. Upon ligand

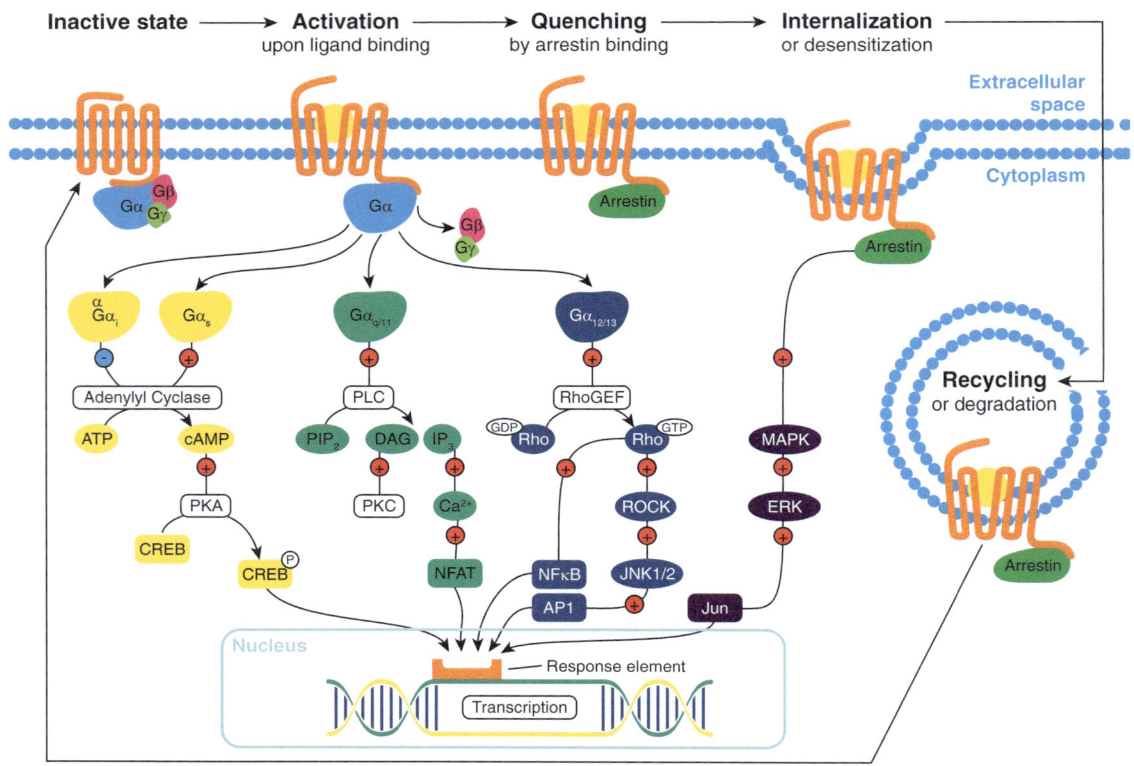

Fig. 1 Schematic diagram of the main GPCR signalling pathways. Activation of a GPCR upon ligand binding leads to the dissociation of G protein subunits. The Gα subunit (e.g. Gα$_i$, Gα$_s$, Gα$_{q/11}$, and Gα$_{12/13}$) activates downstream second messengers (e.g. cAMP or Ca^{2+}) which eventually bind to response elements of target genes and thereby regulate transcription of these genes. GPCR signalling is quenched by the recruitment of β-arrestins to the GPCR. β-arrestins internalize the receptors to either be recycled back to the cell surface or targeted for degradation

binding, a conformational change of the receptor induces the exchange of GDP for GTP at the Gα subunit. The G-protein complex is no longer bound to the receptor, and the GTP-bound Gα subunit dissociates from the Gβγ dimer and initiates an intracellular signalling cascade. The Gα subunit possesses intrinsic GTPase activity causing hydrolysis of GTP back to GDP, and thereby reconstitution of the now inactive heterotrimer.

$G\alpha_i$ and $G\alpha_s$ Signalling

$G\alpha_i$ and $G\alpha_s$ are opposites in their effect on adenylyl cyclases, a group of enzymes that convert ATP into cyclic AMP (cAMP). Whereas activation of the $G\alpha_i$ ("i" for inhibition) family of Gα proteins inhibits adenylyl cyclases, $G\alpha_s$ stimulates their activity ("s" for stimulation). The resulting intracellular cAMP activates protein kinase A (PKA) and exchange protein activated by cAMP (EPAC). These proteins mediate the physiological effects of cAMP, such as alterations in transcription through phosphorylation of cAMP response element binding protein (CREB) [14]. CREB is an example of a transcription factor, a protein that binds the DNA and modulates gene expression. Finally, cAMP binds cyclic nucleotide-gated ion channels, playing a role in the regulation of membrane potential in neurons and of other physiological processes [15].

Defects in $G\alpha_s$ signalling, for example by pathogenic variants in *GNAS*, can therefore cause monogenetic obesity because it impacts downstream receptor signalling, such as MC4R signalling. However, as $G\alpha_s$ mediates signalling of other GPCRs as well, patients with pathogenic *GNAS* variants also present additional phenotypes, such as delayed growth and developmental delays [16].

$G\alpha_{q/11}$ Signalling

$G\alpha_{q/11}$ proteins activate phospholipase C (PLC)-β. This enzyme catalyses the synthesis of diacylglycerol (DAG) and inositol-1, 4, 5-triphosphate (IP_3). DAG, in turn, activates protein kinase C (PKC). PKC is a serine-threonine kinase that phosphorylates a range of proteins that are involved in cellular function. IP_3 binds its receptor on the endoplasmic reticulum (ER), resulting in the release of Ca^{2+} from the ER [17]. This increase in cytoplasmic Ca^{2+} concentration, as well as PKC activity, results in changes in transcription through the activation of the transcription factor nuclear factor of activated T cells (NFAT).

$G\alpha_{12/13}$ Signalling

$G\alpha_{12/13}$ proteins affect a multitude of signalling pathways, of which Rho activation has been best described [18]. Activated $G\alpha_{12/13}$ directly activates Rho-guanine nucleotide exchange factors (Rho-GEFs), which, in turn, regulate Rho activity.

Rhos are a family of GTPases, of which RhoA is the main member involved in $G\alpha_{12/13}$ signalling. Signaling via this pathway regulate energy homeostasis and glucose metabolism contribute to the physiology and pathogenesis of metabolic disease [19, 20].

Non-canonical Gα Signalling

Besides triggering their canonical signalling cascades, such as cAMP or calcium (Fig. 1), GPCRs can signal via other routes. For example, in addition to activating PLC, GPCR activated Gq signaling can lead to the activation of the mitogen-activated protein kinase (MAPK)/extracellular regulated-signal kinase (ERK) pathway [21, 22]. Gq can also interact with $G\alpha_{12/13}$ signalling by activating RhoGEFs [23]. Finally, $G\alpha_{12/13}$ subunits can activate not only RhoA, but also PLC, adenylyl cyclase, and MAPK/ERK signalling pathways [18]. This overlap between canonical and non-canonical signalling of the different Gα subfamilies, presents an additional layer of complexity in GPCR signalling. This complexity emphasizes the value of functionally assessing multiple pathways when analysing the impact of variants in GPCRs.

1.1.4 Termination of Signalling and β-Arrestins

To terminate signalling, GPCR kinases (GRKs) phosphorylate the receptor. The effects of this phosphorylation are two-fold: (1) it desensitizes the receptor, and (2) it enables β-arrestins to bind the GPCR. These β-arrestins block G proteins from interacting with the receptor, simply by physical obstruction. In addition, β-arrestins also activate various signalling pathways on their own, such as RhoA. Through these pathways, β-arrestins alter the transcriptional activity of cells [24].

1.1.5 Internalization and Recycling

Termination of GPCR signaling is accompanied by receptor phosphorylation and β-arrestin-binding which initiates their internalization (Fig. 1). During internalization, receptors are transported back into the cell through endocytosis: i.e. the cell forms vesicles, which will detach from the plasma membrane, taking the receptor along into the cell. Here, the content of the endocytotic vesicles, including the GPCRs, are sorted by Rab proteins. These proteins will designate the GPCR for degeneration in lysosomes or for recycling to the membrane. Recycled receptors are dephosphorylated prior to membrane allocation, to allow ligand-induced re-activation [25].

2 Functional Analysis of GPCR Signalling

One of the key players in the regulation of body weight and energy expenditure is MC4R. Pathogenic variants in *MC4R* are the most common cause of monogenetic obesity and numerous variants in *MC4R* have been reported. Because *MC4R* encodes a GPCR, the second part of this chapter will provide an overview of recent methodologies used to study the function of GPCRs, emphasizing assays used to study the impact of receptor variants on ligand binding, cell surface expression, G protein interaction, intracellular second messengers levels, and β-arrestin recruitment, as summarised in Fig. 1.

2.1 Expression Plasmids and Mutagenesis

In vitro cell based models require expression of the WT or variant receptor together with appropriate reporter genes. Therefore, one of the first steps to functionally analyse GPCR gene variants is to insert a cDNA of the gene into a plasmid that is capable of expressing the protein in mammalian cells. Plasmids that are capable of doing this carry a constitutively active promoter sequence upstream of the gene, such as the cytomegalovirus (CMV) promoter. Plasmids such as pcDNA3.1 are commonly used for this purpose. Next, it is necessary to introduce the variant into the wild type receptor cDNA using site-directed mutagenesis [26]. The modified genes are then verified by Sanger sequencing of the isolated plasmid DNA.

Depending on the cell-based assay used, the wild type and variant receptor cDNAs may need to be cloned into plasmids that tag the expressed protein with specific fluorescent or luminescent proteins. Epitope tags (short amino acid sequences recognised by commercially available antibodies, such as FLAG and HA) can also be added to the gene at this stage to allow, for example, localisation of the receptor within the cell. Tags can also be added that allow assessment of protein-protein interactions, for example recruitment of β-arrestins by a receptor. These include, for example, split fluorescent or luminescent peptides, which will become functional if the expressed proteins come into close contact with each other in or at the surface of the cell or in response to binding of a signalling molecule such as cAMP.

2.2 Expression in Mammalian Cells

Screening of GPCR function relies for a large part on cell-based assays that assess changes in intracellular levels of second messengers upon ligand binding to the receptor. Once the relevant plasmid constructs have been prepared, they can then be introduced into mammalian cells using a process called transfection [27, 28]. These methods allow for the transient expression of WT and mutated genes in cells.

Human immortalized cell lines, such as the human embryonic kidney cell line (HEK293), are common *in vitro* cell models to study GPCR signalling [28]. HEK293 cells are easy to transfect and express the downstream GPCR machinery necessary for GPCR signalling, but do not express many of the obesity-related GPCRs. This makes them a suitable model to compare signalling of the wild type and variant receptor upon transfection. A limitation of this method is that transfection may result in levels of expression of the GPCR that are considerably greater than found *in vivo*. A further limitation of such a cell model is that it may not fully represent the tissue-specific environment of obesity-related GPCRs and thus lack important cofactors that modulate GPCR signalling. However, human hypothalamic cell lines are not available, and therefore HEK293 cells are commonly used, also in the analysis of MC4R variants.

2.3 Assessment of Receptor-Ligand Binding

2.3.1 Radio-Labelled Ligands

Radioligand binding assays are used to determine GPCR expression, affinity of the receptor for ligands, as well as the kinetics of binding. These assays require the radioactive labelling of the ligand. The concentration of unlabelled ligand to replace 50% of the specific binding of the radioligand (IC50) can be used to determine the affinity of ligand for the receptor. By comparing WT and variant receptor it can be determined whether a variant alters the affinity. For MC4R, a fixed concentration of radiolabelled ^{125}I-NDP-MSH is used to be competed off with increasing concentrations of unlabelled α-MSH. Iodinated NDP-MSH is used because iodination of α-MSH disrupts receptor binding. For the MC4R D126Y variant, it was shown that this variant completely disrupts ligand binding, while there are also variants (D146N) that cause reduced maximal binding and increased affinity [29].

Radioligand binding assays have been the gold standard for GPCR binding assays. However, radiolabelling can destabilize the ligand through radiolysis or prevent receptor binding, as has been shown for α-MSH. Furthermore, radioactive compounds are hazardous, requiring safety measures and appropriate disposal procedures.

2.3.2 Fluorescent and Luminescent Labelled Ligands

The development of fluorescence and luminescence-based methods has provided good alternatives to radioligand binding assays, and are better approaches for high-throughput screening of experimental ligands or variant receptors since optical microplate readers can be used to measure output of these assays in high density plate formats [30, 31]. Fluorescently tagged ligands allow a number of different approaches to be used to assess their ability to bind to GPCRs such as MC4R including fluorescence anisotropy [28], fluorescence polarization [32], and other more quantitative methods [33, 34].

Tagging the receptor with either fluorescent (eg. green fluorescent protein) or bioluminescent (eg. nanoluciferase /Nanoluc) proteins allows an alternative, more specific, approach that uses the physical effect of resonance energy transfer (fluorescence and bioluminescence energy transfer, or FRET and BRET) [31]. On ligand binding, energy from the tag on the receptor, emitted either as fluorescence or bioluminescence, is transferred to the fluorescent tag on the ligand causing light emission at a different wavelength that can be detected in a plate reader or by microscopy. A BRET-based approach has been used to assess binding of a fluorescently labelled α-MSH analogue to MC4R tagged at its N-terminus with Nanoluc [35]. The CRISPR/Cas9 system can also be used to tag endogenous receptors with Nanoluc preserving natural levels of expression of the GPCR and allow assessment of binding of a fluorescently labelled ligand [36].

The split Nanoluc (NanoBiT) system has also been used to examine ligand binding to the ghrelin receptor (GHSR), variants of which have been associated with obesity [37]. It consists of two fragments (SmBiT and LgBiT) of Nanoluc which are tagged onto different proteins. When they come into close proximity, as occurs when a ligand binds to a receptor, the luminescent properties of Nanoluc are reconstituted. SmBiT and LgBiT have low affinity for each other to prevent non-specific recombination from occurring. In this example the ligand ghrelin was labelled with SmBiT and GHSR was tagged at its extracellular N-terminus with LgBiT. The amount of ghrelin bound was proportional to the level of bioluminescence from the reconstituted Nanoluc.

2.3.3 Label-Free Methods

As previously alluded to, the tagging of ligands can have an impact on their binding properties. To try to circumvent this problem a number of biophysical methods have been developed to assess the binding of untagged ligands to their receptors. For example, these include methods such as surface plasmon resonance and related approaches, mass spectrometry, nuclear magnetic resonance and thermodynamic binding assays. These approaches tend to require specialist expensive equipment and are therefore less commonly used.

2.4 Cell Surface Expression and Intracellular Trafficking

2.4.1 Epitope-Tagged Receptors

A commonly used approach to determine levels of expression of receptors at the cell surface is to express the receptor with an epitope tag on the extracellular N-terminus. Epitope tags are short peptide sequences that are recognised with high specificity by commercially available monoclonal antibodies [38]. Cells expressing N-terminally tagged receptors can be grown in, for example, 96-well plates and fluorescently labelled antibodies are used to measure levels of cell surface receptor by flow cytometry or in a microplate reader [26, 39]. A similar approach can be used to examine trafficking of receptors, with either an epitope tag and fluorescently labelled antibodies [40] or a fluorescent protein tag [41], into cells following ligand treatment using confocal microscopy.

2.4.2 Nanoluciferase-Based Approaches

The split Nanoluc approach described in Sect. 2.3.2 can also be used to measure cell surface expression of receptors. In this approach Nanoluc fragments with high affinity for each other are used: HiBiT, which is used to tag the receptor, and LgBiT, which is added to the cells to reconstitute bioluminescent Nanoluc on binding to HiBiT on the receptors. LgBiT cannot enter intact cells, thus ensuring that reconstituted Nanoluc is only detectable at the cell surface [42, 43]. The level of luminescence generated is proportional to the amount of HiBiT-fused target GPCR present in the cell membrane [42]. Because LgBiT cannot enter the cell, it is possible to follow ligand-induced internalisation of the receptor from the cell surface by continuously measuring luminescence following treatment of the cells with ligand. Additionally, lysis of the cells with detergent allows access of LgBiT to both surface and intracellular receptors allowing the measurement of total levels of receptor expression using this system. Such an approach has been used to assess cellular localisation of variants of MC4R [6, 44].

2.4.3 Bystander BRET

An approach to monitor the position of the receptor in the cell is bystander BRET [45]. As described briefly in Sect. 2.2 of this chapter, BRET occurs when energy is transferred from a receptor tagged with a bioluminescent donor, such as Nanoluc, to a fluorescent acceptor such as green fluorescent protein (GFP). Bystander BRET uses luminescent donors and fluorescent acceptors that have moderate affinity for each other, which improves energy transfer and signal to noise ratio. Tagging the acceptor fluorophore with a peptide sequence that localises them in specific membrane compartments allows one to monitor the proximity of receptors in the same subcellular compartment. Such tags include the CAAX box of KRas which localises specifically to the plasma membrane and the FYVE domain of endofin which localises in intracellular vesicles. Therefore, this approach can be used to assess cell surface levels of receptor as well as ligand-induced trafficking into the cell, as has been shown for MC4R [6, 46].

2.5 Gα-Protein–Receptor Interactions and Activation

The split luciferase NanoBiT system has been developed not only to examine ligand-receptor interactions (Sect. 2.2) but also to study the interaction between GPCRs and the G proteins [47, 48]. For example, Laschet et al. fused SmBiT into the C terminus of GPCRs and LgBiT at internal sites or at the N-terminus of several members of the family of Gα proteins and demonstrated their ligand-induced recruitment to a variety of GPCRs [48, 49]. Brouwers et al. used this approach to assess agonist-dependent binding of $G\alpha_s$ to variants of MC4R [6].

In addition, several BRET-based assays have been developed to assess G-protein recruitment by GPCRs, including MC4R. In this assay the receptor is tagged with a bioluminescent energy donor, such as *Renilla* luciferase (RLuc), and the G protein is tagged with a fluorescent acceptor based on GFP, such as Venus [50, 51]. Recruitment of the G protein by the receptor allows BRET to occur and the level of fluorescence correlates with the degree of interaction.

Ligand binding to a GPCR leads to separation of Gα from the dimeric G-βy complex bound to its cytoplasmic tail. This property of dissociation of the trimeric G-protein complex has been exploited to produce biosensors of G protein activation. Recently, a set of BRET-based G protein activity sensors for all four major families of G proteins were developed, known as the G-CASE (G protein tricistronic activity sensors). G-CASE consists of a single plasmid that expresses all three G protein subunits, which improves sensitivity and removes the need to co-transfect several plasmids into the cells [48, 52]. The Gα subunit is tagged with Nanoluciferase as the energy donor, and the Gγ subunit is tagged with the variant GFP, cpVenus [52]. At basal state (no stimulation), the G proteins form a trimeric complex allowing BRET to occur. However, upon ligand stimulation of the receptor the complex dissociates which decreases the BRET signal, indicating activation of GPCR signalling.

2.6 Second Messenger Assays

2.6.1 cAMP Reporter Systems

Agonist-induced cAMP levels in cells can be measured using many different techniques and initially was measured directly using antibodies in cell lysates by radioimmunossay and ELISA. Immunoassays using time resolved fluorescence energy transfer (TR-FRET; Lance), homogeneous time resolved fluorescence (HTRF) and amplified luminescent proximity homogeneous assay (Alphascreen) are also available from Perkin-Elmer. Although these assays are designed for high-throughput applications, they can be scaled down, exemplified by a study of MC4R variants using the Alphascreen assay [44].

A different method to measuring cAMP is to use a plasmid-based reporter gene approach. A common example of a reporter gene is insect luciferase whose coding region is joined to a promoter element that responds transcriptionally to cAMP, in this case the cAMP response element (CRE). Once expressed in cells, the bioluminescent enzymatic activity of the luciferase reporter can be measured in the presence of its substrate luciferin [53, 54]. The level of cAMP correlates with the measured bioluminescent output, and this approach has been used extensively to assess the activity of variants of MC4R (e.g [55]). The possible disadvantage of this approach is that several hours of treatment are required to allow sufficient production of the luciferase for its agonist-induced activity to become measurable.

Finally, bioluminescent biosensors of agonist-induced cytosolic cAMP responses are available which, unlike the previously described approaches, have the advantage of being able to measure the kinetics of the cAMP response in real-time immediately following activation of a receptor by its ligand. An example of this type of biosensor is the GloSensor cAMP assay (Promega). It is based on firefly luciferase which has been engineered to contain the cAMP binding domain of the regulatory subunit of protein kinase A, which without cAMP is in an inactive state [56]. On binding cAMP the binding domain undergoes a conformational shift reconstituting the luciferase activity and catalysing the oxidation of the substrate luciferin, generating luminescence. Here, the level of cAMP in the cell corresponds with the magnitude of luminescence signal. This biosensor has been used to assess ligand-induced cAMP responses of MC4R variants in several studies (e.g [6, 46, 57]).

Gαs/cAMP is the main signalling pathway for MC4R making the cAMP response the first endpoint to measure when assessing the effects of MC4R variants. Many obesity-associated MC4R variants are frameshift or missense variants, mostly resulting in a partial or complete loss of cAMP signalling. For example two MC4R variants identified in patients with obesity, N97D and R165Q, resulted in a complete and partial loss of cAMP response respectively [58]. The low levels of cAMP response seem to be linked with the obesity phenotype of the patients, indicating that disruption of this pathway could lead to obesity. Although MC4R signals mainly through the Gαs/cAMP pathway, studies have suggested that MC4R can also signal through other G proteins. MC4R increases calcium levels through the Gq-dependent signalling pathway in GT1–1 cells, a mouse hypothalamic cell line [59], and in other immortalized cell lines such as HEK293 cells [44]. MC4R variants associated with a lean phenotype, V103I and H158R, showed an increase in $G\alpha_q$ signalling *in vitro* [44]. MC4R variants associated with obesity have also shown normal $G\alpha_s$ signalling, but impaired $G\alpha_q$ activation, suggesting that $G\alpha_q$ signalling may also be an important aspect of MC4R signalling for the regulation of body weight [35]. The following procedures are used to measure the downstream signalling of $G\alpha_q$ protein.

2.6.2 Calcium-Reporter Assays

As described in the Introduction, a wide variety of GPCRs couple with $G\alpha_q$ proteins that lead to signalling through mobilisation of the second messenger, Ca^{2+}, from stores in the ER.

A relatively direct approach to measuring changes in mobilisation of intracellular calcium stores induced by stimulation of GPCRs is to load cells with one of the many available small molecule calcium indicators, each one providing different benefits. Recently developed indicators, such as Rhod-2 and Fluo-4 [60], provide a number of advantages over earlier versions including better signal to noise ratios and improved cell permeability and stability. Fluorescence levels correlate with intracellular Ca^{2+} levels and fluorescence can be captured using either a plate reader or fluorescence microscopy. This approach has been used to measure calcium responses generated by variants of MC4R [61].

Like cAMP, there are also luciferase-reporter plasmids available that respond to changes in cytoplasmic Ca^{2+} and can be used to measure their levels. The most commonly used version of these contains the NFAT response element, as has been reported for MC4R [35, 44, 54].

An alternative approach is to measure Ca^{2+} levels using genetically encoded biosensors, of which there are several [62–64]. In this chapter we will focus on one of these, the photoprotein aequorin which has, for example, been used to examine GHSR signalling [40, 41, 65]. Aequorin is a Ca^{2+}-sensitive photoprotein that was first isolated from the bioluminescent jellyfish *Aequorea victoria* [66]. When complexed with the cofactor coelenterazine it emits blue light when bound Ca^{2+} ions with a stoichiometry that allows accurate measurement of intracellular calcium [67]. Aequorin can be expressed in mammalian cells using transfected plasmid expression constructs (the protein form of aequorin is called apoaequorin, and its complex with coelenterazine is known as aequorin). Interestingly, constructs are available in which aequorin has been tagged with peptides that direct it to different compartments of the cell, such as the plasma membrane and mitochondria, so that site-specific changes in Ca^{2+} can be measured [68]. Mitochondrially directed aequorin is often used for studies with Ga_q-coupled GPCRs [40]. Unlike fluorescent indicators, Ca^{2+}-bound aequorin can be detected without illuminating the sample, thereby eliminating interference from autofluorescence. The response of Ca^{2+} upon ligand stimulation is rapid and transient (seconds after ligand stimulation), therefore an immediate measurement is necessary requiring the use of a microplate reader with an injector. This allows measurement of the bioluminescence immediately following injection of ligand onto cells transfected with a receptor and an aequorin expression construct. This can also be performed in reverse, by injecting transfected cells into a ligand-containing buffer.

$G\alpha_q$ protein signalling can also be analysed by measuring IP1 (see Introduction, $Ga_q/11$ signalling). IP1 is a relatively stable metabolite of inositol trisphosphate (IP3) which stimulates release of Ca^{2+} from stores in the ER. The accumulation of IP1, for example following treatment of cells with agonist, can be measured using a commercially available homogeneous time resolved fluorescent assay (IPOne HTRF, Perkin-Elmer) [69]. This assay is a reliable and stable technique for assessing Gq/11 activation that has been used for assessing variants of MC4R and function of GHSR [70].

2.6.3 Measuring MAP Kinase Levels and Activity

Since specific high affinity antibodies are available for both total (will detect both phospho and non-phospho forms) as well as phosphorylated forms of ERK (e.g. from Cell Signaling Technology), one of the most direct ways to assess effects of variants on signalling through this pathway is to use antibody-based approaches. Of the available methods, Westerns are most commonly used for low-throughput applications. Westerns involve the isolation of proteins from cells transfected with receptor that have been treated with ligand for specific periods of time. The proteins are then separated electrophoretically on polyacrylamide gels and transferred to membranes that can be screened using anti-ERK antibodies using either luminescent or fluorescent methods. Scanners are available to measure the level of luminescence/fluorescence to assess the level of phospho- and non-phospho ERK. The ratio of phospho/total ERK gives an estimate of the degree of activation. This approach has been used for several types of GPCRs, including MC4R [6, 71, 72].

Another approach, which is more quantitative than Westerns as well as being more high-throughput, is to use a reporter-luciferase plasmid construct, as described for cAMP and Ca^{2+} measurements. These constructs make use of the serum response element (SRE) promoter to drive luciferase expression [54].

2.6.4 Beta-Arrestin Recruitment

As described in the Introduction, ligand-induced cellular internalisation, or endocytosis, is an important regulator of receptor responsiveness through alteration of cell surface density. Arrestins are master regulators of GPCR endocytosis, acting as bridges between the receptor and proteins that facilitate cellular internalisation. The recruitment of arrestins to the receptor is therefore an important step in this process, and this can be measured in several ways including BRET and Nanoluc-complementation (NanoBiT) based methods [44, 73, 74]. Direct co-localisation of fluorescently tagged receptor and β-arrestin by confocal microscopy can also be used, since β-arrestin can show a change in distribution from the cytoplasm to the plasma membrane on treatment of cells with agonist [73]. This is a direct way of looking at β-arrestin localisation/recruitment but is less easy to quantify and is of low throughput.

BRET-based approaches are very similar to those described in Sects. 2.2 and 2.4 for ligand-receptor and G-protein-receptor interactions. They involve co-expression in cells of the (variant) receptor tagged at the C-terminus with a bioluminescent energy donor, such as Nanoluc, and either β-arrestin-1 or β-arrestin-2 tagged with an energy acceptor, usually a GFP variant such as Venus [74]. Similarly, the NanoBiT-based β-arrestin recruitment assay requires co-expression of C-terminal NanoBiT tagged receptor and either C- or N-terminally NanoBiT tagged β-arrestin. The orientation of tagging (N- or C-terminal on β-arrestin) and the use of LgBiT or SmBiT on the receptor or β-arrestin may have to be assessed empirically, although for several receptors, including MC4R [6], this is already described in the literature. Importantly, both BRET and luciferase complementation techniques allow assessment of agonist dose-dependent responsiveness of variant receptors which provides quantitative data on the effects of variants. Moreover, they also give the opportunity to make real-time measurements of β-arrestin recruitment following agonist treatment which can provide clues to possible mechanisms by which variants could modulate β-arrestin recruitment [75].

Studies have identified MC4R variants that alter β-arrestin recruitment. β-arrestin recruitment of MC4R variants has been associated with leanness in the general population. V103I, a common European MC4R variant, showed significantly increased levels of β-arrestin-2 recruitment (as well as cAMP response and cell surface expression) and has been associated with a lean phenotype. However, many MC4R variants show decreased levels of β-arrestin-2 recruitment alongside low levels of cAMP response, for example the pathogenic variant V95I which has been associated with obesity. Interestingly, studies have identified MC4R variants, for example L325F and R236C, with normal cAMP production and low recruitment of β-arrestins, suggesting an important role for β-arrestin-2 in MC4R signalling [46]. Furthermore, the findings indicate the importance of the interaction between the receptor and the β-arrestins in the regulation of food intake and body weight [46].

3 Limitations and Future Perspectives

This chapter is not an exhaustive review of GPCR signalling and methodology. However, some of the methods summarised here are described in more detail in a recent compilation by Martins et al. [28].

The methods described in this chapter have shown some limitations that need to be acknowledged. Tagging the target proteins with relatively large proteins such as green fluorescent protein and its derivatives, could affect the interaction dynamics of the receptor with G protein and/or β-arrestin recruitment [76]. Furthermore, genetically encoded biosensors, such as the Ca^{2+} indicators, may cause deleterious and off-target effects in cells, by inhibiting cellular survival, signalling, and metabolism [77]. These limitations indicate the importance of validating the findings and a second method is obligatory in order to confirm the findings.

The investigation of exogenous GPCRs in immortalized cell lines has limitations as well. Immortalized cell lines are a useful model system to study GPCR signalling because they contain all the necessary components of GPCR signalling but lack most of the receptors of interest in obesity research. This means one can relatively easily examine the effects of variants of a receptor using plasmid transgenes without interference from endogenously expressed receptors. Moreover, these cell lines are easy to maintain and transfect. However, in recent years, many questions have arisen about the use of exogenous uncontrolled overexpression of target receptors which may lead to false positive measurements, particularly since many of these receptors are expressed at relatively low levels *in vivo* [78]. Investigating the signalling of hypothalamic GPCRs, such as MC4R in HEK293 cells has the additional limitation that they can lack important components for the proper regulation of GPCR signalling. MC4R has been shown to be regulated by an accessory protein known as melanocortin 2 receptor accessory protein 2 (MRAP2). Immortalized cell lines may have low or zero amounts of MRAP2 expression, lacking an important component for the regulation of MC4R [44]. Furthermore, these immortalized cell lines also have a homogeneous genetic background [78], therefore the genetic background of patients with the investigated disease is not properly represented.

The limitations of immortalized cell lines point to the need for new scientific technologies to study GPCR signalling and diseases caused by variants in genes that encode these GPCRs. A significant breakthrough in science is the use of induced pluripotent stem cells (iPSCs). These have been used for disease modelling, cell therapy development, and drug discovery [79]. iPSCs are produced from somatic cells and have the capacity to generate almost any cell type. These cells can be used to generate human disease models in-a-dish by obtaining patient-derived iPSCs containing the disease-causing variant [79]. Importantly, this allows the study and measurement of GPCR signalling at their natural expression levels [78]. iPSCs could prove to be a powerful tool to develop personalized medicine for people with obesogenic variants of GPCRs, since they can mimic the characteristics of cells within the patient [80].

4 Conclusion

In this chapter, we show the importance of experimental approaches for the identification and characterization of pathogenic variants in GPCRs through *in vitro* studies. These approaches not only aid in the identification of pathogenic variants in different aspects of GPCR signalling but also enable future personalized treatment using existing drugs or through drug discovery.

Conflict of Interest J.A.V. has received royalties from AMH assays, paid to the institute/laboratory with no personal financial gain.

A. V. R. R., K.P., and P.J.D.D. have no conflict of interest.

References

1. De Smet F, Christopoulos A, Carmeliet P. Allosteric targeting of receptor tyrosine kinases. Nat Biotechnol. 2014;32(11):1113–20.
2. Zhu Y, Yang J, Yeh F, Cole SA, Haack K, Lee ET, Howard BV, Zhao J. Joint association of nicotinic acetylcholine receptor variants with abdominal obesity in American Indians: the Strong Heart Family Study. PLoS One. 2014;9(7):e102220.
3. Serra-Juhe C, Martos-Moreno GA, Bou de Pieri F, Flores R, Gonzalez JR, Rodriguez-Santiago B, Argente J, Perez-Jurado LA. Novel genes involved in severe early-onset obesity revealed by rare copy number and sequence variants. PLoS Genet. 2017;13(5):e1006657.
4. Liu T, Ji RL, Tao YX. Naturally occurring mutations in G protein-coupled receptors associated with obesity and type 2 diabetes mellitus. Pharmacol Ther. 2022;234:108044.
5. Wade KH, Lam BYH, Melvin A, Pan W, Corbin LJ, Hughes DA, Rainbow K, Chen JH, Duckett K, Liu X, Mokrosinski J, Morseburg A, Neaves S, Williamson A, Zhang C, Farooqi IS, Yeo GSH, Timpson NJ, O'Rahilly S. Loss-of-function mutations in the melanocortin 4 receptor in a UK birth cohort. Nat Med. 2021;27(6):1088–96.
6. Brouwers B, de Oliveira EM, Marti-Solano M, Monteiro FBF, Laurin S-A, Keogh JM, Henning E, Bounds R, Daly CA, Houston S, Ayinampudi V, Wasiluk N, Clarke D, Plouffe B, Bouvier M, Babu MM, Farooqi IS, Mokrosiński J. Human MC4R variants affect endocytosis, trafficking and dimerization revealing multiple cellular mechanisms involved in weight regulation. Cell Rep. 2021;34(12):108862.
7. He Y, Brouwers B, Liu H, Liu H, Lawler K, Mendes de Oliveira E, Lee DK, Yang Y, Cox AR, Keogh JM, Henning E, Bounds R, Perdikari A, Ayinampudi V, Wang C, Yu M, Tu L, Zhang N, Yin N, Han J, Scarcelli NA, Yan Z, Conde KM, Potts C, Bean JC, Wang M, Hartig SM, Liao L, Xu J, Barroso I, Mokrosinski J, Xu Y, Sadaf FI. Human loss-of-function variants in the serotonin 2C receptor associated with obesity and maladaptive behavior. Nat Med. 2022;28(12):2537–46.
8. Mafi A, Kim SK, Goddard WA 3rd. The mechanism for ligand activation of the GPCR-G protein complex. Proc Natl Acad Sci U S A. 2022;119(18):e2110085119.
9. Hilger D, Masureel M, Kobilka BK. Structure and dynamics of GPCR signaling complexes. Nat Struct Mol Biol. 2018;25(1):4–12.
10. Breit A, Buch TR, Boekhoff I, Solinski HJ, Damm E, Gudermann T. Alternative G protein coupling and biased agonism: new insights into melanocortin-4 receptor signalling. Mol Cell Endocrinol. 2011;331(2):232–40.
11. Tennakoon M, Senarath K, Kankanamge D, Ratnayake K, Wijayaratna D, Olupothage K, Ubeysinghe S, Martins-Cannavino K, Hebert TE, Karunarathne A. Subtype-dependent regulation of Gbetagamma signalling. Cell Signal. 2021;82:109947.
12. Ulloa-Aguirre A, Zarinan T, Gutierrez-Sagal R, Tao YX. Targeting trafficking as a therapeutic avenue for misfolded GPCRs leading to endocrine diseases. Front Endocrinol (Lausanne). 2022;13:934685.
13. Weis WI, Kobilka BK. The molecular basis of G protein-coupled receptor activation. Annu Rev Biochem. 2018;87:897–919.
14. Glas E, Muckter H, Gudermann T, Breit A. Exchange factors directly activated by cAMP mediate melanocortin 4 receptor-induced gene expression. Sci Rep. 2016;6:32776.

15. Ostrom KF, LaVigne JE, Brust TF, Seifert R, Dessauer CW, Watts VJ, Ostrom RS. Physiological roles of mammalian transmembrane adenylyl cyclase isoforms. Physiol Rev. 2022;102(2):815–57.
16. Mendes de Oliveira E, Keogh JM, Talbot F, Henning E, Ahmed R, Perdikari A, Bounds R, Wasiluk N, Ayinampudi V, Barroso I, Mokrosinski J, Jyothish D, Lim S, Gupta S, Kershaw M, Matei C, Partha P, Randell T, McAulay A, Wilson LC, Cheetham T, Crowne EC, Clayton P, Farooqi IS. Obesity-associated GNAS mutations and the melanocortin pathway. N Engl J Med. 2021;385(17):1581–92.
17. Litosch I. Decoding Galphaq signaling. Life Sci. 2016;152:99–106.
18. Guo P, Tai Y, Wang M, Sun H, Zhang L, Wei W, Xiang YK, Wang Q. Galpha12 and Galpha13: versatility in physiology and pathology. Front Cell Dev Biol. 2022;10:809425.
19. Rasheed SAK, Subramanyan LV, Lim WK, Udayappan UK, Wang M, Casey PJ. The emerging roles of Galpha12/13 proteins on the hallmarks of cancer in solid tumors. Oncogene. 2022;41(2):147–58.
20. Yang YM, Kuen DS, Chung Y, Kurose H, Kim SG. Galpha(12/13) signaling in metabolic diseases. Exp Mol Med. 2020;52(6):896–910.
21. Villaseca S, Romero G, Ruiz MJ, Perez C, Leal JI, Tovar LM, Torrejon M. Galphai protein subunit: a step toward understanding its non-canonical mechanisms. Front Cell Dev Biol. 2022;10:941870.
22. Kwon Y, Mehta S, Clark M, Walters G, Zhong Y, Lee HN, Sunahara RK, Zhang J. Non-canonical beta-adrenergic activation of ERK at endosomes. Nature. 2022;611(7934):173–9.
23. Aittaleb M, Boguth CA, Tesmer JJ. Structure and function of heterotrimeric G protein-regulated Rho guanine nucleotide exchange factors. Mol Pharmacol. 2010;77(2):111–25.
24. Jiang H, Galtes D, Wang J, Rockman HA. G protein-coupled receptor signaling: transducers and effectors. Am J Physiol Cell Physiol. 2022;323(3):C731–48.
25. Martinez-Morales JC, Solis KH, Romero-Avila MT, Reyes-Cruz G, Garcia-Sainz JA. Cell trafficking and function of G protein-coupled receptors. Arch Med Res. 2022;53(5):451–60.
26. Delhanty PJ, Bouw E, Huisman M, Vervenne RM, Themmen AP, van der Lely AJ, van den Akker EL. Functional characterization of a new human melanocortin-4 receptor homozygous mutation (N72K) that is associated with early-onset obesity. Mol Biol Rep. 2014;41(12):7967–72.
27. Kim TK, Eberwine JH. Mammalian cell transfection: the present and the future. Anal Bioanal Chem. 2010;397(8):3173–8.
28. Martins SAM, Prazeres DMF (eds). G protein-coupled receptor screening assays: methods and protocols. Humana Press, New York, NY; 2021.
29. Wang ZQ, Tao YX. Functional studies on twenty novel naturally occurring melanocortin-4 receptor mutations. Biochim Biophys Acta. 2011;1812(9):1190–9.
30. Owicki JC. Fluorescence polarization and anisotropy in high throughput screening: perspectives and primer. J Biomol Screen. 2000;5(5):297–306.
31. Lohse MJ, Nuber S, Hoffmann C. Fluorescence/bioluminescence resonance energy transfer techniques to study G-protein-coupled receptor activation and signaling. Pharmacol Rev. 2012;64(2):299–336.
32. Do EU, Jo EB, Choi G, Piao LZ, Shin J, Seo MD, Kang SJ, Lee BJ, Kim KH, Kim JB, Kim SI. Melanocortin 4 receptors interact with antimicrobial frog peptide analogues. Biochem Biophys Res Commun. 2006;343(4):1094–100.
33. Breen CJ, Raverdeau M, Voorheis HP. Development of a quantitative fluorescence-based ligand-binding assay. Sci Rep. 2016;6:25769.
34. Teerapanich P, Pugniere M, Henriquet C, Lin YL, Chou CF, Leichle T. Nanofluidic Fluorescence Microscopy (NFM) for real-time monitoring of protein binding kinetics and affinity studies. Biosens Bioelectron. 2017;88:25–33.
35. Heyder NA, Kleinau G, Speck D, Schmidt A, Paisdzior S, Szczepek M, Bauer B, Koch A, Gallandi M, Kwiatkowski D, Burger J, Mielke T, Beck-Sickinger AG, Hildebrand PW, Spahn CMT, Hilger D, Schacherl M, Biebermann H, Hilal T, Kuhnen P, Kobilka BK, Scheerer

P. Structures of active melanocortin-4 receptor-Gs-protein complexes with NDP-alpha-MSH and setmelanotide. Cell Res. 2021;31(11):1176–89.
36. White CW, Johnstone EKM, See HB, Pfleger KDG. NanoBRET ligand binding at a GPCR under endogenous promotion facilitated by CRISPR/Cas9 genome editing. Cell Signal. 2019;54:27–34.
37. Wang JH, Li HZ, Shao XX, Nie WH, Liu YL, Xu ZG, Guo ZY. Identifying the binding mechanism of LEAP2 to receptor GHSR1a. FEBS J. 2019;286(7):1332–45.
38. Terpe K. Overview of tag protein fusions: from molecular and biochemical fundamentals to commercial systems. Appl Microbiol Biotechnol. 2003;60(5):523–33.
39. Bruysters M, Verhoef-Post M, Themmen AP. Asp330 and Tyr331 in the C-terminal cysteine-rich region of the luteinizing hormone receptor are key residues in hormone-induced receptor activation. J Biol Chem. 2008;283(38):25821–8.
40. Evron T, Peterson SM, Urs NM, Bai Y, Rochelle LK, Caron MG, Barak LS. G protein and beta-arrestin signaling bias at the ghrelin receptor. J Biol Chem. 2014;
41. Delhanty PJ, van Kerkwijk A, Huisman M, van de Zande B, Verhoef-Post M, Gauna C, Hofland LJ, Themmen AP, van der Lely A. Unsaturated fatty acids prevent desensitization of the human growth hormone secretagogue receptor by blocking its internalization. Am J Physiol Endocrinol Metab. 2010;299(3):E497–505.
42. Promega Corporation. Nano-Glo® HiBiT Extracellular Detection System. Technical Manual. https://www.promega.com/-/media/files/resources/protocols/technical-manuals/500/nano-glo-hibit-extracellular-detection-system-technical-manual.pdf?la=en
43. Boursier ME, Levin S, Zimmerman K, Machleidt T, Hurst R, Butler BL, Eggers CT, Kirkland TA, Wood KV, Friedman Ohana R. The luminescent HiBiT peptide enables selective quantitation of G protein-coupled receptor ligand engagement and internalization in living cells. J Biol Chem. 2020;295(15):5124–35.
44. Paisdzior S, Dimitriou IM, Schope PC, Annibale P, Scheerer P, Krude H, Lohse MJ, Biebermann H, Kuhnen P. Differential signaling profiles of MC4R mutations with three different ligands. Int J Mol Sci. 2020;21(4)
45. Namkung Y, Le Gouill C, Lukashova V, Kobayashi H, Hogue M, Khoury E, Song M, Bouvier M, Laporte SA. Monitoring G protein-coupled receptor and beta-arrestin trafficking in live cells using enhanced bystander BRET. Nat Commun. 2016;7:12178.
46. Lotta LA, Mokrosiński J, Mendes de Oliveira E, Li C, Sharp SJ, Ja L, Brouwers B, Ayinampudi V, Bowker N, Kerrison N, Kaimakis V, Hoult D, Stewart ID, Wheeler E, Day FR, Perry JRB, Langenberg C, Wareham NJ, Farooqi IS. Human gain-of-function MC4R variants show signaling bias and protect against obesity. Cell. 2019;177(3):597–607.e599.
47. Dixon AS, Schwinn MK, Hall MP, Zimmerman K, Otto P, Lubben TH, Butler BL, Binkowski BF, Machleidt T, Kirkland TA, Wood MG, Eggers CT, Encell LP, Wood KV. NanoLuc complementation reporter optimized for accurate measurement of protein interactions in cells. ACS Chem Biol. 2016;11(2):400–8.
48. Laschet C, Dupuis N, Hanson J. A dynamic and screening-compatible nanoluciferase-based complementation assay enables profiling of individual GPCR-G protein interactions. J Biol Chem. 2019;294(11):4079–90.
49. Laschet C, Hanson J. Nanoluciferase-based complementation assay to detect GPCR-G protein interaction. Methods Mol Biol. 2021;2268:149–57.
50. Wan QW, Okashah N, Inoue A, Nehme R, Carpenter B, Tate CG, Lambert NA. Mini G protein probes for active G protein-coupled receptors (GPCRs) in live cells. J Biol Chem. 2018;293(19):7466–73.
51. Kim H, Baek IY, Seong J. Genetically encoded fluorescent biosensors for GPCR research. Front Cell Dev Biol. 2022;10:1007893.
52. Schihada H, Shekhani R, Schulte G. Quantitative assessment of constitutive G protein-coupled receptor activity with BRET-based G protein biosensors. Sci Signal. 2021;14(699):eabf1653.
53. Shan Q, Storm DR. Optimization of a cAMP response element signal pathway reporter system. J Neurosci Methods. 2010;191(1):21–5.

54. Cheng Z, Garvin D, Paguio A, Stecha P, Wood K, Fan F. Luciferase reporter assay system for deciphering GPCR pathways. Curr Chem Genom. 2010;4:84–91.
55. Lubrano-Berthelier C, Dubern B, Lacorte JM, Picard F, Shapiro A, Zhang S, Bertrais S, Hercberg S, Basdevant A, Clement K, Vaisse C. Melanocortin 4 receptor mutations in a large cohort of severely obese adults: prevalence, functional classification, genotype-phenotype relationship, and lack of association with binge eating. J Clin Endocrinol Metab. 2006;91(5):1811–8.
56. Wang FI, Ding G, Ng GS, Dixon SJ, Chidiac P. Luciferase-based GloSensor cAMP assay: temperature optimization and application to cell-based kinetic studies. Methods. 2022;203:249–58.
57. Moore BS, Mirshahi T. Genetic variants help define the role of the MC4R C-terminus in signaling and cell surface stability. Sci Rep. 2018;8(1):10397.
58. Farooqi IS, Keogh JM, Yeo GS, Lank EJ, Cheetham T, O'Rahilly S. Clinical spectrum of obesity and mutations in the melanocortin 4 receptor gene. N Engl J Med. 2003;348(12):1085–95.
59. Tao YX. The melanocortin-4 receptor: physiology, pharmacology, and pathophysiology. Endocr Rev. 2010;31(4):506–43.
60. Okumura W, Kozono T, Sato H, Matsui H, Takagi T, Tonozuka T, Nishikawa A. Jaw1/LRMP increases Ca2+ influx upon GPCR stimulation with heterogeneous effect on the activity of each ITPR subtype. Sci Rep. 2022;12(1):9476.
61. Kumar SS, Ward ML, Mountjoy KG. Quantitative high-throughput assay to measure MC4R-induced intracellular calcium. J Mol Endocrinol. 2021;66(4):285–97.
62. Whitaker M. Genetically encoded probes for measurement of intracellular calcium. In: Methods Cell Biol, vol. 99; 2010. p. 153–82.
63. Perez Koldenkova V, Nagai T. Genetically encoded Ca(2+) indicators: properties and evaluation. Biochim Biophys Acta. 2013;1833(7):1787–97.
64. Ma Q, Ye L, Liu H, Shi Y, Zhou N. An overview of Ca(2+) mobilization assays in GPCR drug discovery. Expert Opin Drug Discov. 2017;12(5):511–23.
65. Kern A, Albarran-Zeckler R, Walsh HE, Smith RG. Apo-ghrelin receptor forms heteromers with DRD2 in hypothalamic neurons and is essential for anorexigenic effects of DRD2 agonism. Neuron. 2012;73(2):317–32.
66. Shimomura O, Johnson FH, Saiga Y. Extraction, purification and properties of aequorin, a bioluminescent protein from the luminous hydromedusan, Aequorea. J Cell Comp Physiol. 1962;59:223–39.
67. Shimomura O. Luminescence of aequorin is triggered by the binding of two calcium ions. Biochem Biophys Res Commun. 1995;211(2):359–63.
68. Bonora M, Giorgi C, Bononi A, Marchi S, Patergnani S, Rimessi A, Rizzuto R, Pinton P. Subcellular calcium measurements in mammalian cells using jellyfish photoprotein aequorin-based probes. Nat Protoc. 2013;8(11):2105–18.
69. Garbison KE, Heinz BA, Lajiness ME. IP-3/IP-1 assays; 2004.
70. Srisai D, Yin TC, Lee AA, Rouault AAJ, Pearson NA, Grobe JL, Sebag JA. MRAP2 regulates ghrelin receptor signaling and hunger sensing. Nat Commun. 2017;8(1):713.
71. He S, Tao YX. Defect in MAPK signaling as a cause for monogenic obesity caused by inactivating mutations in the melanocortin-4 receptor gene. Endocr Rev. 2014;35(3)
72. Mousseaux D, Le Gallic L, Ryan J, Oiry C, Gagne D, Fehrentz JA, Galleyrand JC, Martinez J. Regulation of ERK1/2 activity by ghrelin-activated growth hormone secretagogue receptor 1A involves a PLC/PKCvarepsilon pathway. Br J Pharmacol. 2006;148:350–65.
73. Moo EV, van Senten JR, Brauner-Osborne H, Moller TC. Arrestin-dependent and -independent internalization of G protein-coupled receptors: methods, mechanisms, and implications on cell signaling. Mol Pharmacol. 2021;99(4):242–55.
74. Ma X, Leurs R, Vischer HF. NanoLuc-based methods to measure β-arrestin2 recruitment to G protein-coupled receptors. Methods Mol Biol. 2021;2268:233–48.
75. Hoare SRJ, Hughes TE. Biosensor assays for measuring the kinetics of G-protein and arrestin-mediated signaling in live cells; 2021.

76. Wouters E, Vasudevan L, Crans RAJ, Saini DK, Stove CP. Luminescence- and fluorescence-based complementation assays to screen for GPCR oligomerization: current state of the art. Int J Mol Sci. 2019;20(12)
77. Bootman MD, Allman S, Rietdorf K, Bultynck G. Deleterious effects of calcium indicators within cells; an inconvenient truth. Cell Calcium. 2018;73:82–7.
78. Chen G, Obal D. Detecting and measuring of GPCR signaling - comparison of human induced pluripotent stem cells and immortal cell lines. Front Endocrinol (Lausanne). 2023;14:1179600.
79. Shi Y, Inoue H, Wu JC, Yamanaka S. Induced pluripotent stem cell technology: a decade of progress. Nat Rev Drug Discov. 2017;16(2):115–30.
80. Moradi S, Mahdizadeh H, Saric T, Kim J, Harati J, Shahsavarani H, Greber B, Moore JBt. Research and therapy with induced pluripotent stem cells (iPSCs): social, legal, and ethical considerations. Stem Cell Res Ther. 2019;10(1):341.
81. Jamaluddin A, Gorvin CM. RISING STARS: targeting G protein-coupled receptors to regulate energy homeostasis. J Mol Endocrinol. 2023;70(4)
82. Kowalski TJ, Spar BD, Weig B, Farley C, Cook J, Ghibaudi L, Fried S, O'Neill K, Del Vecchio RA, McBriar M, Guzik H, Clader J, Hawes BE, Hwa J. Effects of a selective melanin-concentrating hormone 1 receptor antagonist on food intake and energy homeostasis in diet-induced obese mice. Eur J Pharmacol. 2006;535(1–3):182–91.

DNA Medication Pass: If Genomics Data Is Available, Why Not Look at Pharmacogenetic Variants Too?

Martina Cornel, Anja Roelofsen, and Loes Kreeftenberg

1 Introduction

Since the publication of the human genome sequence in 2000, many new genetic tests have been developed, enabling an increasing number of DNA-tests, amongst others, for patients with developmental problems and/or severe obesity. The indication of the DNA-test is that a genetic or syndromal origin is suspected. Whether or not a syndrome is diagnosed, many patients will need medication sooner or later in life. It might be useful to report not only the gene variants that might cause developmental problems or severe obesity, but also the pharmacogenomic variants. Genetic counselling on developmental problems and severe obesity is done by clinical geneticists, often specialized in dysmorphology or developmental problems. The expertise in pharmacogenomics often lies with (clinical) pharmacists. Sharing expertise between these professionals is essential to move the implementation of pharmacogenomics in daily medical care forward. A recent publication of the Global Alliance for Genomics & Health (GA4GH) can be seen as a bridge between these fields [1].

M. Cornel (✉) · A. Roelofsen · L. Kreeftenberg
Department of Human Genetics, Section Community Genetics and Amsterdam Public Health Research Institute, Amsterdam University Medical Center, Vrije Universiteit Amsterdam, Amsterdam, The Netherlands
e-mail: mc.cornel@amsterdamumc.nl

M. van Haelst, E. van den Akker (eds.), *Clinical Obesity Genetics*,
https://doi.org/10.1007/978-3-032-04095-4_19

2 How Can Information on DNA-Variants Guide Prescription?

Medication is often metabolized by the liver. Liver enzymes can metabolize a pro-drug to the active metabolite. In other cases, the breakdown and excretion take place via liver enzymes. If an enzyme is less active in one person compared to many other persons, then the drug would be less effective, or it might stay active for a much longer period. With a DNA medication pass we can offer personalized prescriptions, tailored to the individual patient's needs. This might imply the need for a different dosage or a different drug.

Liver enzymes are proteins encoded in genes in the DNA. Genes can contain variations, which may be small, e.g. a single nucleotide variant, and lead to a protein with somewhat increased or decreased activity. Apart from these small variations, genes coding for enzymes can harbour copy number variants: different people can have different numbers of gene copies. The usual number of gene copies is two (one copy of the gene at each chromosome), however, four, three, one or none also occurs. More copies of the gene implies more enzyme activity, while less copies implies less enzyme activity. Depending on the copy number and the variants patients can be stratified to poor, intermediate, normal, rapid and ultra-rapid metabolizers [2]. A person with more than two copies of an active gene variant could be an (ultra-)rapid metabolizer. If the gene is involved in modifying a pro-drug to an active metabolite, the effect in an (ultra-)rapid metabolizer would be fast and occur already at a relatively low dose. A person with gene variants that are less active could be a poor metabolizer, who would not experience a rapid effect, and might need a higher dose or a different drug.

In pharmacogenetics the gene variants are often indicated with stars. The first few variants recognized, often rather frequent variants, are indicated with *1 and *2. The combination of variants found in two alleles (on two chromosomes) is a combination of (at least) two star numbers. The numbers do not have a meaning but simply refer to a list of known variants for a specific gene. In this list the activity of the variants can be annotated.

Pharmacogenetic tests can be ordered at different moments in relation to the prescription of (new) medication. If it is ordered right before prescription or delivery of a specific drug, it is a companion diagnostic (Fig. 1) [3]. If it is ordered after an adverse effect, it is a reactive test. For pre-emptive testing, the test results are

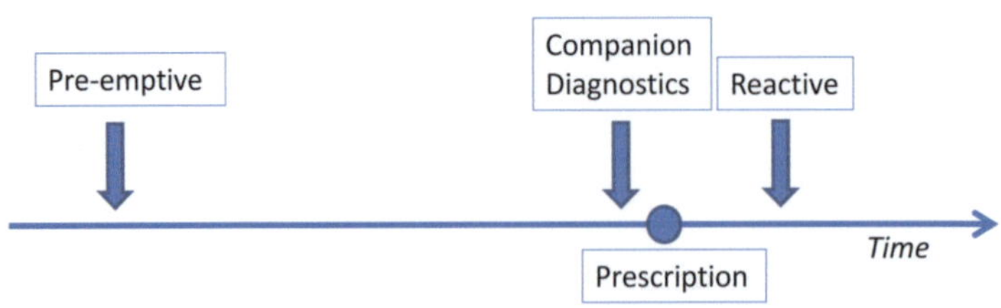

Fig. 1 Possible timing of pharmacogenetic testing in relation to prescription [3]

generated independently of a prescription, so that the information is available at any moment in the future when medication is needed. Using sequencing information to generate a report on secondary pharmacogenomic variants will often be independent of a prescription and, therefore, be pre-emptive testing. Maintaining the information in the health record of the patient is important.

3 Examples of Medication Frequently Used in Paediatrics

For some drugs that are frequently used in paediatric patients with syndromes, drug labels already include pharmacogenetic advice. The genes involved however differ. The tests are now often ordered as a companion diagnostic.

4 Omeprazole

Proton pump inhibitors such as omeprazole may be prescribed in children for the indication of gastro-esophageal reflux. The regulatory authorities from four regions around the world (the US Food and Drug Administration (FDA), Health Canada (HC), European Medicines Agency (EMA), and Pharmaceuticals and Medical Devices Agency in Japan) all consider that pharmacogenetics information about CYP2C19 is relevant for the dosage of omeprazole [1]. If the patient is a rapid metabolizer, they may be at risk for therapeutic failure at standard doses, and increasing the dose by 50–100% should be considered. If the patient is a poor metabolizer, a 50% lower dose should be considered after efficacy has been achieved to minimize the risk of adverse effects [4].

5 Valproic Acid

Persons with genetic syndromes causing epilepsy often get antiepileptic drugs prescribed. Hepatotoxicity potentially leading to liver failure may occur if children carry certain *POLG* variants and receive valproic acid [5]. Acute hyperammonaemia may occur due to valproic acid in patients with ornithine transcarbamylase (OTC) deficiency. Testing for specific *POLG* variants is required by FDA and a diagnosis of OTC deficiency is considered "actionable pharmacogenomics".

6 Carbamazepine

Carbamazepine is an antiepileptic drug for which HLA-B*15:02 and HLA-A*31:01 testing is required or recommended by the FDA, HC and EMA. These specific star alleles of the HLA genes are associated with specific side effects. Patients positive for HLA-B*15:02 may be at increased risk of severe skin reactions such as Stevens Johnson syndrome/toxic epidermal necrolysis [6]. HLA-A*31:01-positive patients are at increased risk for carbamazepine-induced hypersensitivity syndrome or maculopapular exanthema.

7 How Can Pharmacogenetic Variants Be Reported and Recorded?

Many health systems have a way to order pharmacogenetic tests, and subsequently report the test-result. The exact procedure differs between countries and health services. Orders from physicians for pharmacogenetic tests may go to a laboratory, followed by a letter back to the ordering physician reporting the results. Such a letter could be uploaded in the Electronic Patient Record. However, to make the information easily accessible, it would be better to create a specific field in the record where medication monitoring is possible. This field might be used, for instance, to generate a pop-up or even an interruptive alert if a relevant genetic variant would require a different prescription [7]. Decision support systems should support physicians when prescribing medication with potential pharmacogenetic advice. Similar systems are in place for allergy information or decreased kidney function.

Since data sharing between Electronic Patient Records in different health services is not optimal, one might also give a DNA medication pass to the patient containing the relevant information. Thus, a patient can show this DNA medication pass at the next prescription and share the information with physicians or pharmacists. Also, they can monitor potential pharmacogenetic effects of their own (new) medication, if their DNA medication pass is linked to a database with variant specific alert texts. The Amsterdam University Medical Center together with Leiden University Medical Center, for instance, use a “mijnDNAmedicatiepas” (my DNA medication pass) which contains a QR code that refers to an online database with pharmacogenetic advice linked to specific gene variants (www.mijndnamedicatiepas.nl). The patient’s gene variants are encrypted in the QR code.

8 From Pharmacogenetic Panel-Based Testing Towards Whole Exome/Genome Sequencing

More than 99% of people carry at least one actionable genomic variant [2]. The implementation of pharmacogenetics in clinical care however progresses slowly. Often applications today are reactive (to explain an adverse effect) or pharmacogenetic tests are used as a companion diagnostic (a specific DNA test at the moment of prescribing a certain drug). Should pre-emptive testing be performed, the results will not be relevant for the person in the short run. Thus, often, the (cost)effectiveness has been questioned.

A recent cluster-randomized trial in adults implemented a 12-gene pharmacogenetic panel [8]. Whenever a drug was prescribed for which a relevant gene should be tested, all 12 genes were reported. The study showed a 30% reduction in the incidence of clinically relevant adverse drug reactions within a 12-week follow-up period. Although a broad analysis of many pharmaco-genes from whole exome/genome sequencing would be even more effective, such studies have not (yet) been performed. Analysis of existing sequencing data might be cheaper, but at the same time, not all relevant variants can be detected by standard sequencing techniques. This is especially true for CYP2D6, which has a repetitive structure [1]. Additional testing might for instance be performed in case of the prescription of codeine.

For patients with obesity whose sequencing data is available, secondary analysis might generate information on pharmacogenetic variants. Clinical geneticists and other clinicians might collaborate with clinical pharmacists to stimulate the secondary use of this data. This information could be provided to (parents of) patients with obesity on a DNA medication pass, and be integrated in the Electronic Patient Record.

9 Conclusion

For children or adults with obesity who undergo whole exome/genome sequencing, data is generated that might also be analyzed to identify pharmacogenomics variants. As long as data in health records are not automatically shared between primary care, hospitals and pharmacies, parents could carry a DNA medication pass for themselves or their child. Thus, they would be empowered to share the information whenever a new drug is prescribed. In due time, decision support systems will be available in the Electronic Patient Records, and data sharing will become more common. But for now, a DNA medication pass may support personalized medicine for patients with obesity.

References

1. Friedman JM, Bombard Y, Carleton B, Issa AM, Knoppers B, Plon SE, Rahimzadeh V, Relling MV, Williams MS, van Karnebeek C, Vears D, Cornel MC, Global Alliance for Genomics and Health Regulatory and Ethics Workstream. Should secondary pharmacogenomic variants be actively screened and reported when diagnostic genome-wide sequencing is performed in a child? Genet Med. 2024;26:101033. https://doi.org/10.1016/j.gim.2023.101033.
2. Pirmohamed M. Pharmacogenomics: current status and future perspectives. Nat Rev Genet. 2023;24:350–62. https://doi.org/10.1038/s41576-022-00572-8.
3. Rigter T, Jansen ME, de Groot JM, Janssen SWJ, Rodenburg W, Cornel MC. Implementation of pharmacogenetics in primary care: a multi-stakeholder perspective. Front Genet. 2020;11:10. https://doi.org/10.3389/fgene.2020.00010.
4. CPIC (Clinical Pharmacogenetics Implementation Consortium). Omeprazole pre and post test alerts. Available from: Omeprazole_Pre_and_Post_Test_Alerts.xlsx (live.com). Accessed 22 February 2024.
5. Saneto RP, Lee IC, Koenig MK, Bao X, Weng SW, Naviaux RK, Wong LJ. POLG DNA testing as an emerging standard of care before instituting valproic acid therapy for pediatric seizure disorders. Seizure. 2010;19:140–6. https://doi.org/10.1016/j.seizure.2010.01.002.
6. Amstutz U, Shear NH, Rieder MJ, Hwang S, Fung V, Nakamura H, Connolly MB, Ito S, Carleton BC, CPNDS clinical recommendation group. Recommendations for HLA-B*15:02 and HLA-A*31:01 genetic testing to reduce the risk of carbamazepine-induced hypersensitivity reactions. Epilepsia. 2014;55:496–506. https://doi.org/10.1111/epi.12564.
7. Wake DT, Smith DM, Kazi S, Dunnenberger HM. Pharmacogenomic clinical decision support: a review, how-to guide, and future vision. Clin Pharmacol Ther. 2022;112:44–57. https://doi.org/10.1002/cpt.2387.
8. Swen JJ, van der Wouden CH, Manson LE, Abdullah-Koolmees H, Blagec K, Blagus T, Böhringer S, Cambon-Thomsen A, Cecchin E, Cheung KC, Deneer VH, Dupui M, Ingelman-Sundberg M, Jonsson S, Joefield-Roka C, Just KS, Karlsson MO, Konta L, Koopmann R, Kriek M, Lehr T, Mitropoulou C, Rial-Sebbag E, Rollinson V, Roncato R, Samwald M, Schaeffeler E, Skokou M, Schwab M, Steinberger D, Stingl JC, Tremmel R, Turner RM, van Rhenen MH, Dávila Fajardo CL, Dolžan V, Patrinos GP, Pirmohamed M, Sunder-Plassmann G, Toffoli G, Guchelaar HJ, Ubiquitous Pharmacogenomics Consortium. A 12-gene pharmacogenetic panel to prevent adverse drug reactions: an open-label, multicentre, controlled, cluster-randomised crossover implementation study. Lancet. 2023;401:347–56. https://doi.org/10.1016/S0140-6736(22)01841-4.

Genome-Wide Association Studies and Polygenic Risk Prediction in Obesity Research

Philip Jansen and Mieke van Haelst

1 Introduction

Research of genetic factors in disease have traditionally focused on finding rare, highly penetrant gene variants with a high risk of disease. For obesity, many such causes have now been identified [1] (Fig. 1). These 'monogenic' causes of obesity are characterised by variants within the coding sequences of the genome (i.e. exons) that often follow a Mendelian inheritance pattern in families (e.g. dominant or recessive, see also Chapter "General Introduction to Obesity Genetics and Genomics"). However, in recent years the scope in the search of genes for obesity has expanded to common genetic variants (i.e. variants present in >1% of the population) through large collaborative *genome-wide association studies* [2] (GWAS). Individual common genetic variants such as *single-nucleotide polymorphisms (SNPs)* have only a minor effect on obesity risk, however their abundance in the population lead to a substantial contribution of these variants to the overall heritability of obesity [3]. Developments in *polygenic risk scoring (PRS)* have provided new tools to capture and quantify an individual's genome-wide risk of disease based on a multitude of risk variants observed in GWAS. These PRS have promising applications in both public health and clinical settings to better understand who is most at risk of obesity and may benefit most from interventions. In this chapter, we discuss the role of common genetic variation in obesity, as has been explored through GWAS. We explain several methods that build forth on GWAS to understand the biological factors involved in obesity, and use information from common variants to understand its causes and consequences, such PRS and *Mendelian Randomization (MR)*.

P. Jansen (✉) · M. van Haelst
Department of Human Genetics, Section Clinical Genetics, Amsterdam University Medical Center, Amsterdam, The Netherlands
e-mail: p.jansen3@amsterdamumc.nl; m.vanhaelst@amsterdamumc.nl

M. van Haelst, E. van den Akker (eds.), *Clinical Obesity Genetics*,
https://doi.org/10.1007/978-3-032-04095-4_20

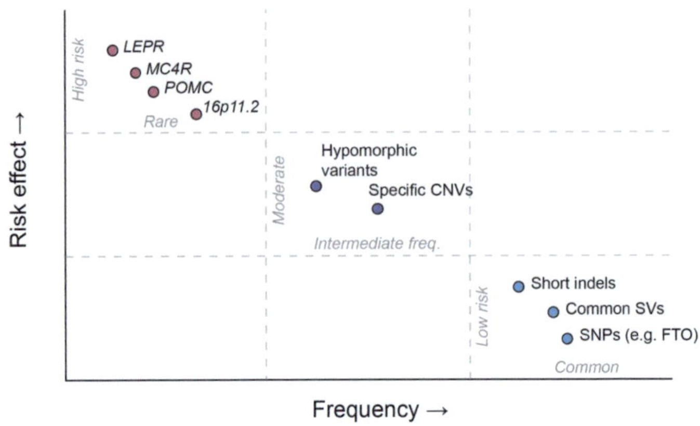

Fig. 1 Overview of the spectrum of frequencies and effect sizes of genetic variation involved in obesity

2 Genome-Wide Association Studies

The predominant focus in (clinical) genetics has historically been on the rare gene variants that an individual carries [4], even though the large majority of the genetic variants are common variants with a population frequency greater than 1%. *Genome-wide association studies* (GWAS) aim to link common genetic variants (also referred to as *single-nucleotide polymorphisms* (SNPs)) to an outcome of interest by statistically testing associations of each variant across the entire genome in a hypothesis-free approach [5, 6]. For each gene variant, it is possible to identify groups in the population: (1) homozygous for the reference allele (often the most common allele); (2) heterozygous for the alternative allele; (3) homozygous for the alternative allele (see Fig. 2). It can then be tested whether an increase in the number of alternative alleles is significantly associated with the outcome of interest (e.g. BMI).

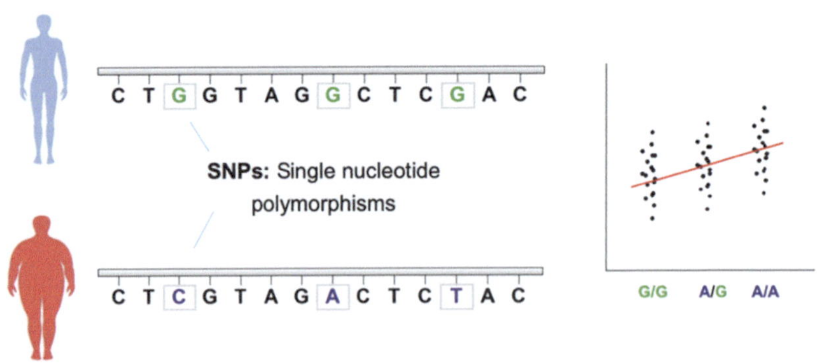

Fig. 2 Methods of a genome-wide association study (GWAS) to identify common genetic variants for obesity. The left side shows three single-nucleotide polymorphisms (SNPs) that differ between individuals. The right side shows linear regression analyses that can be carried out per SNP, calculating an effect on a continuous outcome of interest (e.g. BMI) per additional copy of the risk allele “A” (0, 1 or 2)

2.1 GWAS of Obesity

Early GWAS studies of obesity, for the first time gathering thousands of participants, pinpointed the *FTO* gene as the first susceptibility locus in 2006 [7]. However, it soon became apparent that much larger samples are necessary to provide sufficient statistical power to detect common variants of small effect. GWAS studies have thus far mainly focused on BMI as an indicator of obesity, since it is an easily obtainable measure and allows for the collection of obesity in large samples required for GWAS. Subsequently, large-scale GWAS studies of BMI have been highly successful in discovering large numbers of genetic variants that predispose to obesity. Collaborative efforts have now found over 700 genetic loci related to BMI through meta-analyses of different cohorts [8]. Effects of these individual variants are typically small, with an increase of 0.1 BMI points (kg per m^2) for each risk SNP[3]. However, the effects of genetic variants from GWAS combined explain around *~14 of the variation in obesity* in the population [8].

2.2 From SNP to Hypothesis

By mapping these GWAS results to various multi-omics data sets, it is possible to identify mechanisms explaining how identified genetic variants influences a phenotype across different biological dimensions (Fig. 3) [9]. SNPs that are significantly associated with obesity in GWAS can first be mapped to genes in which they are located (or closely located to). This enables the analysis of whether genes are enriched for certain gene-functions or pathways using gene-set analysis [10]. Moreover, it can be tested whether these genes are higher or lower expressed in certain organs, tissues or cell-types such as neurons by using gene-expression

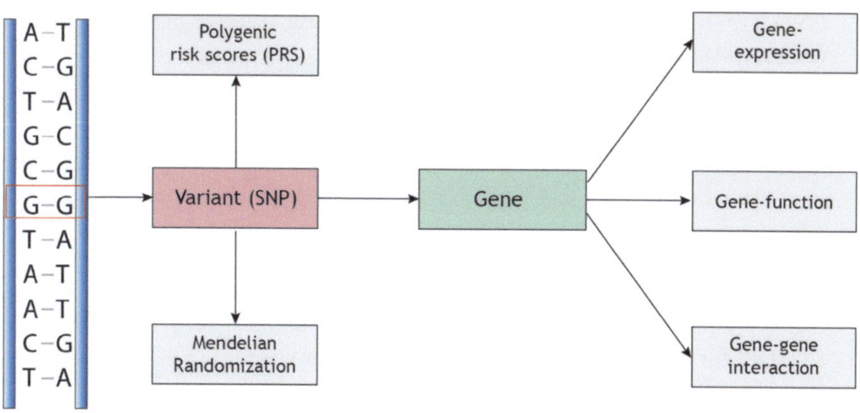

Fig. 3 GWAS analysis and possible follow-up analyses using different types of omics data

analyses, or whether their expression interacts with other genes at the protein level, by using protein-protein interaction (PPI) data. A couple of notable finding from GWAS studies are that obesity-associated genes are highly enriched for gene expression in the brain [1, 3], and less so in other organs, suggesting that common variants have an effects through brain-related mechanisms. Identified regions confirm known brain areas of importance, such as the hypothalamus and pituitary, but also areas involved in cognition, including the hippocampus and frontal cortical areas [1, 3]. On an even more fine-grained resolution, studies using single-cell RNA sequencing (scRNA-seq) have been able to find links of obesity genes with specific brain cell types of the hypothalamus, subthalamus and midbrain, among others [11].

3 Polygenic Risk Scores (PRS)

Among the many applications of GWAS results is the identification of individuals who are genetically most at risk of developing obesity, and who may thus benefit from prevention and personalized intervention plans. Based on recent large GWAS, it has become possible to estimate an individuals' overall genetic predisposition based on large sets of genetic variants observed in GWAS. *Polygenic risk scores (PRS)* are scores that include the cumulative effects of large number of risk variants found in GWAS [12, 13]. The rationale of PRS is that individual GWAS variants only explain a fraction of risk, but since obesity is in most cases a highly 'polygenic' trait, these effects combined in a genome-wide score more accurately reflect its complex polygenic architecture.

In its simplest form, a PRS is a score that indexes how many risk variant an individual carries in total, weighted by the size of the effect of the risk variant [14]. Calculation of PRS is a relatively straightforward process that includes three important steps (Fig. 4):

1. Obtain statistics of associations of genetic variants (effect sizes, P-values) from GWAS studies of a trait of interest (e.g. BMI). These are often publicly available or obtainable through consortium websites.
2. Obtain SNP genotype data of participants in whom PRS should be calculated.
3. Run one of the many PRS algorithms that are available [15].

For interpretability, PRS can be subsequently standardised to have a zero mean and standard deviation of 1 (i.e. Z-scored), as the resulting PRS often approach a normal distribution in a sufficiently large sample.

A PRS can then be tested for an association with any outcome of interest in a statistical model, by either including PRS as a continuous variable, or by stratifying groups in low and high genetic risk (e.g. through percentiles). PRS has shown to be a value tool for studying genetics of obesity across a wide array of possible study designs [16]. We here highlight several domains where PRS can provide a valuable tool to study obesity (Fig. 5).

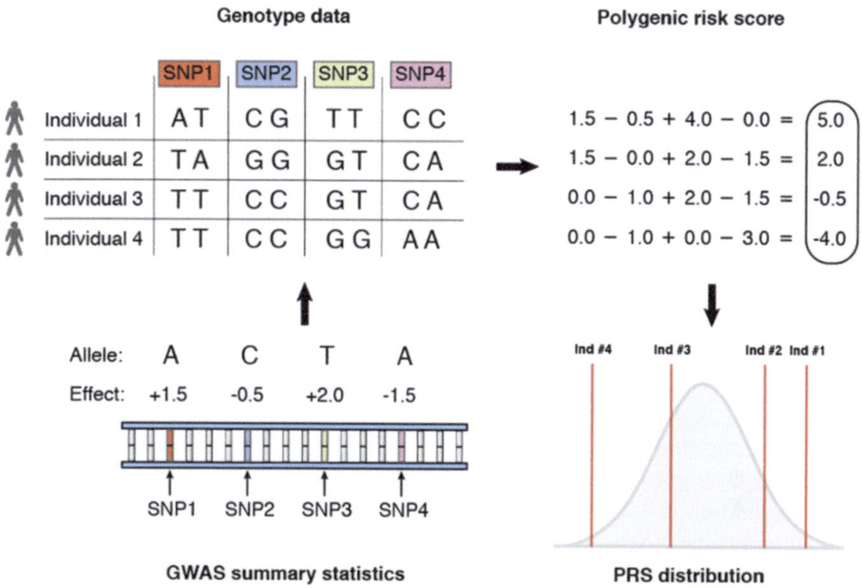

Fig. 4 Steps required for the calculation of polygenic risk scores (PRS)

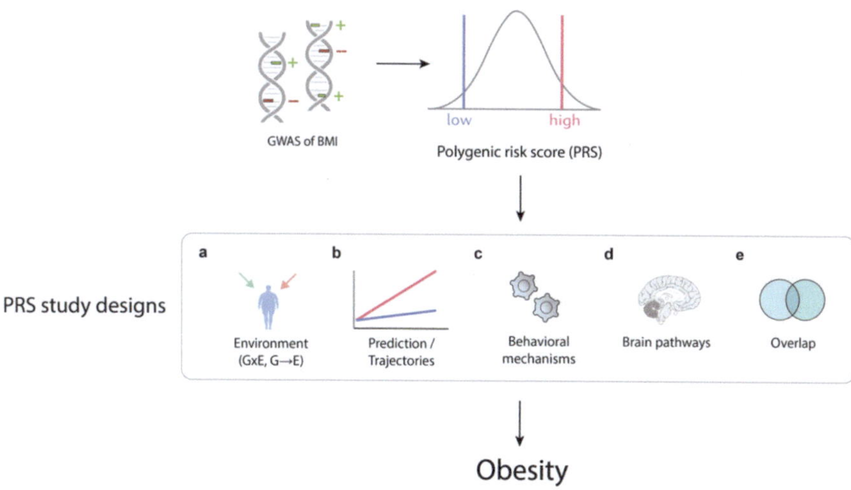

Fig. 5 Possible applications of obesity PRS in various study designs. G: genes; E: environment; GxE: gene-environment interaction

3.1 Predicting Obesity

It is estimated that the current best predicting PRS can explain almost 15% of the variation in BMI in the population [8]. This estimated is expected to increase as more SNPs for BMI are discovered. This means that PRS of BMI is among the best predicting PRS of any human phenotype. PRS of BMI can be used to investigate a link between genes and *weight trajectories* across the lifespan, that may not be captured by a cross-sectional design. These data can identify specific time windows where the influence of genetic predisposition is the strongest, and during which targeted intervention may be most beneficial. Such longitudinal analyses showed that differences in BMI at baseline were relatively small in different PRS groups, but during a multi-year follow-up, young adults in the high BMI PRS group had over 15% risk of developing severe obesity over time, compared to only ~1% in the low PRS group (lowest vs highest 10% of PRS) [17]. Interestingly, studies investigating weight trajectories within PRS categories for adult obesity (i.e. adult BMI PRS) in children, found that children with a higher PRS gain weight more rapidly in their early years (between 0 and 10 years [18, 19]) than those with more favourable PRS profiles. This shows that weight trajectories in different PRS groups diverge as early as in the preschool age. Moreover, studies found that an unfavorable BMI PRS relates to a more chronic and persistent trajectory of obesity during life, and half of the PRS-obesity association at an adult age is shown to be mediated by adiposity that is already present during childhood [20].

3.2 Gene-Environment Interaction

Recognizing that genes do not operate in a vacuum is fundamental to the study of gene-environment interactions (G × E) [21], which takes environmental influences that modulate genetic risk into account. PRS provide a useful tool to study G × E interactions, which can be tested as statistical interactions between the PRS and the environment on obesity outcomes. These interactions provide information about the context in which these genetic effects are attenuated or enhanced [22]. Distinguishing between G × E interactions and G × E correlations (correlation between genetic risk and environmental factors) in obesity research can be challenging. For example, individuals with a high obesity PRS may show a stronger association with a high BMI specifically in those who are less physically active. While this pattern could reflect a gene–environment interaction (physical activity attenuating the expression of genetic risk) it might also result from gene–environment correlation, if the same genetic factors that increase obesity risk also reduce an individual's predisposition to engage in physical activity.

PRS G × E studies show an important role of 'obesogenic' environments that can influence the phenotypic expression of obesity-associated risk variants: individuals with a higher obesity PRS are more sensitive to obesity-related environmental stimuli, such local fast-food chains near the home environment [23] with the PRS having a stronger association with BMI when these factors are present. Such modulating interactions have previously been observed for various other environmental factors, including healthy lifestyle factors [24], environmental air pollution [25], stress exposure during childhood [26], socioeconomic background [27] and immigration [28]. Such modulation may suggest a relevant role for epigenetics which can influence gene-expression based on the presence of (harmful) environmental factors.

Furthermore, G × E interaction effects are not confined to external factors but can exist with comorbid conditions as well. Conditions such as depressive symptoms [29] and sleep deprivation [30] have been shown to interact with the effects of PRS on obesity, showing stronger PRS-obesity associations when these conditions are indeed present. This highlights the complex interaction between polygenic predisposition to obesity, the environment and concurrent conditions (Fig. 6).

3.3 *Endophenotypes*

Beyond prediction of obesity, PRS offers a powerful tool to find mechanisms that bridge genetic predisposition to the manifestation of obesity, by relating genetic risk to potential mediating factors. By combining genetic and neuroimaging data, previous studies have investigated what neuronal mechanisms explain how genetic predispositions for obesity leads to a more obesity-prone brain [31]. MRI research suggests that higher polygenetic risk for BMI relates to lower cortical volume and thickness in the frontal [31] and temporal areas [32] compared to lower PRS

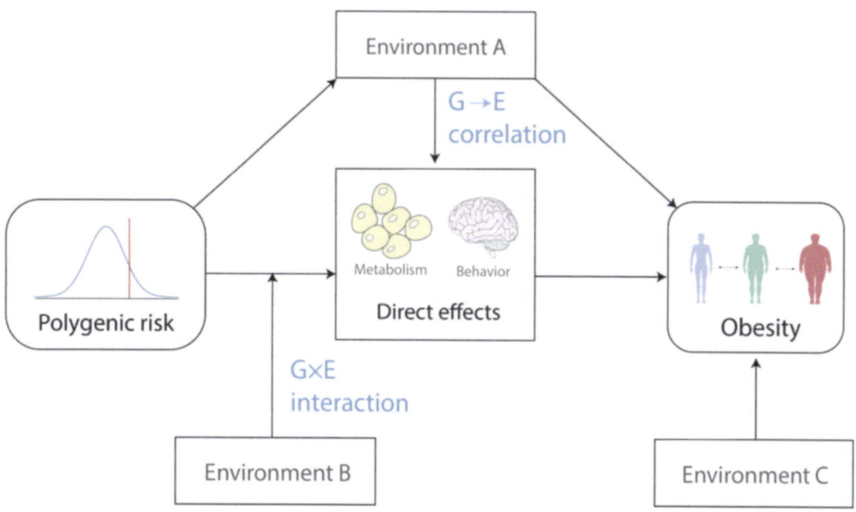

Fig. 6 Diagram showing the complex links between PRS, the environment and obesity outcomes. (From Jansen et al. 2024)

individuals. These brain areas play a fundamental role in executive function, reward processing, and control of eating behavior and cognitive processes previously linked to eating patterns and weight regulation [33]. On a behavioral level, the effects of PRS are shown to be partially mediated by more unhealthy eating behavior, as well as through obesogenic environments that provoke weight gain. Adolescents with a more unfavorable obesity PRS are more likely to show frequent snacking [34], overeating [35] and binge eating [36], suggested to result from a loss of control in eating behavior [35] and/or an altered satiety response [37]. Conversely, a healthy diet can mitigate the effects of PRS on obesity measured in young individuals [38]. In adults, higher rates of snacking behaviour [34], fried-food intake [39] and poorer workplace food choices [40] are observed in individuals with higher BMI PRS, underlining the potential of targeted interventions on these behaviors to mitigate the consequences of a high polygenetic risk.

3.4 Clinical Applications

The potential to predict obesity from genetic data when obesity is not (yet) present, suggest that PRS may be a useful clinical tool to stratify high and low risk individuals [12], contributing to personalizing prevention and treatment. Such clinical implementation may be within reach across several (pre)clinical settings:

- *Personalized prevention:* PRS associations with obesity trajectories within specific time windows allow the development of individualized health advice and follow-up plans based on PRS, which can optimize prevention and management strategies in those that have not (yet) developed obesity (e.g. in general practitioner settings). Given decreasing costs of SNP genotyping for PRS (as low as 20–30$ [41]) combined with the potential savings through more effective prevention of obesity and its health consequences, PRS in such a prevention setting may thus prove to be cost-effective.
- *Personalized treatment:* in those that have developed obesity, PRS may contribute in predicting persistent or refractory obesity, and identify those most likely to benefit from early (pharmacological) treatment. New pharmacological anti-obesity treatments such as GLP-1 agonist (Liraglutide, Semaglutide) are promising, yet can sometimes only be prescribed in the Dutch healthcare system if strict criteria are met, such as the identification of a proven monogenic cause (See also Chapter "General Introduction to Obesity Genetics and Genomics"). Given comparable relative risks of monogenic disease forms and unfavorable PRS [17], one may argue that policies from monogenic disease risk should be extended to unfavorable polygenic disease risk as well.
- *Predicing therapy response:* PRS has been explored as a predictor of persistent weight-loss during follow-up after bariatric surgery. These studies showed that the predictive value of PRS for therapy response is mixed, as some studies indicate that obesity-related PRS do not predict weight loss after gastric bypass surgery, nor are they associated with weight regain post-surgery [42, 43].

However, other research found that a higher BMI and waist-hip ratio (WHR) PRS negatively impacts weight loss post-procedure and during follow-up [44, 45]. Further, one study revealed that a lower obesity PRS was associated with improved metabolic outcomes, such as lower glycemia, triglycerides, and total cholesterol following bariatric surgery [46]. As such, while these results are promising, more research is needed to clarify the role of PRS in stratifying post-surgical outcomes, alongside clinical predictors [47].

- *Diagnostic testing:* PRS can be a useful addition to the arsenal of clinical diagnostic testing (e.g. array testing, next-generation sequencing) for patients referred to a clinical geneticist for a suspected genetic obesity. In a significant number of cases where a monogenic cause is suspected but not found, an unfavorable PRS, consistent with multiple risk variants, may offer an alternative explanation. At our national expertise center for genetic obesity (Amsterdam UMC/Erasmus MC, the Netherlands) [48], we indeed found a significantly higher BMI PRS in clinically referred patients suspected for a genetic obesity disorder, who were tested negative for a monogenetic cause, (unpublished data). This may provide an alternative explanation for their obesity. Moreover, we observed that individuals with explanatory monogenic obesity gene variants identified by sequencing tests have a significantly lower PRS compared to those without an identified pathogenic obesity gene variant. This may mean that a PRS as a first-tier test could select patients in whom costly and time-consuming sequencing is most likely to identify a genetic cause.

4 Mendelian Randomization

Mendelian Randomization (MR) is a powerful analytical tool to infer causal relationships between phenotypes using genetic variants as input. This technique uses the natural random assortment of alleles during gamete formation as an instrumental variable [49], thereby circumventing reverse causation that often complicates epidemiological studies. By comparing the occurrence of obesity-related traits across different genetic profiles, MR enables researchers to isolate causal effects of specific factors on obesity and vice versa, providing insights into (potential preventable) risk factors and underlying mechanisms. These methods use genetic variants found in GWAS of e.g. BMI as instrumental variables. Developments in these statistical methods have allowed causal inference between traits based on GWAS data alone (Fig. 7).

Variants that show clear pleiotropy (i.e. significant associations between a variant and both the risk factor (R) and disease (D)) are removed from the analyses. Also, variants used as instrumental variable should not influence the outcome through a confounder (C). All effects of the variant on the outcome of interest are then through the causal risk factor (R).

MR analyses have been used to explore causal relationships in previously identified epidemiological associations between obesity and various health outcomes. Through MR, it has been found that obesity is a suggested causal factor for type 2

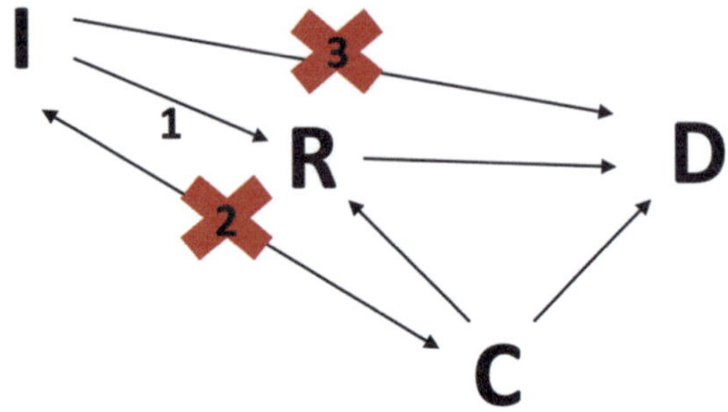

Fig. 7 Assumptions in Mendelian Randomization (MR) analysis based on GWAS data. I: instrumental variable; R: risk factor; D: disease; C: confounder

diabetes and coronary artery disease [50], cardiac rhythm disturbances [13], kidney disease [51], certain types of cancers [52] whereas no causal link was found with stroke [53]. Moreover, MR analyses have found previously less explored relationships including BMI predisposing to multiple sclerosis (MS) [54]. For non-disease phenotypes, it was found that a higher educational level causally reduces the risk of obesity [55] as well as coffee consumption [56]. Although developments in statistical methods to derive causality are ongoing rapidly, it is important to note that experimental validation is still required to prove causality. Also, most MR methods cannot distinguish between direct causal effects between phenotypes and the possibility of confounders that associate with both. By making use of genetic variants related to certain biochemical markers, such as metabolite levels, blood markers, and proteins, MR studies are able to identify (suggested) causal biological mechanisms related to obesity. For example, it has been shown that BMI causally lowers vitamin D levels [57], but no such causal link was found of vitamin D levels influencing BMI .

5 Limitations and Future Directions

While ongoing developments in GWAS and PRS have strongly improved understanding of obesity etiology, several challenges remain:

- *Euro-centered:* Current PRS are derived predominantly from populations of European ancestry [58], raising concerns about their applicability in other ethnic groups and limiting insights into genetic factors across diverse populations. In the latest GWAS of BMI, all approximately 700,000 investigated participants were of European ancestry [8], showing the need for expanding such investigations to include diverse ancestries in these studies. Newer generation population biobanks, such as the All of Us [59] program, are designed with the aim to prioritize diversity and reflect the multiethnic makeup of the population, promising to further close this knowledge gap.
- *Modest predictive power:* the modest predictive power of the obesity PRS [60, 61] indicates that a large proportion of the variation in obesity remains unexplained (i.e. 'missing heritability' [62]). However, it is important to realize that,

akin to many other types of DNA-tests, PRS should not be viewed as a single definitive test for developing obesity; rather, it can serve as a biomarker that helps stratifying low and high-risk individuals and help identifying those most at risk. Beyond merely including signal from common variants, integration of information from both common (through PRS) and rare variants (through sequencing and/or chromosomal tests) in a single risk model is expected to lead to more optimal predictions, as was recently shown in a large exome sequencing study combining common and rare variants [1]. With increasingly lower costs, whole-genome sequencing (WGS, including copy number variant (CNV) analysis) [63] will become more readily available, which can capture the whole spectrum of both rare coding variants and common non-coding variants in a single assay, leading to most precise risk estimates.

- *Integrating genes/environment:* current prediction accuracies of obesity PRS contain noise due to a lack of insight into the complex gene-environment interactions and correlations, including their potential to amplify or attenuate the effects of PRS, requiring more complex statistical models and larger and more diverse datasets than currently available.
- *Integrating genetics/epigenetics:* Along these lines, PRS and epigenetics (typically influenced by environmental factors) may also be integrated, as a higher BMI prediction has been obtained by the combined use of PRS and epigenetics than either data type alone [64], and the addition of epigenetics to genetics should be investigated more thoroughly.

Importantly, while PRS of obesity show promise for personalized medicine, caution is necessary in their clinical application in daily practise, given the ethical implications, and its potential for misinterpretation, misuse [65] or even discrimination [66].

6 Conclusion

The study of common variants has emerged as invaluable area in genetic obesity research in the past years, enabling a better understanding of the causes and consequences of obesity through a wide array of study designs. Despite current limitations, the clinical potential of PRS to inform personalized interventions is on the near horizon. As these areas of analysis continue to evolve, they have the potential to significantly advance both mechanistic insights and eventually (personalized) strategies for managing obesity.

References

1. Akbari P, et al. Sequencing of 640,000 exomes identifies GPR75 variants associated with protection from obesity. Science (80-.). 2021;373:eabf8683.

2. Loos RJF. 15 years of genome-wide association studies and no signs of slowing down. Nat Commun. 2020;11:5900.
3. Locke AE, et al. Genetic studies of body mass index yield new insights for obesity biology. Nature. 2015;518:197–206.
4. Claussnitzer M, et al. A brief history of human disease genetics. Nature. 2020;577:179–89.
5. Visscher PM, et al. 10 years of GWAS discovery: biology, function, and translation. Am J Hum Genet. 2017;101:5–22.
6. Abdellaoui A, Yengo L, Verweij KJH, Visscher PM. 15 years of GWAS discovery: realizing the promise. Am J Hum Genet. 2023;110:179–94.
7. Fawcett KA, Barroso I. The genetics of obesity: FTO leads the way. Trends Genet. 2010;26:266–74.
8. Yengo L, et al. Meta-analysis of genome-wide association studies for height and body mass index in~ 700000 individuals of European ancestry. Hum Mol Genet. 2018;27:3641–9.
9. Uffelmann E, Posthuma D. Emerging methods and resources for biological interrogation of neuropsychiatric polygenic signal. Biol Psychiatry. 2021;89:41–53.
10. de Leeuw CA, Neale BM, Heskes T, Posthuma D. The statistical properties of gene-set analysis. Nat Rev Genet. 2016;17:353–64.
11. Timshel PN, Thompson JJ, Pers TH. Genetic mapping of etiologic brain cell types for obesity. elife. 2020;9:e55851.
12. Torkamani A, Wineinger NE, Topol EJ. The personal and clinical utility of polygenic risk scores. Nat Rev Genet. 2018;19:581–90.
13. Chatterjee NA, et al. Genetic obesity and the risk of atrial fibrillation: causal estimates from Mendelian randomization. Circulation. 2017;135:741–54.
14. Lewis CM, Vassos E. Polygenic risk scores: from research tools to clinical instruments. Genome Med. 2020;12:1–11.
15. Ni G, et al. A comparison of ten polygenic score methods for psychiatric disorders applied across multiple cohorts. Biol Psychiatry. 2021;90:611–20.
16. Torkamani A, Topol E. Polygenic risk scores expand to obesity. Cell. 2019;177:518–20.
17. Khera AV, et al. Polygenic prediction of weight and obesity trajectories from birth to adulthood. Cell. 2019;177:587–96.
18. Steinsbekk S, Belsky D, Guzey IC, Wardle J, Wichstrøm L. Polygenic risk, appetite traits, and weight gain in middle childhood: a longitudinal study. JAMA Pediatr. 2016;170:e154472.
19. Craig SJC, et al. Constructing a polygenic risk score for childhood obesity using functional data analysis. Econom Stat. 2021;
20. Belsky DW, et al. Polygenic risk, rapid childhood growth, and the development of obesity: evidence from a 4-decade longitudinal study. Arch Pediatr Adolesc Med. 2012;166:515–21.
21. Hunter DJ. Gene–environment interactions in human diseases. Nat Rev Genet. 2005;6:287–98.
22. Plomin R, Gidziela A, Malanchini M, Von Stumm S. Gene–environment interaction using polygenic scores: do polygenic scores for psychopathology moderate predictions from environmental risk to behavior problems? Dev Psychopathol. 2022;34:1816–26.
23. Mason KE, Palla L, Pearce N, Phelan J, Cummins S. Genetic risk of obesity as a modifier of associations between neighbourhood environment and body mass index: an observational study of 335 046 UK Biobank participants. BMJ Nutr Prev Health. 2020;3:247–55.
24. Dashti HS, et al. Interaction of obesity polygenic score with lifestyle risk factors in an electronic health record biobank. BMC Med. 2022;20:1–12.
25. Furlong MA, Klimentidis YC. Associations of air pollution with obesity and body fat percentage, and modification by polygenic risk score for BMI in the UK Biobank. Environ Res. 2020;185:109364.
26. Sun Y, et al. Polygenic differential susceptibility to cumulative stress exposure and childhood obesity. Int J Obes. 2018;42:1177–84.
27. Hüls A, et al. Polygenic risk for obesity and its interaction with lifestyle and sociodemographic factors in European children and adolescents. Int J Obes. 2021;45:1321–30.

28. McArdle CE, et al. Findings from the Hispanic Community Health Study/Study of Latinos on the importance of sociocultural environmental interactors: polygenic risk score-by-immigration and dietary interactions. Front Genet. 2021;12:720750.
29. Clarke TK, et al. Major depressive disorder and current psychological distress moderate the effect of polygenic risk for obesity on body mass index. Transl Psychiatry. 2015;5:e592.
30. Fu J, et al. Childhood sleep duration modifies the polygenic risk for obesity in youth through leptin pathway: the Beijing Child and Adolescent Metabolic Syndrome cohort study. Int J Obes. 2019;43:1556–67.
31. Opel N, et al. Prefrontal gray matter volume mediates genetic risks for obesity. Mol Psychiatry. 2017;22:703–10.
32. Morys F, et al. Neuroanatomical correlates of genetic risk for obesity in children. Transl Psychiatry. 2023;13:1.
33. Shott ME, et al. Orbitofrontal cortex volume and brain reward response in obesity. Int J Obes. 2015;39:214–21.
34. Masip G, et al. The genetic architecture of the association between eating behaviors and obesity: combining genetic twin modeling and polygenic risk scores. Am J Clin Nutr. 2020;112:956–66.
35. Sardahaee FS, Holmen TL, Micali N, Kvaløy K. Effects of single genetic variants and polygenic obesity risk scores on disordered eating in adolescents–the HUNT study. Appetite. 2017;118:8–16.
36. Micali N, Field AE, Treasure JL, Evans DM. Are obesity risk genes associated with binge eating in adolescence? Obesity. 2015;23:1729–36.
37. Llewellyn CH, Trzaskowski M, van Jaarsveld CHM, Plomin R, Wardle J. Satiety mechanisms in genetic risk of obesity. JAMA Pediatr. 2014;168:338–44.
38. Fang J, et al. Polygenic risk, adherence to a healthy lifestyle, and childhood obesity. Pediatr Obes. 2019;14:e12489.
39. Park S, et al. Interactions between polygenic risk scores, dietary pattern, and menarche age with the obesity risk in a large hospital-based cohort. Nutrients. 2021;13:3772.
40. Dashti HS, et al. Polygenic risk score for obesity and the quality, quantity, and timing of workplace food purchases: a secondary analysis from the ChooseWell 365 randomized trial. PLoS Med. 2020;17:e1003219.
41. Puckett EE. Variability in total project and per sample genotyping costs under varying study designs including with microsatellites or SNPs to answer conservation genetic questions. Conserv Genet Resour. 2017;9:289–304.
42. Aasbrenn M, et al. Genetic markers of abdominal obesity and weight loss after gastric bypass surgery. PLoS One. 2021;16:e0252525.
43. Käkelä P, et al. Genetic risk score does not predict the outcome of obesity surgery. Obes Surg. 2014;24:128–33.
44. Bandstein M, et al. A genetic risk score is associated with weight loss following Roux-en Y gastric bypass surgery. Obes Surg. 2016;26:2183–9.
45. Katsareli EA, et al. A genetic risk score for the estimation of weight loss after bariatric surgery. Obes Surg. 2020;30:1482–90.
46. Nicoletti CF, et al. The genetic predisposition score of seven obesity-related single nucleotide polymorphisms is associated with better metabolic outcomes after Roux-en-Y gastric bypass. Lifestyle Genom. 2017;9:222–30.
47. van der Meer R, et al. Genetic variants associated with weight loss and metabolic outcomes after bariatric surgery: a systematic review. Obes Rev. 2023;
48. Kleinendorst L, et al. Identifying underlying medical causes of pediatric obesity: results of a systematic diagnostic approach in a pediatric obesity center. PLoS One. 2020;15:e0232990.
49. Davey Smith G, Ebrahim S. 'Mendelian randomization': can genetic epidemiology contribute to understanding environmental determinants of disease? Int J Epidemiol. 2003;32:1–22.
50. Riaz H, et al. Association between obesity and cardiovascular outcomes: a systematic review and meta-analysis of Mendelian randomization studies. JAMA Netw Open. 2018;1:e183788.

51. Kjaergaard AD, et al. Obesity and kidney function: a two-sample Mendelian randomization study. Clin Chem. 2022;68:461–72.
52. Fang Z, Song M, Lee DH, Giovannucci EL. The role of Mendelian randomization studies in deciphering the effect of obesity on cancer. JNCI J Natl Cancer Inst. 2022;114:361–71.
53. Marini S, et al. Mendelian randomization study of obesity and cerebrovascular disease. Ann Neurol. 2020;87:516–24.
54. Mokry LE, et al. Obesity and multiple sclerosis: a mendelian randomization study. PLoS Med. 2016;13:e1002053.
55. Böckerman P, et al. Does higher education protect against obesity? Evidence using Mendelian randomization. Prev Med (Baltim). 2017;101:195–8.
56. Nordestgaard AT, Thomsen M, Nordestgaard BG. Coffee intake and risk of obesity, metabolic syndrome and type 2 diabetes: a Mendelian randomization study. Int J Epidemiol. 2015;44:551–65.
57. Vimaleswaran KS, et al. Causal relationship between obesity and vitamin D status: bi-directional Mendelian randomization analysis of multiple cohorts. PLoS Med. 2013;10:e1001383.
58. Martin AR, et al. Clinical use of current polygenic risk scores may exacerbate health disparities. Nat Genet. 2019;51:584–91.
59. All of Us Research Program Investigators, et al. The "All of Us" research program. N Engl J Med. 2019;381:668–76.
60. Belsky DW, et al. Development and evaluation of a genetic risk score for obesity. Biodemography Soc Biol. 2013;59:85–100.
61. Damavandi N, Soleymaniniya A, Bahrami Zadegan S, Samiee Aref MH, Zeinali S. Development of a genetic risk score for obesity predisposition evaluation. Mol Gen Genomics. 2022;297:1495–503.
62. Manolio TA, et al. Finding the missing heritability of complex diseases. Nature. 2009;461:747–53.
63. Mantere T, Kersten S, Hoischen A. Long-read sequencing emerging in medical genetics. Front Genet. 2019;10:426.
64. Shah S, et al. Improving phenotypic prediction by combining genetic and epigenetic associations. Am J Hum Genet. 2015;97:75–85.
65. Wehby GL, Domingue BW, Ullrich F, Wolinsky FD. Genetic predisposition to obesity and medicare expenditures. J Gerontol A. 2018;73:66–72.
66. Cuevas AG, Mann FD, Krueger RF. Discrimination exposure and polygenic risk for obesity in adulthood: testing gene-environment correlations and interactions. Lifestyle Genom. 2023;16:90–7.

MIX
Papier aus verantwortungsvollen Quellen
Paper from responsible sources
FSC® C105338

If you have any concerns about our products,
you can contact us on
ProductSafety@springernature.com

In case Publisher is established outside the EU,
the EU authorized representative is:
Springer Nature Customer Service Center GmbH
Europaplatz 3, 69115 Heidelberg, Germany

Printed by Libri Plureos GmbH
in Hamburg, Germany